Deconstructing Stigma in Mental Health

Brittany A. Canfield
Southern New Hampshire University, USA

Holly A. Cunningham
CPES Inc., USA

A volume in the Advances in
Psychology, Mental Health, and
Behavioral Studies (APMHBS) Book
Series

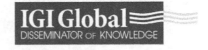

Published in the United States of America by
    IGI Global
    Medical Information Science Reference (an imprint of IGI Global)
    701 E. Chocolate Avenue
    Hershey PA, USA 17033
    Tel: 717-533-8845
    Fax: 717-533-8661
    E-mail: cust@igi-global.com
    Web site: http://www.igi-global.com

Library of Congress Cataloging-in-Publication Data

Names: Canfield, Brittany, editor. | Cunningham, Holly A., 1980- editor.
Title: Deconstructing stigma in mental health / Brittany A. Canfield and
   Holly A. Cunningham, editors.
Description: Hershey, PA : Medical Information Science Reference, [2018] |
   Includes bibliographical references.
Identifiers: LCCN 2017022183| ISBN 9781522538080 (hardcover) | ISBN
   9781522538097 (ebook)
Subjects: | MESH: Mental Health | Mental Disorders | Mentally Ill Persons |
   Social Stigma
Classification: LCC RC455 | NLM WM 101 | DDC 616.89--dc23 LC record available at https://
lccn.loc.gov/2017022183

This book is published in the IGI Global book series Advances in Psychology, Mental Health, and Behavioral Studies (APMHBS) (ISSN: 2475-6660; eISSN: 2475-6679)

British Cataloguing in Publication Data
A Cataloguing in Publication record for this book is available from the British Library.

All work contributed to this book is new, previously-unpublished material.
The views expressed in this book are those of the authors, but not necessarily of the publisher.

For electronic access to this publication, please contact: eresources@igi-global.com.

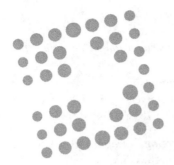

Advances in Psychology, Mental Health, and Behavioral Studies (APMHBS) Book Series

ISSN:2475-6660
EISSN:2475-6679

Editor-in-Chief: Bryan Christiansen, Global Research Society, LLC, USA & Harish C. Chandan, Argosy University, USA

MISSION

The complexity of the human mind has puzzled researchers and physicians for centuries. While widely studied, the brain still remains largely misunderstood.

The **Advances in Psychology, Mental Health, and Behavioral Studies (APMHBS)** book series presents comprehensive research publications focusing on topics relating to the human psyche, cognition, psychiatric care, mental and developmental disorders, as well as human behavior and interaction. Featuring diverse and innovative research, publications within APMHBS are ideally designed for use by mental health professionals, academicians, researchers, and upper-level students.

COVERAGE

- Human Behavior
- Developmental Disorders
- Human Interaction
- Psychiatry
- Personality Disorders
- Treatment & Care
- Trauma & Stress
- Eating Disorders
- Anxiety
- Cognition

IGI Global is currently accepting manuscripts for publication within this series. To submit a proposal for a volume in this series, please contact our Acquisition Editors at Acquisitions@igi-global.com or visit: http://www.igi-global.com/publish/.

Titles in this Series

For a list of additional titles in this series, please visit:
https://www.igi-global.com/book-series/advances-psychology-mental-health-behavioral/110200

Social, Psychological, and Forensic Perspectives on Sexual Abuse
Rejani Thudalikunnil Gopalan (Gujarat Forensic Sciences University, India)
Information Science Reference • ©2018 • 374pp • H/C (ISBN: 9781522539582) • US $195.00

Raising Mental Health Awareness in Higher Education Emerging Research and Opportunities
Melissa Martin (State University of New York at Plattsburgh, USA) Jean Mockry (State University of New York at Plattsburgh, USA) Alison Puliatte (State University of New York at Plattsburgh, USA) Denise A. Simard (State University of New York at Plattsburgh, USA) and Maureen E. Squires (State University of New York at Plattsburgh, USA)
Medical Information Science Reference • ©2018 • 136pp • H/C (ISBN: 9781522537939) • US $175.00

Web-Based Behavioral Therapies for Mental Disorders
Sitwat Usman Langrial (Sur University College, Oman)
Medical Information Science Reference • ©2018 • 310pp • H/C (ISBN: 9781522532415) • US $255.00

Measuring the Psychological and Electrophysiological Attributes of Human Personality ...
Sanja Tatalović Vorkapić (University of Rijeka, Croatia)
Information Science Reference • ©2017 • 242pp • H/C (ISBN: 9781522522836) • US $130.00

Emerging Research in Play Therapy, Child Counseling, and Consultation
Rheta LeAnne Steen (Loyola University New Orleans, USA)
Information Science Reference • ©2017 • 436pp • H/C (ISBN: 9781522522249) • US $205.00

Workforce Development Theory and Practice in the Mental Health Sector
Mark Smith (Te Pou o te Whakaaro Nui: National Workforce Center for Adult Mental Health, Addiction and Disability, New Zealand) and Angela F. Jury (Te Pou o te Whakaaro Nui: National Workforce Center for Adult Mental Health, Addiction and Disability, New Zealand)
Information Science Reference • ©2017 • 378pp • H/C (ISBN: 9781522518747) • US $190.00

For an entire list of titles in this series, please visit:
https://www.igi-global.com/book-series/advances-psychology-mental-health-behavioral/110200

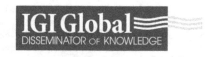

701 East Chocolate Avenue, Hershey, PA 17033, USA
Tel: 717-533-8845 x100 • Fax: 717-533-8661
E-Mail: cust@igi-global.com • www.igi-global.com

Table of Contents

Detailed Table of Contents

Katrina Y. Billingsley, South University – High Point, USA
Donté R. Corey, South University – High Point, USA

This chapter seeks to deconstruct racial stigma of mental illness held by counselors within the therapeutic relationship. The authors will provide counselors with practical tools that will help them work through their own prejudices, discriminations, and stereotypes about people of color and mental illness. This chapter will provide background information on stigma, specifically racial stigma, the process for incorporating theoretical variation in clinical work, and its importance. Additionally, the authors will explore best practices that will help counselors obtain the knowledge and skills needed to effectively work with a variety of clients who are racially and ethnically diverse.

Stephen Gichuhi Kimotho, United States International University –
Africa, Kenya

Besides health and social costs, mentally ill, often, are also victims of stigma and discrimination, among many communities in Africa. Cultural beliefs, stereotypes are some of the social constructions used to perpetuate mental illness stigma. The purpose of this study was to describe the nature of stigma communication associated with mental illness, beliefs and stereotypes underpinning mental illness stigma. Generally, the findings indicate nature of mental illness stigma communication is an intersection of stigma messages, cultural beliefs, and stereotypes associated with mental illness. Cultural beliefs associated with mental illness are inextricably intertwined with the perceived causes of mental illness (which include curses, witchcraft, cultural misdemeanor, and possession by spirits or demons). Symptoms of mental illness (mainly aggression and nudity) mark the mentally ill as different and expose them to labeling by the rest of the community. Generally, the mentally ill are stereotyped as aggressive, symbol of shame, and unpredictable.

Chapter 3
Sudeep Uprety, Tribhuvan University, Nepal
Rajesh Ghimire, Tribhuvan University, Nepal

This chapter attempts to unfold the trend and nature of mainstream and social media coverage on mental health issues in Nepal through suicide case of Yama Buddha, a popular musician. Using the securitization theory and concepts of threat construction and threat neutralization, major findings through content analysis and key informant interviews reveal reputed mainstream media following cautious route towards threat neutralization and therefore, maintaining a level of journalistic professionalism. However, especially in the other online media, blogs, and other social media, there were sensationalist words and tone used to attract the audience, triggering various sorts of emotional responses, thereby fulfilling the act of securitization. Major recommendations from this chapter include more awareness and understanding about the nature and type of mental health problems; capacity building of journalists and media professionals to better understand and report on mental health problems; development and proper implementation of media guidelines on reporting mental health issues.

Chapter 4
Ben Tran, Alliant International University, USA

Mental health stigma can be defined as the display of negative attitudes, based on prejudice and misinformation, in response to a marker of illness. Stigma creates mental distress for individuals, which furthers stigmatizing attitudes, thereby making it a relentless force and as incompetent in achieving life goals such as living independently or having a good job. Over the years, researchers have consistently highlighted the problem of mental health service underutilization within the Asians and Asian-Americans communities. As such, understanding the cultural contexts that facilitate good outcomes may offer a lever or stigma reduction. Thus, the purpose of this chapter is to understand and address the sociocultural and psychological paradigms of the stigma in mental health within Asians and Asian-Americans. This chapter will cover the history of stigma within the Asian culture, Asian's mental health, mental health services utilization within the Asian culture, and methods of addressing the stigma within the Asian culture to promote the utilization of mental health services.

This chapter is concerned with the impact of practitioner biases on the experience of a meaningful life for individuals who live with serious mental illness (SMI). Professional biases, systemic biases that originate in societal fear and lack of knowledge, and internalized stigma taken on by the consumer affect life decisions. Following a history of treatment initiatives experienced by consumers as abusive, it is important to understand how a system envisioned to protect and treat was often experienced as harmful. In the 1980s a movement emerged to transform the nature of mental health treatment to a client-centered, recovery-oriented model. In 1999, the Surgeon General proclaimed that all agencies serving this population should be recovery oriented. Yet, the shift to this approach to understanding people with SMI has not been complete. While there are many explanations why practitioners may not fully embrace this perspective, this chapter introduces the concept of "schemas" from cognitive behavioral theory as a way of examining professional biases in the field of SMI.

This chapter will discuss action research conducted in Tuscany to fight stigma surrounding mental illness. Public mental health services (PMHS) in Italy are perceived as ascribing a mentally ill label to individuals who utilize these programs. Local associations, especially sports associations, can be used to fight this stigma. This chapter will present key aspects and results of a community social innovation intervention jointly performed by a PMHS and the University of Florence. The research will explore perceptions surrounding the role and value of the community sports association, participants' perceived improvements, effects of sports participation, and the role of the sports association as an instrument to promote mental health. Results will show that the sports association is perceived as an agent of social capital to reduce social barriers emerging from mental illness. In addition, stigma is deconstructed through improvements to individual and social wellbeing.

Chapter 7

Tatiana Davidson, Medical University of South Carolina, USA
Angela Moreland, Medical University of South Carolina, USA
Brian E. Bunnell, Medical University of South Carolina, USA
Jennifer Winkelmann, Medical University of South Carolina, USA
Jessica L. Hamblen, National Center for PTSD, USA
Kenneth J. Ruggiero, Medical University of South Carolina, USA

The authors present the use of digital storytelling with two populations that have been consistently shown to be at increased risk for developing mental health disorders: veterans and firefighters. Despite efforts to increase access to evidence-based mental health programs, stigma remains a major barrier to care. AboutFace and Firefighters Helping Firefighters are two DST resources designed to help recognize the symptoms of posttraumatic stress disorder (PTSD) and related mental health symptoms, and to encourage help-seeking. These web-based video galleries introduce the viewer to 70+ peers who have experienced PTSD and have received formal treatment. These sites use the shared bonds of service to educate and help normalize common reactions that they may have due to the stressful nature of their occupations. Visitors to the site can "meet" peers and hear how mental illness has affected them through unscripted, authentic personal stories and can learn about common symptoms, struggles regarding decisions to seek care, and detailed descriptions of what treatment was like.

Chapter 8

Sara Bender, Central Washington University, USA
Karlie Hill, Central Washington University, USA

Misconceptions regarding the cause(s) of sexually transmitted infections (STIs) has led to a number of prejudices against those with such diagnoses. A fear of being the object of prejudicial attitudes and behaviors leaves many individuals concerned about the social stigma of a STI diagnosis. This, in turn, may leave people unwilling to get tested or hesitant to disclose their diagnosis to others, which may fuel the spread of such infections. In addition to the numerous medical concerns associated with STIs, the psychological consequences of STIs are notable as well. Understanding the stigma related to STIs is an important step towards improving the mental health of people with such diagnoses. This chapter provides the reader with an overview of STI diagnoses, and an explanation of their physical and mental health consequences. The chapter continues by examining the three types of stigma as well as their components. Finally, the chapter offers a number of suggestions regarding how to combat STI stigma, which may be extrapolated to combat other forms of stigma affecting mental health.

Chapter 9

This research was conducted with a view to ascertaining the perceptions, feelings, and thoughts of the women who care for patients with schizophrenia regarding the challenges they face and stigma. This research was conducted by using qualitative research method. To this end, in-depth interviews were made with 10 women who care for schizophrenia patients. As a result of the research, it was found out that the women who care for patients often care of the patient on their own, and thus, they have some psychosocial challenges. The disease negatively affects family relationships, but some families, on the contrary, have positive changes in their relationships. The parents accuse themselves as they are the cause of the disease and they are accused by the social circles. The women who care for patients are exposed to stigma during almost the all processes of the disease and some women internalize being stigmatized and they mostly tend to hide the disease in order to cope with the stigma.

Preface

OVERVIEW OF SUBJECT MATTER

Despite the good intentions of the mental health community, stigma continues to play an integral role in the multifaceted issues facing mental health. While identifying a clear operational definition of stigma has been a challenge in the field, the issues related to stigma as a whole include ignorance, prejudice, and discrimination. These issues transfer into the daily practices within mental health via the clinicians, educators, researchers and policy makers, which grossly effects not only the mental health population but society as a whole. In *Deconstructing Stigma in Mental Health*, the collaborative nature of the text highlights the ingenuity and interdisciplinary attention necessary for reducing and preventing the systematic stigmatization of mental health.

DESCRIPTION OF TOPIC IN THE WORLD TODAY

Stigma

As Byrne (2000) so poignantly describes, "Stigma has become a marker for adverse experiences." In recent years, research has served to uncover the impact stigma has on individuals' experiencing mental health issues, society's view of mental health that maintains stigmatized views are often generated in media, and the very attitudes and beliefs held by professionals in the mental health field that directly or indirectly perpetuate stigma. The presence of stigma creates a "disconnection" from mental health services and as Corrigan (2004) indicates, an "avoidance of the label of mental illness and harm it brings." Stigma impacts the individual on multiple levels and can impede treatment before services are sought as a result of the individual's depreciated self-esteem and social opportunities that are no longer seen as available (Corrigan, 2004).

As was said, ignorance, prejudice, and discrimination are the guiding drives of stigma and in the case of mental health; this triumvirate contributes to the private and public shame experienced by those impacted by mental health issues. When shame invalidates the presence of serious mental illness symptoms, secrecy becomes an adaptive response (Byrne, 2000), thus generating self-stigmatization and a barrier to seek or obtain services within an already isolated support network. Hence, stigma and discrimination negatively impact the course and outcome of mental illness and are then compounded by aspects including the very labeling of mental illness, the associated symptoms and behaviors, and physical appearance (Corrigan, 2000). Further, Gary (2009) notes that the very "potency" of the stigma defines the barrier of seeking or participating in services. As one of the primary pillars of stigma, discrimination and discriminatory practices are experienced across "every aspect of social and economic existence" (Fink & Tasman, 1992; Heller et al., 1996; Read & Reynolds, 1997; Byrne, 1997; Thompson & Thompson, 1997; as Cited in Byrne, 2000).

In Gary's (2009) research on mental health stigma among ethnic minorities proposes the "double stigma," a stacking of discriminations, due to the pre-existing experience of prejudice and discrimination is compounded by the burdens of mental illness. Ethnic marginalization and the presence of stigma can negatively impact treatment attempts and overall wellbeing, which produce "preventable and treatable mortalities and morbidities" (Gary, 2009). It need be said that the concept of "double stigma" does not exclusively relate to ethnic marginalization. Meyer's (2003) research highlights the component of minority stress among the LGBTQ community, which for the time of Meyer's research did not include Transsexual and Queer, yet provides the opportunity to greater focus on the impact of stigma as it relates to minority stress. In this research, the "stress processes" are noted to describe the experience of stigma, prejudice, and discrimination events, the process of hiding and concealing, anticipated rejection, internalized homophobia, and coping processes (Meyer, 2003). Exacerbating the issue, stereotypes help perpetuate the culture of dismissal and thus create distance between the "stigmatizer" and those being stigmatized (Byrne, 2000). This distance is the very construction of the *other*, a creation of an "us and them" mentality, thereby allowing the stigmatizer the ability to disown a sense of personal responsibility and placing the burden of responsibility on the subjected.

The societal acceptance of and complicit participation in stigma can be understood by the history of mental illness by our treatment, social segregation, and depictions of mental illness in art, literature, film, and the media; the very devices used to create and challenge social norms, maintain the status quo, and act as a mirror for the collective and individual aspects of society. The media averts the unease of mental illness by its polarized treatment of the narratives representative of those impacted by it: this polarization is typified by psych-thrillers, comedic tragedies, or romantic rescuing, thus aiding in the stigmatized portrayals of mental illness. Byrne (1997) discusses the use of mental illness in comedic form, an act that participates in the "them and us" strategy, which also includes "highly charged negative connotations of self-infliction, an excuse for laziness and criminality."

Criminalization of Mental Illness

The relationship between stigma and the process of criminalization of mental illness is one that creates a system of neglect and consequently, a failure, for those individuals experiencing and impacted by mental illness. The criminalization of mental illness begins with criminal intervention by service agencies not equipped to provide intervention. Bernstein and Seltzer (2003) describe criminalization as the process of arrest, booking, and incarceration of individuals with mental illness, which has far reaching ramifications upon their release to include limited opportunities for mental health services and access to equal housing. This means, the stigmatization of mental health begins on a medico-legal level. Further, criminalization also occurs by holding the belief that reconnecting individuals with mental health services alone will decrease their risk for arrest (Fisher, Silver, & Wolff, 2006), as opposed to addressing the reconnection of services as a working part in a much larger mechanism.

TARGET AUDIENCE

This text is intended for mental health administrators and clinicians, researchers, educators, policy makers, social advocates and activists, social services, and intersectionality studies to include gender, race and class. Potential uses include: new research on stigma and its role in mental health; the perpetuation of stigma; barriers to reducing and/or preventing stigma; methods to reduce the perpetuation of stigma in mental health; and the intersectionality of stigma to include gender, race and class. *Deconstructing Stigma in Mental Health* will serve as an educational and practical resource for educators, researchers, and practitioners in the field of psychology but also in the intersectional fields related to culture and the human experience. The value of this publication is three-fold: (1) to provide historical context of stigma in the mental health field; (2) through intersectional collaboration, current issues and resolution attempts will be explored to reduce stigma in multiple settings as they relate to mental health issues; and (3) serve as a platform for intersectional problem solving and collaboration for the deconstruction of stigma in mental health.

DESCRIPTION AND IMPORTANCE OF CHAPTERS

The chapters in *Deconstructing Stigma in Mental Health* address a spectrum of topics and issues currently relevant to the construct of stigma. This text opens a discourse in a range of social and therapeutic issues, to include research, theory, and practice on understanding, reducing, and combating the issues of race, sex, gender, class, age, and type of mental illness affected by stigma. Each chapter, unique in its approach to stigma, provides detailed backgrounds on the research and the history of the topic are explored while also challenging current power structures and offering methods of stigma reduction.

In Chapter 1, Billingsley and Corey seek to deconstruct racial stigma within therapeutic relationships and survey literature on racial stigma and incorporate theoretical variation in clinical settings. The authors provide therapeutic tools to address practitioners' prejudice, discrimination, and stereotypes of ethnic minorities and mental illness.

Chapter 2 covers the expansive topic of communication, of all types, in mental illness, cultural beliefs and stereotypes in Africa. Kimotho examines cultural beliefs that serve as the perceived causes of mental illness within African culture and the social impact these beliefs have on individuals experiencing mental illness.

Authors Uprety and Ghimire explore mainstream and social media coverage on mental health issues in Nepal in Chapter 3. The authors utilize the suicide case of Yama Buddha, a popular musician, to address the negative impact of the media in the creation of stigma. The Securitization Theory and concepts of both threat construction and threat neutralization function as the primary foundation of analysis of this case and the media's impact on social awareness and understanding of mental health.

In Chapter 4, the sociocultural and psychological paradigms of mental health stigma in Asians and Asian Americans are examined. Tran covers the history of stigma within Asian culture, mental health, mental health utilization, and methods of addressing the stigma within Asian culture to promote mental health service utilization.

Chapter 5 places focus on recovery perspectives and the barriers to practitioners' endorsement therein. Kram-Fernandez utilizes the concept of "schemas" from cognitive behavioral theory to examine professional biases in the field of Serious Mental Illness (SMI). The author posits that the presence of professional biases, systemic biases, and internalized stigma influence life decisions made by consumers.

Bosco and Authors examine action research for fighting stigma in mental illness realized in Tuscany, Italy. Chapter 6 addresses the utilization of sports associations to combat public and self-stigma of mental illness. The chapter describes action research from the University of Florence in Italy and the Public Mental Health

Service (PMHS) of Tuscany, Italy on the perceptions of the value and roles of sports associations within the community as a tool to address mental illness, reduce barriers, and deconstructing stigma.

Davidson and authors discuss the utilization of digital storytelling in the reduction of stigma in mental health in Chapter 7. The authors place focus on veterans and firefighters due to their increased risk for developing mental health disorders and the use of digital storytelling to reduce stigma. Due to stigma acting as a primary barrier to care for veterans and firefighters, the process of digital storytelling is described as a direct method of stigma reduction in order to gain access to mental health services.

In Chapter 8, Bender contributes a special issue on stigma and mental health issues found in Sexually Transmitted Infections (STIs) diagnoses. Background information is provided on STIs, additional medical concerns, and the psychological consequences that contribute to STI and mental health stigma.

GÖK and ÇiFCi present research on stigmatization stories of women who care for patients with schizophrenia in Chapter 9. Using a qualitative research method, the authors conducted ten in-depth interviews with women to ascertain their perceptions, feelings, and thoughts regarding the challenges they face and mental health stigma relevant to these narratives. Authors GÖK and ÇiFCi offer an introspective look at the secondary experience of mental illness and illuminate a subsection of the mental health field often not discussed. With primary focus tending toward psychiatrists, therapists, psychologists and mental health nurses, a unique perspective is offered by GÖK and ÇiFCi's research.

CONCLUSION

In this book, the authors will discuss stigma from multiple frameworks, utilizing multiple devices that span global perspectives on the subject. Stigma is addressed in each chapter discussing the prevalence of this construct in various aspects of mental health. Intersectional issues on stigma are examined from a cross-cultural context to identify mediating factors of stigma, barriers to treatment and reduction of stigma, combating stigma within communities, highlighting special issues and populations impacted by stigma, and presenting new perspectives on reducing stigma in mental health. Collaboratively, this book challenges the very language responsible for the perpetuation of stigma and draws attention to the multi-level participation that is required from community members, mental health professionals, and extending to the criminal justice system.

REFERENCES

Bernstein, R. & Seltzer, T. (2003). Criminalization of people with mental illnesses: The role of mental health courts in system reform. *University of the District of Columbia Law Review, 143*.

Byrne, P. (1997). Psychiatric stigma: Past, passing and to come. *Journal of the Royal Society of Medicine*, *90*(11), 618–620. doi:10.1177/014107689709001107 PMID:9496274

Byrne, P. (2000). Stigma of mental illness and ways of diminishing it. *Advances in Psychiatric Treatment*, *6*(1), 65–72. doi:10.1192/apt.6.1.65

Corrigan, P. (2004). How stigma interferes with mental health care. *The American Psychologist*, *59*(7), 614–625. doi:10.1037/0003-066X.59.7.614 PMID:15491256

Corrigan, P. W. (2000). Mental health stigma as social attribution: Implications for research methods and attitude change. *Clinical Psychology: Science and Practice*, *7*(1), 48–67. doi:10.1093/clipsy.7.1.48

Fink, P. J., & Tasman, A. (1992). *Stigma and Mental Illness*. Washington, DC: American Psychiatric Press.

Fisher, W. H., Silver, E., & Wolff, N. (2006). Beyond criminalization: Toward a criminologically informed framework for mental health policy and services research. *Administration and Policy in Mental Health*, *33*(5), 544–557. doi:10.100710488-006-0072-0 PMID:16791518

Gary, F. A. (2009). Stigma: Barrier to mental health care among ethnic minorities. *Issues in Mental Health Nursing*, *26*(10), 979–999. doi:10.1080/01612840500280638 PMID:16283995

Read, J., & Reynolds, J. (1997). *Speaking Our Minds—An Anthology*. London: MacMillan.

Thompson, M., & Thompson, T. (1997). *Discrimination Against People with Experiences of Mental Illness*. Wellington: Mental Health Commission.

Chapter 1

Deconstructing Racial Stigma in the Therapeutic Relationship

Katrina Y. Billingsley
South University – High Point, USA

Donté R. Corey
South University – High Point, USA

ABSTRACT

This chapter seeks to deconstruct racial stigma of mental illness held by counselors within the therapeutic relationship. The authors will provide counselors with practical tools that will help them work through their own prejudices, discriminations, and stereotypes about people of color and mental illness. This chapter will provide background information on stigma, specifically racial stigma, the process for incorporating theoretical variation in clinical work, and its importance. Additionally, the authors will explore best practices that will help counselors obtain the knowledge and skills needed to effectively work with a variety of clients who are racially and ethnically diverse.

INTRODUCTION

Unfortunately, stigma is not a new concept. In 1963, Erving Goffman's book *Stigma: Notes on the Management of Spoiled Identity* took a look at the stigma of character traits. The stigma of character traits as outlined by Goffman (1963) are the "blemishes of individual character perceived as weak will, domineering, or unnatural

DOI: 10.4018/978-1-5225-3808-0.ch001

passions" possessing "treacherous and rigid beliefs", and favor "dishonesty". These characteristics are "being inferred from a known record of, for example, mental disorder, imprisonment, addiction, alcoholism, homosexuality, unemployment, suicidal attempts, and radical political behavior" (p.2). The stigma of mental illness is historically wide spread. Stigma for individuals struggling with mental illness robs them of what is perceived as a "quality life: good job, safe housing, satisfactory health care, and affiliation with a diverse group of people" (Corrigan and Watson, 2002, p. 16). Stigma related to mental illness exists in the workplace, in homes and within families, in the education systems and, most surprisingly, in the practice of therapy. Two types of stigma are prevalent in the literature, public stigma and self-stigma. Public stigma "is the reaction that the general population has to people with mental illness" (Corrigan & Watson, 2002, p. 16). Public stigma includes discrimination, stereotypes and prejudices. Racial stigma emerged in the literature and will be explored to better understand its impact on clients of color in the therapeutic relationship within the United States.

Howarth (2006) references Goffman's view of stigma as being seen as a way to reduce the whole person to a "tainted, discounted one" (p.442). Racial stigma emerged as spotlighting what happens when stigma is applied to minority groups of people. Racial stigma is recognized in a variety of settings including the media, education and in the field of medicine. The authors suggest that racial stigma is also present in the therapeutic counseling relationship. Racial stigma "reduces the identity and the potential of those seen as *raced;* they are spoiled or blemished by the racist gaze" (Howarth, 2006, p.442). Howarth (2006) suggests that, "racial others" are individuals with skin that is brown and black who are seen as "less than, different from, unequal to the realizing, normatively white other" (p.442). Howarth (2006) also suggests that "race produces and sustains inequalities and is anchored in histories of prejudice, exclusion and poverty" (p.442). Howarth (2006) further explains that race, as stigma must be understood in order for it to be deconstructed. The authors suggest processing this understanding in order to help counselors become more aware and educated when working with individuals who are different; individuals who are also perceived as being so different that they are not considered normal. Additionally, race as stigma highlights how race reduces one's identity and potential. Howarth (2006) speaks to the fact that race is institutionalized and has historical implications. It is important to understand the impact and legacy negatively associated with race.

Education and awareness are critical to helping counselors engage whole-heartedly and authentically with clients who identify racially and ethnically different from the counselor. It is the intent of this chapter to provide practical ways to help counselors acknowledge and work through their own personal prejudices, discriminatory views and stereotypical behaviors related to racial and ethnic minorities with mental illness. The terms counselor and clinician will be used interchangeably as the terms differ

2

according to therapeutic setting. This chapter highlights the theoretical orientation, Relational-Cultural Theory and will provide therapeutic applications that will help counselors engage clients in a harmless, productive and harmonious way. This chapter is designed to assist current counselors or clinicians in becoming efficient in working with people of color in therapy. In addition, this chapter serves as an additional training guide for counselors-in-training to be utilized in counseling programs.

BACKGROUND

Due to the various levels of stigma, individuals do not seek out the assistance they need to reduce their mental health symptoms leading to the public's prejudicial fear and negative perception (Corrigan and Rao, 2012). Challenges faced by those who have mental illness are diverse and may include the struggle to: understand their illness, gain insight into how the illness effects their lives, understand treatment options, deal with society and how this leads to stereotyping, prejudices and discrimination. Within the counseling setting, it is important to ensure that clinicians are prepared to work with any person seeking their clinical help. Historically, people of color and other marginalized groups have opted out of therapy. Black/African Americans have been prone to not engage in therapy for a variety of reasons including the cost, religious views and the stigma associated with counseling. Only about one quarter of African Americans seek mental health treatment compared to 40% of White Americans (NAMI). With this known history, it is important that counselors are aware of their own stigmas towards Black/African Americans and other people of color (POC). The 2014 American Counseling Association (ACA) Code of Ethics, known as *the Code*, "serves as an ethical guide designed to assist members in constructing a course of action that best serves those utilizing counseling services and establishes expectations of conduct with a primary emphasis on the role of the professional counselor" (p.3).

Therapeutic Relationship

As stated above, clinicians should be mindful of ethical standards when working with clients. However, what makes a relationship therapeutic goes beyond ethical standards. Several theorists began defining a therapeutic relationship as a working alliance that includes unconditional positive regard, empathy, honesty, and acceptance. "Unconditional positive regard implies that clients are the best authority on their own experiences" (Sommers-Flanagan & Sommers-Flannagan, 2017, p. 222). "The authors also suggest that a therapist's judgments are always based on inadequate information because we have not lived our client's lives or their experiences, so we do not know their internal motives" (Sommers-Flanagan & Sommers-Flannagan, 2017, p. 222).

"For Carl Rogers, unconditional positive regard was based on the belief that consistent warmth, acceptance, and encouragement of clients enhanced clients' growth toward their potential" (Sommers-Flanagan & Sommers-Flannagan, 2017, p. 222). Another word that can be used in the place of unconditional positive regard is *respect*. Respect is universally understood. "According to quantitative and qualitative research and clinical anecdotes, it appears safe to say that clients from all minority groups respond better when they have unequivocal respect from members of the dominant culture" (Farber & Doolin, 2011). However, respect can be shown and perceived very differently depending on one's racial background and this is why multicultural awareness and competence is necessary.

Another important aspect of the traditional therapeutic relationship is empathy. Clinicians should not only be skilled listeners, they should be empathetic listeners. Rogers (1980) defined empathy as the counselor's sensitive ability and willingness to understand the client's thoughts, feelings, and struggles from the client's point of view. This is different from sympathy. The counselor should not treat the client in such a way that causes her/him to feel sorry for the client. Being empathetic requires the counselor to put her/himself in the client's shoes and imagine what it is like to experience the experience.

A relationship is not therapeutic without an element of a *working alliance*. In 1979, Bordin introduced a three-dimensional model referred to as the working alliance. The model consisted of goal consensus or agreement, collaborative engagement in mutual tasks, and development of a relational bond. Collaboration is key in the therapeutic relationship. Research shows that clients who have a collaborative bond with their clinicians presents with the most improvement.

Others have supported this view:

What remains in question is how clinicians can best foster a working alliance with culturally diverse clients. A good beginning is to provide clients with a clear statement of purpose individualized to specific cultural orientations. For example, with a client who has a collectivist orientation: "My goal is to provide the best help I can to you and your family" (Sommers-Flannagan & Sommers-Flannagan, 2017, p. 252).

Effective counseling is likely to occur when there is a working alliance and that alliance will not be developed without trust. That trust includes the therapist's ability to understand the client and his/her level of competence.

Others have reinforced this opinion:

Competence encompasses practicing from a theoretical evidence-based approach. Theory is the lens through which the counselor gains a perspective on the client, however theory is useless without a counselor. The clinician, however, comes with her or his own experience. Ideally, there should be a good fit between the clinician's own eyes or worldview and the theoretical lens she or he chooses (Sullivan, 2005, p. 283).

Racial Identity Models

When trying to deconstruct racial stigma in the therapeutic relationship, clinicians must be aware of the idea of racial identity development. A person's perception and worldview depends on her/his racial identity development. How a person understands her/himself and how one relates to others is also a part of racial identity development. Counselors should not only be aware of their development but should also be aware and understanding of clients' development.

In 1990, Sue and Sue proposed a seven-phase process that integrates many characteristics that explain White racial identity in their White Racial Identity Development Descriptive Model. The first phase is known as naiveté and occurs during early childhood (3-5 years). During this phase, individuals may notice differences but awareness of social meaning is absent or minimal. In the next phase, conformity, minimal awareness of self as a racial/cultural being and characteristics of the naiveté phase are maintained. For example, the individual believes that cultural differences are not important so as a result they "do not see color". In the dissonance phase, obliviousness breaks down when the person becomes aware of inconsistencies in their day-to-day experiences. For instance, the individual may have the belief that "all men are created equal" yet see POC being treated as second class citizens (Sue & Sue, 2016). Individuals become increasingly conscious of Whiteness and may experience dissonance, resulting in feelings of guilt, depression, helplessness or anxiety.

The fourth phase is known as resistance and immersion. In this stage, White individuals begin to realize what racism is all about and begins to question and challenge their own racism. For example, the individual's awareness of racism is enhanced as they see evidence in media, written materials, etc. In the fifth phase of introspection, individuals no longer deny being White, honestly confront their racism, understand the concept of White privilege, and feel increased comfort in relating to people of color. In the sixth phase of integrative awareness, the individual understands and appreciates self as a racial/cultural being while shifting focus from trying to change people of color to changing self and other White people.

The final phase is the commitment to antiracist action and is characterized by social action. When individuals get to this phase, they see things that they perceive as wrong and actively work to make them "right". This is done by objecting to racist jokes, trying to educate family, friends, and coworkers about racial issues and taking direct action to eradicate racism in schools, in the workplace, etc. As clinicians working with diverse clients, progression into the final phase is necessary to maintain the therapeutic relationship. In this phase, the clinician not only has an awareness and understanding of self, there is also an awareness and understanding of others' worldviews and sensitivity to racial issues that impact experience, growth and development.

In 1999, Sue and Sue developed the Racial/Cultural Identity Model. This five-stage model depicts identity development among minority groups. The first stage is the conformity stage which is marked by the desire to assimilate and acculturate and believing in White superiority and minority inferiority. A minority individual in this stage spends a large amount of time trying to "fit in" with the majority group. Unconscious and conscious desire to escape one's own racial heritage is presented in this stage. Physical and cultural characteristics identified with one's own racial/cultural group are perceived negatively, as something to be avoided, denied, or changed. Reports show that Asian women have undergone surgery to reshape their eyes to conform to White female standards of beauty may (but not in all cases) typify this dynamic (Sue & Sue, 2016).

The second stage, dissonance, is when the person of color experiences a breakdown of her/his denial system. Dominant-held views of minority strengths and weaknesses begin to be questioned and the individual begins to realize that attempts to assimilate or acculturate may not be fully allowed by the larger society. For example, a Latino adolescent boy tries to befriend a group of his White peers at school but is met with racial slurs. Individuals in this stage begin to become aware of racism, racial microaggressions and covert gestures of oppression. In resistance and immersion, the third stage, individuals begin to understand social-psychological forces associated with prejudice and discrimination. Members of the dominant group are viewed with suspicion and there is considerable anger and hostility directed toward White society.

Stage four is known as the introspection stage. The POC begins to spend more and more time and energy trying to sort out aspects of self-identity and begins to increasingly demand individual autonomy. For example, the individual spends a large amount of time trying to disconnect from White society instead of attempting to understand one's cultural heritage. In the final stage, integrative awareness, the individual develops an inner sense of security as conflicts between new and old identities are resolved. The individual begins to perceive himself or herself as an individual who is unique, a member of one's own racial-cultural group, a member of a larger society, and a member of the human race. At this stage, the POC finds comfort in being a part of all of these systems and takes pride in her/his diverse uniqueness.

Relational-Cultural Theory

Having a strong theoretical foundation is important in working with all clients. However, it is imperative when working with clients who differ from the counselor to be aware of their worldview and how those differences may impact their interaction with and care for the client. It is the belief of the authors that counselors should revisit their theoretical orientation as they prepare to engage in a therapeutic relationship with diverse clients. Relational Cultural Theory (RCT) is an alternative theory that has emerged as a framework for working with racially and ethnically different clients because it an act of social change and an emphasis on movement out of isolation (Jordan, 2009). Although RCT was initially developed to address the concerns of women it has advanced and is applicable to a more diverse population. RCT was developed to "better understand the importance of growth-fostering relationships in people's lives" seeking to "lessen the suffering caused by chronic disconnection and isolation whether at an individual or societal level, to increase the capacity for relational resilience, and to foster social justice" (Jordan, 2009, p.23). Maureen Walker (2002) suggests that the connections and disconnections in relationships are characterized in a context that has been "raced, engendered, sexualized, and stratified along dimensions of class, physical ability, religion, or whatever constructions carry ontological significance in the culture" (Jordan, 2008, p.23). As a good first step to ensuring one will openly engage in the counseling process, beginning with RCT is a way to become more introspective.

There are seven key components of RCT that will help counselors frame how and why utilizing a theoretical framework such as RCT can help nurture the therapeutic relationship in a more meaningful and developmental way. The key components according to Jordan (2002) include understanding that: people grow throughout the lifespan because of relationships in their lives; mature functioning occurs because of movement toward mutuality not when separation occurs; the differences between individuals and the elaborations of those who are in relationship together create growth for those involved. As counselors, being able to acknowledge the differences between oneself and one's clients can be used as a tool to foster growth for both parties. Additionally, mutual empathy and empowerment, along with authenticity are necessary for the development and prospering of healthy relationships. The relationship is not a one-way endeavor but takes both individuals to foster development. It will take courage for the counselor to go beyond what is the norm for them and reach out to create a therapeutic relationship that will help clients grow. Engaging in the tenets of RCT, requires counselors to live outside of their comfort zone and garner a relationship with someone who may hold many differences than they do. Committing to clients in such a way means committing to the process of establishing an authentic relationship.

MAIN FOCUS OF CHAPTER

Issues, Controversies and Problems

Being aware of and understanding why racial stigma may exist in the therapeutic relationship is a very significant part of assisting clients. However, knowledge and awareness is only the first step. Clinicians need to take an active role in deconstructing racial stigma in the therapeutic relationship. This is important for a few reasons. Firstly, minorities are not seeking out treatment for their mental health needs. Secondly, minorities that are getting treatment do not always feel safe, supported or understood by the public, and more importantly clinicians.

"Public stigma is the most prominent form observed and studied, as it represents the prejudice and discrimination directed at a group by the larger population" (Corrigan and Rao, 2012). Most times, public stigma develops due to how mental illness is portrayed in the media. People of color are already discriminated against because of the color of their skin and the assumptions that surround their racial identity. Thus when they are experiencing a mental illness, this adds to the negative perception that the public has about this population; racially and mentally.

Self-stigma has been a term coined to describe how an individual struggling with mental illness experiences self-hate, low self-esteem, and a lack of self-efficacy due to how they are perceived by others. This self-perception is detrimental and can cause counter-productivity within the person's life and the counseling process. Self-stigma can also cause additional pathologies such as depression and may lead to suicide attempts and suicide completion. As reported by the Office of Minority Mental Health (2016), suicide was the leading cause of death for American Indian/ Alaska Native girls between the ages of 10 and 14 in 2014. Due to these varying levels of stigma, people of color are not receiving the assistance that they need to reduce their symptoms which causes an increase in the person's symptomology and the public's negative perception.

Although mental health professionals do not intentionally practice a level of stigma when working with clients, several discriminating factors play a role in the counselor-client relationship if the counselor is not self-aware. Certain cues can be very debilitating for an individual experiencing mental illness and can have a negative impact on the therapeutic relationship as well as future attempts for the client to seek help. Microaggressions and non-verbal communication signals can affect this therapeutic relationship.

"For effective therapy to occur, the therapist and client must be able to send and receive both verbal and nonverbal messages appropriately and accurately" (Sue & Sue, 2016, pp. 258). Clinicians are continuously observing and assessing their clients so that they do not miss anything of importance. The same way that counselors watch and observe clients, clients at times are also watching the counselor. Counselors must be aware of the types of messages that are being sent when nothing has been said. For some clients, any small gesture from the counselor, for example a head tilt, can be misinterpreted by a client. Nonverbal communication varies from culture to culture, so counselors need to be aware, culturally competent, culturally sensitive and aware while engaging with clients.

Some nonverbal behaviors are microaggressions. Microaggressions are "brief and commonplace daily verbal or behavioral indignities, whether intentional or unintentional, that communicate hostile, derogatory, or negative racial slights and insults that potentially have a harmful or unpleasant psychological impact on the target person or group" (Sue, Bucceri, Lin, Nadal, & Torino, 2007). One common example of a microaggression is clutching a purse tighter while passing by a young Black male on the sidewalk. This action signifies the notion that all Black men are dangerous and will steal purses when walking by others. Another example is asking an Asian American individual where they are from. This last example sends the message that the Asian American individual is not American even if he/she was born in the United States. Microaggressions can also be delivered environmentally through the physical surroundings of target groups, where they are made to feel unwelcome, isolated, unsafe, and alienated (Sue & Sue, 2016, pp. 179).

Based on the literature, although all forms of racism can be hurtful and traumatic, there are different levels of oppression. These different levels can be seen within three different types of microaggressions. The three different types of microaggressions are micro-assault, microinsult, and microinvalidation.

The term microassault refers to a blatant verbal, nonverbal, or environmental attack intended to convey discriminatory and biased sentiments" (Sue & Sue, 2016, pp. 179). Microassaults are overt and are intended to purposely violate and hurt a person or group of people. For example, calling a Latino individual a *spic* is highly offensive and derogatory.

"Microinsults are unintentional behaviors or verbal comments that convey rudeness or insensitivity or demean a person's racial heritage/identity, gender identity, religion, ability, or sexual orientation identity" (Sue & Sue, 2016, pp. 188). An example of a microinsult is assuming that an Latino male should be placed in remedial classes due to one failed test. This assumption would be solely based on his racial background and gender. Microinvalidations are verbal comments or behaviors that exclude, negate, or dismiss the psychological thoughts, feelings, or experiential reality of the target group (Sue & Sue, 2016, pp. 189). "Colorblindness" is an example of a microinvalidation.

Deconstructing racial stigma also includes counselor competence. Counselors have a responsibility to their clients to not only be competent but to be culturally competent. There are several ways a counselor can enhance competency. When counselors lack self-awareness, are not culturally competent, and lack exposure/experience they can unintentionally create racial stigma in the therapeutic relationship. Baruth and Manning (2003) state that it is often easier to rely on stereotypical beliefs about others than to learn about cultures and to get to know people on a first-hand basis. Stereotyping can result both from a counselor's personal prejudices and biases as well as from a lack of factual information about cultures and individuals. "Just as a European American counselor might hold stereotypical perceptions about African-American, Asian-American, Hispanic American, and American Indian clients, a counselor from any of these cultural groups might hold stereotypical perceptions about European American clients" (Baruth & Manning, 2003).

Within counselor competence, there is also a need for theoretical approach variation. All clients are not created equally; meaning, counselors cannot treat all clients the same by using the same theoretical approaches for every client. A common issue that maintains stigma in mental health is counselors' lack of theoretical variation. It is an expectation that counselors learn a variety of approaches for all individuals and be able to utilize any of these approaches, when necessary. RCT therapy requires counselors to understand the vulnerabilities that many clients come with and foster a nurturing relationship that allows the therapeutic alliance to develop. Being empathetic and authentic allows clients to feel seen and heard. This level of acceptance fosters allows for growth within the therapeutic relationship.

Self-exploration is a main part of every counselor's educational program, however after one graduates the exploration should not stop. White counselors may be: unintentional racists; unaware of their biases, prejudices, and discriminatory behaviors; and using therapeutic approaches to multicultural populations that are likely to be more harmful (unintentionally) than helpful (Sue & Sue, 2016). "An important part of the solution to deconstructing racial stigma in clinical practice is that White clinicians need to examine the contexts of power and privilege that pervade every encounter with a client or colleague of color" (Lee, 2005, p. 96). A large part of understanding a client's worldview and life situation, is first understanding our own.

A current controversial misconception is that just because the counselor and client share the same racial background, means that the counselor can identify with the client. Race is only one part of an individual's world. Even if they have race or ethnicity in common, the client may experience comfort due to that commonality, however, this can affect the therapeutic relationship, negatively or positively. Building rapport with the client and showing genuine concern is key. Baruth and Manning (2003) stated that regardless of the client's native communication and cultural backgrounds, building rapport during counseling sessions depends significantly on communication between the counselor and client.

Lack of self-awareness and exploration, most times, comes with a lack of exposure/experience. Racial stigma can develop due to counselors not engaging in opportunities that will enhance their understanding of people of color. When new counselors enter into the world of counseling, they come with only the experiences that they had while in their graduate programs. This experience is limited and most times lacks culture.

A significant part of being culturally competent is being exposed to different cultures to enhance knowledge. According to the 2016 CACREP annual report, 61.12% of students graduating at the master's level are White. The likelihood that people of color seeking counseling services will be seen by someone who does not identify culturally as the client is very high. As stated earlier, identity development is the driving force of one's perception of self. Oftentimes, a counselor does not know where a client is regarding identity development. This lack of information can promote racial stigma due to the client feeling that the counselor does not understand her/him. Another part of cultural competence is understanding a client's acculturation level. For example, whether a 60-year-old Latino man has lived in the United States all his life or only a few years makes a difference when attempting to understand behaviors, values, and family dynamics.

SOLUTIONS AND RECOMMENDATIONS

Counselors must engage in professional development that will challenge their positions of privilege and help them understand their position of power within the therapeutic relationship. It is important that practitioners deconstruct their stigma towards a particular group by becoming aware of differences that could set them apart from engaging at an authentically human level with a client. This process begins with re-education to set the tone of what can be the start of a culturally competent and sensitive counseling relationship.

To increase awareness and re-educate counselors should begin by becoming active in the profession. Being active in a professional organization will give counselors an additional layer of support and education they would not normally receive. Additionally, being involved in a professional organization will provide insight into new, cutting edge information. As apart of the larger network there are divisions or special interest groups that address specific interests and needs of counselors allowing individuals to connect with colleagues who have similar interests.

A counselor's approach to therapy and how they relate to the client is key in ensuring a successful therapeutic relationship. This is extremely important when engaging with people of color. As stated previously, counselors who are engaging in therapy should be aware of their theoretical orientation and have a toolbox in which to pull from. Each client, whether a POC or otherwise is different with varying needs, wants and desires. Thus, the counselor should be able to diversify their clinical approach to therapy to help the person before them. There are many therapies that can be utilized to address a variety of needs for clients.

One specific therapeutic approach the authors feel would enhance the counselor's skill level for working with persons of color is Relational Cultural Theory (RCT) therapy. RCT is an advanced treatment guided by one's desire "to lessen the experience of isolation, increase the capacity for self-empathy and empathy for others, and develop an appreciation for the power of context and limiting cultural/relational images" (Jordan, 2008, p.35). RCT therapy is most concerned with the attitudes and the quality of mutual engagement as opposed to the types of interventions and techniques used in the counseling process. Changing the clinical approach to focus on relationship building rather than fixing or correcting a client can produce a change in the life of the client that may not be quantifiable.

As with all treatment modalities, RCT therapy begins with an assessment by gathering the usual demographic information. However, with RCT therapy close attention is paid to significant past and current relationships. It is the intent of the counselor to ensure what the client's goals are for seeking assistance. RCT clinicians do not focus solely on the pain that brings clients into treatment but on their strengths and coping skills and how effective they have been. It is important for counselors to assess the resiliency of clients and to determine if they have a community in which the client feels they matter and/or belong. It is also important to assess whether or not a client can engage in constructive conflict. Engaging in constructive conflict will allow the client and counselor to pursue authentic dialogue and create a trusting relationship. It is important, also, to assess if the client can present their needs and views to others even if those views may conflict with the other person's perspective. Additionally, it is also important to understand how the client disengages from others when in conflict. The goals of assessment in RCT therapy are to "identify the sources and functions of the relational images, including controlling societal images, and coping strategies that have shaped the client's experience and to establish the basis for the therapeutic relationship" (Jordan, 2009, p. 37). Gathering such information allows the counselor to effectively meet the client's needs while engaging in the therapeutic process.

It is also of much importance for the counselor to "develop an awareness of their own strategies of disconnection, including when they get activated and how they affect each particular therapy relationship" (p. 38). It is recommended that the counselor develop self-awareness. Being able to identify the signs of disconnection in therapy will help keep the therapeutic relationship authentic. Checking in with the client if the counselor feels a shift in the energy or tone is essential to creating an environment in which sensitivity and awareness are evident. Being sensitive and aware of what the counselor is feeling about their client or the therapeutic relationship will help to build against isolation and disempowering cultural forces. RCT therapy builds the client's desire for connection and is about building "networks and community" (Jordan, 2009, p. 41). RCT therapy emphasizes the utilization of empathy. Exhibiting empathy towards a person of color in the therapeutic relationship reflects that the counselor is authentically engaged and wholly present with the client.

Another recommendation for counselors that would help with becoming culturally aware is to engage in a service learning opportunity. Although service learning is a concept that is usually applicable to secondary education and undergraduate curriculum, the authors propose that utilizing service learning in the field of counseling will increase the awareness and education of counselors working with diverse clients. The incorporation of a service learning experience in the re-education of counselors would be helpful and beneficial to changing how a counselor engages with individuals who are persons of color. Service learning is known for incorporating a community service activity into the instruction of a particular discipline. Being able to apply theory in a real world setting would be beneficial in exposing counselors to a world they may not be familiar with. In return, counselors gain a valuable perspective that would help them engage empathetically with clients who are racially and ethnically different from them. Additionally, communities would gain much from the service provided. For example, if counselors enroll in continuing education courses on diversity this framework can be useful when a counselor engages in a service opportunity with a Black or African American church that is raising monies to support HIV/AIDS research. Immersion in this type of engagement creates a sense of community between the counselor and that population allowing the counselor to shift her paradigm on what she initially thought about Black Americans.

It is a recommendation of the authors that counselors become active and engaged in the larger community as change agents. By engaging in resistance against stigma and racist activities and posturing oneself as an anti-racist counselor is a powerful stance to take. This stance creates a safe zone within one's office space. Positioning oneself as anti-racist could create a steady flow of clients who would feel safe engaging with them in therapy. This position allows counselors to be collaborative with like-minded colleagues helping to de-stigmatize race in the therapeutic relationship.

As mentioned, counselors are required to have an appropriate level of self-awareness including but not limited to one's biases, cultural understanding and ethical standards when working in the mental health field. Exposure (contact) to diverse people and situations will enhance this self-awareness. Counselors should learn about people of color from sources within the group such as clients and colleagues. Purposeful experiences such as travel and venturing out of one's own community will allow counselors to not only learn about other cultures but will also allow them to experience their feelings regarding being around people of color.

Another way to be self-aware is to be mindful of types of communication being used and received in day-to-day living. Being aware of your own microaggressions and nonverbal communications that may be perceived as racially stigmatizing promotes change personally and professionally. Understanding communication of others that could be based on cultural style is also important. Owen, Jordan, Turner, Davis, Hook and Leach's work (as cited in Sue & Sue, 2016) supports the idea that clients' perceptions of racial microaggressions are negatively associated with therapeutic alliance.

Certain types of nonverbal communication such as proxemics, kinesics, and paralanguage can also play a part in creating a therapeutic disconnection. Proxemics refers to perception and use of personal and interpersonal space (Sue & Sue, 2016). For example, a White counselor that is comfortable with close spacing could cause an Asian client to withdraw and feel awkward. Kinesics refers to body movements such as facial expressions and hand gestures. A Japanese smile may mean discomfort (Sue & Sue, 2016). Paralanguage is known as vocal cues including pauses and silences. A counselor could misinterpret a Black client as being angry when speaking loudly about something she or he is passionate about.

As cited earlier, self-awareness includes understanding where one is in their development of identity. Counselors may need to ask themselves, "What does my race mean to me?". This question should generate some exploration into cultural biases, values, beliefs, and the counselor's worldview. Baruth and Manning (2003) found that common barrier in counseling occurs when counselors only expect (perhaps unconsciously) clients to conform to the counselor's cultural standards and expectations. "For example, expecting African American women to emulate European American standards of beauty (or vice versa) has a demoralizing effect and can create racial stigma in the therapeutic relationship" (Baruth & Manning, 2003, pp. 59).

Counselors also need to be aware of what their race may mean to other people, especially their clients. Oftentimes, clients already look at their counselors as experts and the counselor's race can also be seen as powerful or even superior. Sue, Capodilupo and Holder (as cited in Sue & Sue, 2016) found that African Americans consistently report that intellectual inferiority is a common communication they receive from Whites in their everyday experiences. Counselors need to be aware of these perceptions and how they are affecting the therapeutic relationship.

Self-awareness can be developed through a variety of avenues and by several different ways. One way to develop self-awareness is through diversity training. It is imperative that all counselors participate in ongoing diversity training. It is a requirement for all licensed counselors to obtain continuing education units to maintain licensure. Diversity training should be a part of this continuing education experience. Not only will diversity training enhance counselor self-awareness but this experience will also increase counselors' understanding of various cultural groups and cultural evidence-based practices.

FUTURE RESEARCH DIRECTIONS

Forward thinking requires that counselors position themselves to continue to advance their own self-awareness and skills for working with people of color. This requires understanding one's own layers of identity as well as their client's multiple identities and how those roles are addressed in the counseling relationship. The term, intersectionality was coined by Kimberlee Crenshaw in 1989 although the issues it addresses have been around since slaves were freed. Intersectionality is when the overlapping of social identities along with their related system of oppression creates an environment for discrimination (Crenshaw, 2016). It is important to frame an understanding of what it means when individuals have multiple social identities and the impact those identities have on their lives. It is not only just about the identities they hold but also about the oppression associated with those identities. Initially, this concept was developed to address concerns faced by Black American women who were confronted with issues of racism and sexism and how the intersection impacted their lives. The judicial system set a precedence that would not allow lawsuits to be brought forth when the plaintiff suggested was being dually discriminated against. Essentially, these Black women had to choose a struggle – gender or race but not both. Just as discrimination against a woman because she is a woman and she is Black is a reality so is stigmatization in the counseling relationship.

However, intersectionality can be applied to any individual who has multiple identities that are the opposite of what society deems as normal, proper or the standard. For example, Asian American gay men have two intersecting identities – race and sexual orientation in which they can face stigma, social injustice and discrimination. Intersectionality is applicable to a variety of groups of people to include people of colors with identities such as LGBTQ and people of color who are not able-bodied, to name a few.

Counselors must understand not only the impact of race when working with a client who is an ethnic or racial minority but also be mindful of the intersectionality of their own multiple identities that cause injustice, oppression and additional stigma. It is also important for counselors to understand their own biases and stigmas related to these varying identities. It is not possible for individuals to separate one identity from another – it is their own identity and they are whole people. Additional research on intersectionality and counseling would help clarify its impact on clients and counselors.

CONCLUSION

Stigma continues to be an issue in our society. Individuals who struggle with mental illness are perceived and judged, at times, based on this mental illness, which leads to developing a negative outlook and self-stigmatization. Due to public stigmatization and self-stigmatization, people are not seeking counseling services or are not benefiting from the services that are being utilized. This stigmatization phenomenon is even more prevalent among people of color because they are not only being perceived by others negatively because of their mental illness, but also because of the color of their skin. Oftentimes, individuals come to counseling due to experiences of racism, discrimination and oppression. The therapeutic relationship is known to be a supportive alliance built on trust, empathy, and respect. Clients come to counseling hoping to find comfort in a safe place. Counselors must be the driving force in deconstructing racial stigma because counselors are the foundation of the therapeutic relationship.

As mentioned, identity development plays a part in understanding one's self as well as understanding others. Counselors must be aware of many aspects of themselves to appropriately serve clients and deconstruct stigma. Being aware includes being educated, competent, and sensitive to culture. Additionally, understanding how a person's race intersects with other identities that are held by the person is valuable because these factors make the person whole and counselors need to understand the wholeness of the individual.

The ACA *Code of Ethics* speaks to counselors' duties regarding multicultural competence, however these guidelines need to be taken a step further when practicing in the counseling field. Counselors must be purposeful in their cultural experiences. Gaining knowledge and competence includes exploring culture by exposing one's self to it. One aspect that is important for counselors to consider when experiencing cultural exposure is being aware of her/his behavior. Microaggressions and non-verbal communication are significant and can make or break the therapeutic relationship.

Lastly, working with people of color means that counselors must have a full clinical toolbox that includes various theoretical approaches and interventions. What works for one client may not work with another, thus being knowledgeable and purposeful when choosing appropriate culture-specific interventions and theoretical approaches is key. The authors suggest RCT therapy because it is a holistic approach that considers the collectivistic nature that most minority groups value. As society continues to develop new roles and aspects of human nature, it is the responsibilities of mental health providers to keep up with this growth in a way that assists in the deconstruction of racial stigma. It is the ethical duty and responsibility of clinicians to appropriately respond to matters of diversity and stigmatization. In summary, this chapter has assisted in identifying practical approaches that counselors can use when deconstructing racial stigma in the therapeutic relationship.

REFERENCES

African American Mental Health. (n.d.). Retrieved from https://www.nami.org/Find-Support/Diverse-Communities/African-American-Mental-Health

American Counseling Association. (2014). *2014 ACA code of ethics: As approved by the ACA governing council*. Retrieved from http://counseling.org/docs/ethics/2014-aca-code-of-ethics.pdf?sfvrsn=4

Baruth, L. G., & Manning, M. L. (2003). *Multicultural counseling and psychotherapy: A lifespan perspective*. Dallas, TX: Pearson.

Bharadwaj, P., Pai, M. M., & Suziedelyte, A. (2015). *Mental health stigma* (National Bureau of Economic Research). Retrieved from http://economics.ucr.edu/seminars_colloquia/201415/applied_economics/Suzie elyte%20paper%20for%206%205%2015%20seminar.pdf

Bordin, E. S. (1979). The generalizability of the psychoanalytic concept of the working alliance. *Psychotherapy (Chicago, Ill.)*, *16*(3), 252–260. doi:10.1037/h0085885

CACREP Annual Reports. (2016). Retrieved from http://www.cacrep.org/about-cacrep/publications/cacrep-annual-reports/

Corrigan, P. W. (1999). Mental health stigma as social attribution: Implications for research methods and attitude change. *Clinical Psychology: Science and Practice*, *7*(1), 48–67. doi:10.1093/clipsy.7.1.48

Corrigan, P. W. (2004). How stigma interferes with mental health care. *The American Psychologist*, *59*(7), 614–625. doi:10.1037/0003-066X.59.7.614 PMID:15491256

Corrigan, P. W., & Penn, D. L. (1999). Lessons from social psychology on discrediting psychiatric stigma. *The American Psychologist*, *54*(9), 765–776. doi:10.1037/0003-066X.54.9.765 PMID:10510666

Corrigan, P. W., & Rao, D. (2012). On the self-stigma of mental illness: Stages, disclosure, and strategies for change. *Canadian Journal of Psychiatry*, *57*(8), 464–469. doi:10.1177/070674371205700804 PMID:22854028

Crenshaw, K. (2016). *The urgency of intersectionality*. Retrieved from https://www.ted.com/talks/kimberle_crenshaw_the_urgency_of_intersectionalityedWomen2016

Goffman, E. (1963). *Stigma: Notes on the Management of Spoiled Identity*. New York, New York: Simon & Schuster.

Howarth, C. (2006). Race as stigma: Positioning the stigmatized as agents, not objects. *Journal of Community & Applied Social Psychology*, *16*(6), 442–451. doi:10.1002/casp.898

Loury, G. C. (2003). Racial stigma: Toward a new paradigm for discrimination theory. *The American Economic Review*, *93*(2), 334–337. doi:10.1257/000282803321947308

Office of Minority Mental Health. (2016). Retrieved from http://minorityhealth.hhs.gov/templates/content.aspx?ID=6476

Rogers, C. R. (1980). *A way of being*. Boston, MA: Houghton Mifflin.

Shrivastava, A., Johnston, M., & Bureau, Y. (2012). Stigma of mental illness – 1: Clinical reflections. *MSM Mens Sana Monographs*, *10*(1), 70–84. doi:10.4103/0973-1229.90181 PMID:22654383

Shrivastava, A., Johnston, M., & Bureau, Y. (2012). Stigma of mental illness – 2: Non-compliance and intervention. *MSM Mens Sana Monographs*, *10*(1), 85–97. doi:10.4103/0973-1229.90276 PMID:22654384

Strkalj-Ivezic, S. (2013). Stigma in clinical practice. *Psychiatria Danubina*, *25*, 200–202. PMID:23995176

Sue, D. W., Bucceri, J., Lin, A. I., Nadal, K. L., & Torino, G. C. (2007). Racial microaggressions and the Asian American experience. *Cultural Diversity & Ethnic Minority Psychology*, *13*(1), 72–81. doi:10.1037/1099-9809.13.1.72 PMID:17227179

Sue, D. W., & Sue, D. (2016). *Counseling the Culturally Diverse: Theory and Practice* (7th ed.). Hoboken, NJ: John Wiley and Sons.

Sullivan, M. A. (2005). Kum Ba Yah: The relevance of family systems theory for clinicians and clients of African descent. In M. Rastogi & E, Wieling (Eds.), Voices of Color (pp. 277-295). London: Sage.

Chapter 2
Understanding the Nature of Stigma Communication Associated With Mental Illness in Africa:
A Focus on Cultural Beliefs and Stereotypes

Stephen Gichuhi Kimotho
United States International University – Africa, Kenya

ABSTRACT

Besides health and social costs, mentally ill, often, are also victims of stigma and discrimination, among many communities in Africa. Cultural beliefs, stereotypes are some of the social constructions used to perpetuate mental illness stigma. The purpose of this study was to describe the nature of stigma communication associated with mental illness, beliefs and stereotypes underpinning mental illness stigma. Generally, the findings indicate nature of mental illness stigma communication is an intersection of stigma messages, cultural beliefs, and stereotypes associated with mental illness. Cultural beliefs associated with mental illness are inextricably intertwined with the perceived causes of mental illness (which include curses, witchcraft, cultural misdemeanor, and possession by spirits or demons). Symptoms of mental illness (mainly aggression and nudity) mark the mentally ill as different and expose them to labeling by the rest of the community. Generally, the mentally ill are stereotyped as aggressive, symbol of shame, and unpredictable.

DOI: 10.4018/978-1-5225-3808-0.ch002

INTRODUCTION

Mental disorder places immense financial, psychological and social burden on family members of the persons with mental illnesses and ultimately have a significant impact on the family's quality of life. WHO estimates that as many as 450 million people suffer from a mental disorder and nearly one million people commit suicide every year around the world. In addition, one in four families has at least one member with a mental disorder (World Health Organization, 2001).

Besides health and social costs, those suffering from mental illnesses, often, are also victims of human rights violations, stigma and discrimination, both inside and outside psychiatric institutions. Such stigmatization manifest through stereotyping, fear, embarrassment, anger, and rejection or avoidance. Among many communities, stigmatization of mentally ill is highly entrenched in the language and communication of the people and in various social interaction contexts. Understanding this, is important because this study is founded on the philosophical assumption that stigma and stigma communication are social constructions through language. Some of these social constructions used to perpetuate stigma associated with mental illness, among the members of different communities include: myths, cultural beliefs, stereotypes and misconceptions associated with mental illness.

Stigma and stigma communication associated with mental illnesses negatively affect the day-to-day lives of persons affected, leading to discrimination and the denial of even the most basic human rights. All over the world, people with mental disorders face unfair denial of employment and educational opportunities, and discrimination in health insurance and housing policies (Lasalvia, et al., 2013). Though a significant amount of research has been done on mental health, many studies have focused on measurement of mental illness (Van Brakel, 2006); coping strategies (Corrigan, & Miller, 2004) and others psychological outcomes. Despite these extensive research on mental health, mental illnesses continue to financially and socially torment millions of people in Africa because of the stigma, beliefs and stereotypes associated with mental illnesses. Nevertheless, little scholarly work has gone into analyzing the nature of stigma communication associated with mental illness or cultural beliefs and stereotypes underpinning such stigma in Africa. This study set out to fill this gap.

BACKGROUND

Mental illness is a silent epidemic throughout most parts of Africa. Owing to structural and systemic barriers such as inadequate health care infrastructure, insufficient number of mental health specialists, and lack of access to all levels of care, mental illness has been characterized as a neglected and increasingly burdensome problem affecting all segments of the population throughout Africa (Monteiro, 2015).

Stigma has been regarded as the most important obstacle to the appropriate treatment and rehabilitation of those suffering from mental illness (Sartorius, 2002). Some of these social constructions used to perpetuate stigma among the members of different communities include: myths, beliefs, stereotypes and misconceptions associated with mental disorders. However, stigma is a fairly elusive concept and scholars from various disciplines have defined and used the term in varied ways and for different purposes (Link, Yang & Phelan, 2004). Although there are some clear indicators of the social origins of stigmatization and the factors that perpetuate it, a generally accepted unitary theory of the origins stigma remains elusive to date. The following section gives a preview of some approaches and theories used to understand the stigma problem in various contexts.

Symbolic Interactionism

The central argument of symbolic interactionism is that human life is lived in the symbolic domain. Symbols are culturally derived social objects having shared meanings that are created and maintained in social interaction. Therefore, language and communication are key to the process of constructing reality because they provide symbols and ultimately the means by which reality is constructed (James, 2003). The key process linking society and the self in this approach is ''taking the role of the other'': we see ourselves as meaningful social objects (who we are) and appraise our goodness, worthiness, and competence (how good we are) through the eyes of significant others and from the standpoint of the wider community. Since the meanings of social objects and social acts are culturally shared (Burke, & Stets, 2009), an undesirable category or label applied by others to the self becomes an undesirable social identity. That identity in turn results in self devaluation (Goffman 1963), or, in more contemporary terms, produces ''self-stigmatization'' (Corrigan and Watson 2002; Corrigan and Calabrese 2009) or ''internalized stigma.''

One salient philosophical assumption underlying this study is that stigmas are social constructions. The social constructionist ontology has its root in the symbolic interactionism tradition, which states that the meanings of social objects, such as people and actions, are social constructs. Social constructionists hold as their cardinal assumption that in a society, people jointly construct their understanding of phenomena in their world and meanings are developed during social interaction.

Social Constructionist Approaches to Stigma

Social constructionist approaches to stigma spring from Goffman's (1963) seminal work, *Stigma: Notes on the Management of Spoiled Identity*, originally published in 1963. Goffman's theory of stigma derived from his analysis of people's lives, for instance, those with mental illness; physically challenged, blind, deaf, prostitutes, and homosexuals. Goffman averred that individuals are categorized by the society on the basis of the anticipated normative values – separating the "normal" from the "deviants" (Goffman, 1963). Stigma, according to Goffman, refers to an attribute that is profoundly degrading, reducing the individual that possesses a particular trait from a whole to an aspersed and discredited one (Goffman, 1963), and consequently the person is socially disregarded. The gist of this approach is the understanding that stigma arises during a social interaction.

By defining stigma as a spoiled identity, which means that a person is somehow not normal or accepted by society because of a physical disability, signs of "immoral" or non-conforming behavior, or membership to a particular group, Goffman cast stigma as a social construction in which society determines which statuses deserve to be stigmatized (Smith, 2009). As such, the creation and maintenance of stigmatizing beliefs and stereotypes about mental illness would be represented in the language as well as the labels used to describe persons with mental illness.

Therefore, stigma is the process whereby society negatively defines a particular mark such as symptom or symptoms of mental illness as "… an attribute that is deeply discrediting…." (Goffman, 1963, p.3). In other words, at its most basic level, stigma, from social constructionists' point of view, is a powerful discrediting and sullying social label that radically alters the way individuals view themselves and are viewed by others as persons. In general, stigmas result from stereotypic labels, which may or may not be true but nonetheless affect a person's social standing and self-image.

Goffman's work has significant implications for this study. Besides, the fact that Goffman's theory supports one of the fundamental claims of this study that stigma is socially constructed. Goffman's work also underscores the importance of the process of communication in creation and maintenance of stigma. Also, in his discussion of the nature of stigma, Goffman's work emphasizes the importance of societal beliefs and stereotypes in the creation and maintenance of stigma in the society. This as well, was important in addressing the main objective of the study that sought to investigate the nature of mental illness stigma.

Finally, Goffman argues that the process of information control is fundamental to the socialization of the personal identity of a stigmatized person in any society. The discreditable person (individuals who have stigmatizing traits but have not yet been discredited, primarily because the traits they possess have not yet been completely revealed) manages information, constantly judging whether or not to reveal their stigmatic traits or quality. Discredited persons (individuals whose stigma is visible, that is, plainly known and seen) are often faced with managing the tension that ensues (Carnevale, 2007). The process of information control described by Goffman relates to the management of the stigma communication process which was beyond the scope of this study.

Goffman's theory has received significant criticism, however, particularly relating to the seemingly helpless role that the theory attributes to people with stigmatized attributes. According to Carnevale (2007), stigmatized people should not be viewed as helpless because recent studies on disabilities have demonstrated various forms of resistance or valued social roles exhibited by the people with disabilities (Carnevale, 2007). In her discussion of stigma management communication, Meisenbach (2010) also faults Goffman's theory as unsystematic and partial. Meisenbach particularly points at the omission of frequently found stigma management communication strategies like social comparison. In addition, Meisenbach argues that except for the re-education strategy, all the other Goffman's strategies do not suggest a proactive stigma management communication approach.

Stigma Communication Theory

From a communication perspective, stigma is a social constructions about other people. Understanding stigma communication as social constructions expressed through language is a critical starting point in understanding stigma communication. Specifically, stigma communication can be defined as the mechanism through which stigma messages are created, reinforced and maintained through a communication process and how such messages spread through communities to teach their members to recognize the disgraced (i.e., recognizing stigmata) and to react accordingly (Smith, 2007). Stigma communication theory argues that stigma messages are constituted of mark, label, responsibility and peril.

Marks, as described by Smith, are imputes (for example skin color, blindness, or eye color) or deviant behaviors (prostitution) used to pick out an individual within a stigmatized group). Smith describes a label as a name made to discern the stigmatized as a different social entity. The label not only draws attention to the group's stigma but also stresses "them" as different and separate from "us" and aids in distinguishing the marked from the "normals" (Smith, 2007).

Responsibility refers to the implied blame, which is carried by the information entailed in messages. Put differently, responsibility points to the argument that those in the stigmatized group are to blame for the choices they made and such choices put the community at risk.

Peril is the information that connects the marked, labelled, responsible individuals to a physical or social danger jeopardizing the community's way of life. Peril is a constant reminder to the community members to avoid the stigmatized.

Stigma communication theory was relevant to the study in several fundamental ways. First, it helped in forming a framework for the description of labels, marks, responsibilities or perils linked to stigma communication associated with mental illness which was core to achieving answers to the first research question of the study described below.

Question 1: What are the components of mental illness stigma communication among African communities?

In addition, the theory addresses the problem of stigma from a communicative point of view and underscores the inextricable nature of communication in stigma formation, maintenance and management. Finally, the theory is founded on social constructionism and thus is aligned with the study's philosophical assumptions.

Finally, though understanding the components stigma messages (mark, label, responsibility and peril) is fundamental to conceptualization of nature of stigma communication, scholars have established that this does not provide the full picture unless cultural beliefs and stereotypes associated with a certain stigma are included as components of stigma communication (Kimotho, Miller, & Ngure, 2015). These two construct cultural (beliefs and stereotypes) were key to answering the other two research questions of this study.

Question 2: What are the cultural belief associated to mental illness in Africa?
Question 3: What are the stereotypes associated to mental illness in Africa?

METHODS

The study employed a descriptive research design, using a qualitative research approach to describe the nature of stigma communication associated with mental illness. A qualitative approach was deemed appropriate for the study because it facilitated in-depth understanding of the issues surrounding mental illness stigma, and afforded flexibility to respond to unexpected and new development in the data (Yin, 1994).

Twelve in-depth interviews (the recommended standard figure by various qualitative scholars including Onwuegbuzie, Dickinson, Leech, & Zoran, 2009), with individuals from different communities around Africa were conducted. The respondents were mainly drawn from Kenya, Uganda, Malawi, Rwanda, Nigeria,

Burundi, Ethiopia, Zambia and South Sudan. The interviews lasted between 45 minutes to one hour. By the time the researcher was interviewing the 11th respondent, the data had reached a clear point of saturation (Creswell, 2003; Onwuegbuzie, Dickinson, Leech, & Zoran, 2009). No new information or themes were coming forth. The purposefully sampled respondents were drawn from different parts of Africa. Eligible participants were above 18 years, had been brought up in Africa and were willing to spend one hour discussing issues about stigma associated with mental illness stigma.

FINDINGS

Nature of Stigma Communication Associated With Mental Illness

The findings largely support Smith, 2007 stigma communication model. Smith (2007) argued that four types of communication content play critical roles not only in eliciting particular cognitive and affective responses but also in shaping the development of a particular stigma, isolating and removing stigmatized people, and sharing the stigma message with others. These four components of stigma messages (mark, label, responsibility and peril) are fundamental to conceptualization of nature of stigma communication associated with mental illness and are explained below.

Marks

Mark refers to a cue that allows someone to identify another person as a member of a stigmatized group. As in many other forms of stigma, the findings indicate that marks associated with mental illness are particularly effective when they include visible and disgusting cues, because these cues are easier to recognize and they evoke the stigma-appropriate action tendency; to remove and isolate stigmatized persons (Smith, 2007).

Five types of marks associated with mental illness emerged: nakedness, unprovoked aggressive or violent behaviors, use of vulgar language, persistent shabbiness or dirtiness, and inability to recognize contexts of socialization. Of all these marks, nakedness was deemed the most certain way of identifying persons with mental illness among all the respondents. In fact, among the communities that classified the persons with mental illness according to perceived seriousness of the mental illness, nakedness was a sure indicator for classifying an individual in this category as alluded in the following sentiment of one of the respondents.

When a mad person runs in to the market naked such an individual's degrees of mental illness are believed to be at all-time high. Now that's a truly mad man or woman. They are called Janiko in Luo community. Many such individuals display eccentricity or oddities including undressing and running naked. In Luo community this category is euphemistically referred to using a phrase Oseringe (One who has ran).

Being aggressive to other members of the community or exhibiting violent behaviors even when unprovoked was consistently mentioned as another way of identifying or marking people who are perceived persons with mental illness. In such cases, the members of the society were socialized to behave in certain ways towards such people as illustrated by one of the respondent.

Mad people are often violent. Yes they are, and as kids my mother would caution us against using certain routes that were frequented by one of the mad man in the village. We feared them because we believed they would beat kids up. We would only use such routes in the company of adults.

According to the respondents interviewed, society expects individuals to correctly recognize the different contexts of socialization and adhere to the set out norms that guide socialization and conversations in such contexts. In ability to recognize such context would make the society judge one as a person with mental health issues. Some specific context mentioned include dowry, wedding and funeral ceremonies. In such ceremonies, respectable people such as parents, uncles, in-laws and guests are expected to attend. As such, members of the society are expected to show respect, avoid using indecent language, be clean, obey conversational turn- taking norms and generally be presentable.

In addition, being persistently shabby or in ability to keep oneself clean and particularly carrying dirty baggage all the time, were also mentioned as marks of mental illness.

Label

A second message choice is the terms used to reference a person with mental illness by the members of the society. Such terms are called labels. The label promotes the cognitive process of entitativity, or perceiving a collection of people as a distinct, actual group, and highlights intergroup differences (Smith, 2007). According to most of the respondents interviewed, there exist two types of labels: polite and derogatory references. In many of the African communities, the polite way of referring to a person with mental illness in the society is "one who is sick in the mind". For instance, among the AGikuyu, a Bantu community from Kenya, mental illness is politely referred as *"murimu wa meciria"* which can be loosely translated as "the disease of the mind." In the same community a person with mental illness could be derogatory referred to as *"Muguruki."* This is a highly stigmatizing term and also used as an insult even on the 'normal' persons, when the user want to underscore the irrational nature of the behavior of the person targeted with the insult. Among the Kalenjin community persons with mental illness are referred to as *chebiywo (kibiywo- singular).* According to the respondent *"this is not a polite name for a person with mental illness. It stigmatizes. You cannot throw such a term to people living with a mental illness."*

Of all the 12 communities represented in this study, the Luo community from Kenya had the most elaborate way of labelling a person with mental illness as illustrated below:

In my community, two levels of insanity are recognized: the first is Raura. Raura is a degree of mental illness above a fool. A person classified in this category is believed to be incapable of making critical judgment. Such a person cannot be relied on and cannot be trusted to undertake common duties or roles in the society. The second category is Janiko. This is an individual whose mental illness is believed to be degrees higher than that of Raura. This is a mad man or woman. They exhibit outrageous behaviors. They are likely to be aggressive and often undress and run naked. In Luo community this category is euphemistically referred as using a phrase Oseringe (One who has ran). This category is typified by two dramatic forms of behavior: stripping naked and running.

Responsibility

A third message choice focuses on responsibility, that is, to what extent the persons with mental illness could be blamed for their condition. Did the persons with mental illness choose to do activities that caused their stigmatizing conditions? If the rest of the community perceive persons with mental illness to be more responsible for their situation, the society is likely to punish them more heavily (Smith, 2007). According to the respondents, responsibility was closely linked to the perceived cause of mental illness. Narrative from all the communities represented in this study yielded four major reasons why the society would attribute responsibility to the persons with mental illness: failure to follow norms, committing a crime again the community, inherited responsibility and gross misconduct.

According to most of the respondents, failure to follow norms and more often the ritualistic norms could result into bad omen which could manifest as mental illness. For instant, among the Kisii and Yoruba in Nigeria, failure to perform some traditional rituals by an individual as per the community expectation may result to retaliation by the ancestors. It is important to note that such failures may not have necessarily been committed by the persons with mental illness; sometimes it could have been their parent's failure. In such situation, this was referred by the respondents as 'inherited responsibility.' The beliefs in punishment from ancestors and that such punishment could manifest in the form of mental illness are still relevant and used as causal explanation for varied mental illnesses among many communities in Africa, to date, as demonstrated by the respondents in their explanations.

Second, is committing a crime that affects the whole society. A good example from Kisii, Gikuyu and many Kalenjin communities is when one steals public utility good like dismantling a critical river bridge between two ridges. The perpetrator of such a crime is condemned by the whole community and many of the communities represented believe that a communal curse may manifest in mental illness on the perpetrator or their children. Closely related to this theme are other forms of misconducts construed to be gross by the community including committing taboo; for instance having sex with a blood relative or acts of rape particularly on elderly.

Peril

The final message choice relates to content that highlights the peril associated with the stigmatized group. Peril content may highlight physical or moral dangers. Focusing on physical dangers, incurable, painful, fatal conditions carry more danger than curable, mildly uncomfortable, temporary ones (Smith, 2012). Two forms of perils associated with mental illness among the African communities were identified: danger of physically harming others, and danger of causing embarrassment. According to all respondents, persons with mental illness were marked as violent or potentially violent individual. Therefore, the sudden emergence of persons with mental illness among the 'normals' triggers an extra sense of caution.

If you mention that a mad man has joined us to a group of people that were chatting happily, everybody turns. Everyone is cautious, particularly if the mad man has any history of violence. Suddenly there would be uneasiness and anxiety among the people.

Cultural Beliefs

Generally speaking culture is people's way of life. It encompasses the cumulative deposit of knowledge, experiences, beliefs, values, attitudes, meanings, hierarchies, religion, notions of time, roles, spatial relations, concepts of the universe, and material objects and possessions acquired by a group of people in the course of generations through individual and group striving (Hofstede, 1997). Like culture, cultural beliefs are systems of knowledge shared by a relatively large group of people.

In this study, cultural beliefs associated with mental illness are inextricably intertwined with the perceived causations of mental illness. African communities have varied beliefs regarding the causes of mental illness. Majorly, five causes emerged from the data: curses, witchcraft, cultural misdemeanor, possession by spirits or demons, and family problem.

- **Curses:** The respondent identified three potent source of curses that could result to mental illness: parental, ancestral, and elders curses. Parental curses among were perceived to be the most serious of all curses. All respondents were categorical that parents rarely cursed their kids and were rarely expected to do so. However, in cases of persistent mistreatment or gross misconduct by one of the children to a parent, parents would utter curses. The individuals targeted with these parental curses in most communities in Africa are preconceived as doomed and are constantly blamed for whatever befell them. According to the respondents, the parental curses at the most adverse levels, could lead to death of the cursed individual. Otherwise such curses, more often than not resorted to mental illness of the cursed individual or their spouses or their children. Almost all the respondents had interesting stories and anecdotes to illustrate the potency of the three types of curses as illustrated in the excerpt below:

In my village there is this window who sacrificed everything she owned to educate her son. Finally, the son became an architect and earned a lot of money. He became very rich, got married and lived a fairly luxurious life in the city of Nairobi, Kenya. He rarely visited the village to see his mother. His mother cried everyday as she struggled in poverty. "After working and sacrificing so much for my only son, he has forgotten me," she complained constantly. The age mates of this young man took the message to him and in retaliation, the son wrote a letter to his mother asking her to compute all expenses she incurred as he was growing up; including school fees, and other compensations she may desire add, and he would settle that in a ransom payment. The mother did not write a reply but kept on complaining bitterly, "Eat your wealth and eat it well. May it not shock you" It was sarcastically put. It was not blessing, it was a curse and a potent one. After sometime, the wife to this son fell ill. She later got mentally ill as well. She died after a short period of sickness. People attributed the mental illness and consequent death to the mother's curse. However, since it was also believed that, this man brought the misfortune upon himself by neglecting the mother, they refused to participate in the funeral ceremony of the wife as it would be traditionally expected.

Ancestral curses and curses from elders were almost as potent as the parental curses according to most of the respondents. Not everyone in the community could curse though, as demonstrated in the excerpt below:

Most potent curses are from elderly close relatives. Curses from younger members of the society are often not potent. People who can yield highly potent curses according to Luo communities are: Parents, uncles and aunties, in-laws. "In fact, your father in law can curse you in a way your brother in law can't curse you. This is because the father or mother in laws in are believed to possess some spiritual authorities that is not shared or owned by other members of the society.

But why would one get cursed with mental illness? Varied reasons were given by the respondents as to why one may get cursed by elderly or the ancestors. Curses come out of conflict, annoyance of the elderly or the ancestors. In all the communities represented in this study, there exists a solid belief that that words from elderly people are not just words; they can yield blessings or curses. Among some communities like the Kalenjin, Meru and Gikuyu from Kenya, oromo of Ethiopia, Nuer of Southern Sudan communities among others, elders could curse people who contravene the norms of the community on behalf of the whole community as illustrated in the excerpt below:

In my community keeping livestock is the lifeline of the community. Therefore, if someone who stole from the community or got into the habit of stealing cattle from the community. The elders would normally call a community meeting at the market place and ask that the thief or thieves identify themselves and request for forgiveness from the community. When the thieves refuse to heed to such calls, the elders then would curse thief. Such curses are deemed serious and sometimes would take effect before the end of the day. These curses often manifest in the form of mental illness.

Many African communities believe in the influence of the ancestors on the living. There were taboos set to safeguard the ancestors' peace and to appease them. Digging up a grave of the departed particularly the parents was deemed a taboo (among many communities in Africa), interfering with ancestral sacrifices or designated 'holy' areas can also earn one a curse from the ancestors according to some communities in Africa.

- **Witchcraft:** Witchcraft is a ubiquitous notion that is prevalent among many African communities. Among many African communities misfortune are often attributed to witchcraft. Mental illness quite often evoke the notion of witchcraft in many African communities. Two major forms of witchcraft emerged from the data: Retaliatory, and envy witchcraft (commonly labeled as "evil eye").

A number of reasons were provided by respondents on why one may get bewitched.

Witchcraft is not always a retaliatory act. Sometimes it cheer pernicious envy that commonly lead people to bewitch others. There are known people in the community who just use their witch power wantonly to suppress the neighborhood. For instance, if you were my neighbor, and your children do so well in school and you succeed as a result of their success, as an envious neighbor I could bewitch your children.

However not everyone has the supernatural power to bewitch or activate witchcraft. According to most of the respondents, those who do not have such powers have to seek for help from witchdoctors and pay them to perform malicious rituals that will affect the target victim. In every community, there are renowned witchdoctors who are approached for such services. They could also be approached for counter witch or an antidote to witchcraft from another witchdoctor. Most of the respondents noted that mental illness is one of the commonest manifestation of witchcraft.

In retaliatory witchcraft, disgruntles individual may seek for revenge by bewitching others, or seeking for such services from the witchdoctors.

Disgruntled women in a failed marriage relationship can cast a witchcraft spell on the man who divorces them. The relatives to such a disgruntled woman can also do the same as a way of revenging for them. The manifestation of such as spells again, can be in varied forms, but more often, as mental illness.

- **Cultural Misdemeanor:** Committing a cultural misdemeanor refers to committing a 'cultural sin' according to the respondents. It is a form of gross violation of the norms of the communities. Most of them such misdemeanors are in the form of violation of some taboos. In this paper taboos are defined as cultural prohibitions by the community. There are many forms of taboos among the African communities. However, the following were mentioned by most of the respondents in this study: incestuous relationship, fighting parents, stealing or violating the rights of the elderly, and disinheriting others their land. One of the respondents captured some of these taboos in the following excerpt:

Some of the taboos in my community are dramatic and interesting. It is believed that violating them could attracts a curse and often such a curse may make one mad. For instance quarrelling with parents to the extent of touching or exposing their genitalia. It is also a taboo to take (grab) land forcefully from a member of the community that is considered as their inheritance (disinherit).

- **Possession by Spirits:** Almost all communities attributed mental illness to possession by some spirits or demons. Generally two kinds of spirits were identified and associated with mental illness: ancestral spirits and malevolent spirits.

Ancestral spirit (supernatural spirits) could come back to possess the people in the society. It emerged from the data that when ancestral spirits possess an individual, they could manifest in form of mental illness. Ancestral spirits would come back and possess an individual for several reasons. Sometimes, it could be because they are demanding for justice; for instance if there were some funeral rites that were not done – as expected by the community; or they (ancestors) want some of your children named after them. The ancestors may also be on a revenge mission as illustrated by the extract below from one of the respondents.

Ancestral spirits could also possess an individual if such an individual offended them grievously when they were alive; or they want you to join them. That means they want you to join the ancestral community. It is an invitation. They want you dead and you have declined to die and therefore they will make you mad. Often such patients with this rare form of madness end up committing suicide.

The second category of spirits were referred to as *non-local malevolent spirits*. The perception of non-local malevolent spirits is particularly prevalent among a number of communities in Africa. According to the respondents such spirits are often imported potent spirits by individuals to use them to attack some perceived enemies. According to the some African communities like the Luo from Kenya, it is commonly believed that such spirits are imported from the coast of Kenya (often call *Jinni* [singular] or *Majinni* [plural]) or from Tanzania (a neighboring country). According to one of the respondents, *Tanzania enjoys a formidable reputation for the supernatural powers. They have the most powerful witchdoctors and medicine men.* It should be noted, however, that for someone to cast such a spell on you they have to travel hundreds of miles, and incur a great deal of expenses. Such spirits are also very difficult to exorcise.

- **Family Problem:** Finally, the other prominent believe that was constantly mentioned by the respondent, was the belief that mental illness was an inherited problem. It was a referred as to "a family thing". The label of madness or insanity is often flashed around when a young man or lady reveal their intentions of marrying from a certain family known to have cases of mental illness. This is how one of the respondent put:

"She may not be sick, but there have been people who have 'run' (had a severe form of mental illness) in that homestead. Do you want to have children who are like that? This is a family thing you must be careful" That is what they are often told. Madness stigma is one of the most difficult traits to overcome and one that has the most adverse effect on families that have persons with mental illness. Mental illness card is also brandished maliciously when a member of such family with known cases of mental illness seek for an elective post in the government or society.

Stereotypes

Stereotypes are overgeneralized set of ideas that people have about what someone or something is like, but often incorrect. Largely, five types of stereotypes emerged from the data. First, persons with mental illness are stereotyped in many African communities as violent or aggressive. This point has been previously addressed under peril. Second, persons with mental illness are seen as symbol of fear. Their very sight evoke fear. This is mainly so because of their physical outlook (often shabby or unkempt hair etc.). Third, persons with mental illness are often perceived and stereotyped as unpredictable. As one of the respondents put it;

They (persons with mental illness) are often shunned in my community because people think they have some uncontrollable impulses that even they, themselves cannot control. They are simply under a spell or influences from supernatural forces like spirits or demons.

Fourth, persons with mental illness are also often stereotyped as socially impure. The source of impurity is mainly contravention of the social norms and subsequently being cursed by the society; or perception that they are possessed by demons or spirits.

Finally, persons with mental illness are also stereotyped as symbols of shame. It is important though to mention that most of the respondents also believe that, the very nature of mental illness (described under marks) makes many of the 'normal' to shy away from those persons with mental illness.

As Goffman (1963) observed stereotyped expectations lead ''normals'' to block labeled individuals from returning to conventional activities and to reward them for behaviors that conform to the mental patient role. Observing themselves acting in accordance with stereotyped expectations, and highly sensitive when in crisis to the cues provided by others, labeled persons conclude that they must be mentally ill and accept the mental patient role as an identity. This point is well illustrated by the excerpt below from one of the respondents.

...this gentleman from my village was a very brilliant person. People belief he was bewitched by people who did not want the family to progress. But now, interesting, when talking to him you may not notice that he has a mental illness. So when you ask him then why he won't bathe or change his clothes, he shrugs off and says that people notice him a lot and make funny calls at him asking him, what is the occasion? Why is he so clean? Where is he going for a party? So to reduce public attention to himself he decided to stay dirty. He says that way, no one bothers him

As can be deciphered from the example above, subsequent episodes of stress further impair labeled individuals' ability to control their behavior, repeatedly validating their own and others' views of their illness or incompetence. In short, labeling, stereotyping and differential treatment by other people produces a ''mentally ill'' identity and self-devaluation (Kowalski, Morgan, & Taylor, 2016).

DISCUSSIONS

The purpose of this study was to establish nature of stigma communication associated with mental illness or beliefs and stereotypes underpinning such stigma among the African communities. The findings of this study largely support Smith's theory of stigma communication which postulates that understanding the components stigma messages (mark, label, responsibility and peril) is fundamental to conceptualization of nature of stigma communication. Generally, the findings indicate that nature of mental illness stigma communication is an intersection of three major components during stigma communication processes. These components are: stigma messages, cultural beliefs, and stereotypes associated with mental illness.

Symptoms of mental illness as described by the respondents (which include aggression or violence, shabbiness, nudity particularly in public) mark the persons with mental illness as different and give them away for labelling by the rest of the community. According to the findings of this study individuals labelled as persons with mental illness are then discursively placed in distinguishable categories so as to accomplish some degree of separation of "us" from "them" (Devine, et al.,

1999). In some communities it is not just uniform separation but there exist degrees of separation according to the classification of mental illnesses. A good case is among the Luo community from Kenya which has two categories which are clearly linguistically labelled: *Raura* (moderately insane) and *Janiko* (the completely insane). More often the separation in many of the communities is effectively attained through activation of cultural beliefs (including beliefs in curses or witchcraft) that related labelled persons to undesirable characteristics and to negative stereotypes (Link & Phelan, 2001).

While cultural beliefs including beliefs about curses from ancestors or parents, beliefs in witchcraft do not feature prominently as components of stigma communication as conceptualized by Smith's model of stigma communication (Smith, 2007), it is important to note that they are key components of stigma communication process among African communities. Of course, the likely explanation is the cultural and ideological difference between the theorist orientation (individualistic societies) and the communities studied (communal societies).

Indeed, as the findings indicate, in many African languages cultural beliefs associated with mental illness were attributive in nature and inextricably intertwined with the perceived causes of mental illness. Five major causes of mental illness associated with the cultural beliefs were identified: curses, witchcraft, cultural misdemeanor, possession by spirits or demons, and family problem.

These causes do not receive similar blanket interpretation from the society. For instance, the belief in curses are not only given a causal attribution to mental illness but also inadvertently perpetuate the constant awareness in the minds of the community members that such individuals are cursed. A curse is a condemnation (Wakanyi-Kahindi, 2012) among many African communities. According to the findings, the rationale used to justify that condemnation, was that people don't just get cursed for no reason (Kimotho, Miller & Ngure, 2015). Rather, they are cursed because they erred at some point in their lives, committed a cultural misdemeanor or violated the social norms and values. A curse is therefore perceived by society as a punishment (Kimotho, Miller & Ngure, 2015).

Most of these cultural beliefs and stereotypes associated with mental illness are then gradually adopted into the communities' linguistic repertoire and manifests in commonly used folklore during social interactions. According to the findings the society possesses well-crafted sayings and proverbs and anecdotes that are often used during stigma communication process to warn people about interacting with cursed individuals in the society.

According to Thoits (2011) once individuals have been classified as persons with mental illness, stereotypes about mental illness become activated in the language and imaginations of other people. These stereotypes are learned early in life and are reinforced over time in ordinary interaction and by caricatures in the media.

In almost all of the communities interviewed, there exist songs, sayings, jokes or anecdotes that capture some of the stereotypes described in the findings.

Where it was believed that the person with mental illness or the family bore responsibility for the illness the folklores were often used to warn the rest of the community on the dangers of breaking. For instance a respondent from the Banyore community in Western Kenya noted:

We have certain ceremonies in our communities and during such ceremonies people who have contravened the social norms and gotten mad, or because of other reason are identified publicly through songs and dances. We want to make the society aware of who they are dealing with. Particularly when they are perceived to have gotten the mental illness because of violating taboos or abuse of drugs like marijuana which is a very common drug.

RECOMMENDATIONS

This study makes several important contributions to the literature on stigma communication associated with mental illness. For instance cultural beliefs and stereotypes about mental illness were found out to be instrumental in creation, maintenance and management of mental illness stigma communication. These cultural beliefs, and stereotypes are apparently sustained by low levels of awareness about etiology mental illness among many African communities. As such they continue to fuel the stings of stigma associated with mental illness among many poor communities in Africa. The aftermath of stigmatization of individuals suffering from mental illness has been their continued discrimination, exclusion and marginalization.

Since the findings suggest that ignorance about the etiology of mental illness is one of the key reasons behind the proliferation of the mental illness stigma; then, culturally (and linguistically) appropriate and sensitive awareness campaigns that would increase knowledge and understanding about the causes of mental illness in many African communities would greatly demystify mental illness.

FURTHER RESEARCH DIRECTIONS

During the study, there were several descriptions by respondents that alluded to the fact that religion could be an important means of understanding mental illness, and even coping with mental illness stigma. While religion, spirituality could be critical in understanding stigma communication management associated with mental illness, analysis of the data indicate there is need to further understand the role of religion and religious beliefs in the understanding of serious mental illnesses. This area is highly recommended for further studies. Additionally, I recommend further studies on experiences of relatives of the persons with mental illness and outcomes of stigma communication on such relatives.

CONCLUSION

In general mental illness stigma remains a serious challenge and impediment to health seeking and utilization of health facilities among many poverty-stricken communities in Africa. Understanding the mechanism through which mental illness stigma messages are created, reinforced and managed through a communication process can greatly help in the minimizing the impact of mental stigma.

REFERENCES

Burke, P. J., & Stets, J. E. (2009). *Identity theory*. Oxford University Press. doi:10.1093/acprof:oso/9780195388275.001.0001

Carnevale, F. A. (2007). Revisiting Goffman's Stigma: The social experience of families with children requiring mechanical ventilation at home. *Journal of Child Health Care*, *11*(1), 7–18. doi:10.1177/1367493507073057 PMID:17287220

Corrigan, P. W., Larson, J. E., & Rusch, N. (2009). Self-stigma and the "why try" effect'' impact on life goals and evidence based practices. *World Psychiatry; Official Journal of the World Psychiatric Association (WPA)*, *8*(2), 75–81. doi:10.1002/j.2051-5545.2009.tb00218.x PMID:19516923

Corrigan, P. W., & Miller, F. E. (2004). Shame, blame, and contamination: A review of the impact of mental illness stigma on family members. *Journal of Mental Health (Abingdon, England)*, *13*(6), 537–548. doi:10.1080/09638230400017004

Corrigan, P. W., & Watson, A. C. (2002). The paradox of self-stigma and mental illness. *Clinical Psychology: Science and Practice*, *9*(1), 35–53. doi:10.1093/clipsy.9.1.35

Creswell, J. W. (2003). *Research design: Qualitative, quantitative, and mixed methods approaches* (2nd ed.). Thousand Oaks, CA: Sage.

Devine, P. G., Plant, E. A., & Harrison, K. (1999). The problem of "us" versus "them" and AIDS stigma. *The American Behavioral Scientist*, *42*(7), 1212–1228. doi:10.1177/00027649921954732

Goffman, E. (1963). *Stigma: Notes on the management of spoiled identity*. Englewood Cliffs, NJ: Prentice Hall.

Hofstede, G. (1997). *Cultures and Organizations: Software of the mind*. New York: McGraw Hill.

James, P. (Ed.). (2003). *International encyclopedia of marriage and family*. New York, NY: Macmillan.

Kimotho, S., Miller, A. N., & Ngure, P. (2015). Managing communication surrounding tungiasis stigma in Kenya. *Communicatio*, *41*(4), 523–542. doi:10.1080/0250016 7.2015.1100646

Kowalski, R. M., Morgan, M., & Taylor, K. (2016). Stigma of mental and physical illness and the use of mobile technology. *The Journal of Social Psychology*, 1–9. PMID:27841705

Lasalvia, A., Zoppei, S., Van Bortel, T., Bonetto, C., Cristofalo, D., Wahlbeck, K., & Germanavicius, A. (2013). Global pattern of experienced and anticipated discrimination reported by people with major depressive disorder: A cross-sectional survey. *Lancet*, *381*(9860), 55–62. doi:10.1016/S0140-6736(12)61379-8 PMID:23083627

Link, B. G., & Phelan, J. C. (2001). Conceptualizing stigma. *Annual Review of Sociology*, *27*(1), 363–385. doi:10.1146/annurev.soc.27.1.363

Link, B. G., Yang, L. H., Phelan, J. C., & Collins, P. Y. (2004). Measuring mental illness stigma. *Schizophrenia Bulletin*, *30*(3), 511–541. doi:10.1093/oxfordjournals. schbul.a007098 PMID:15631243

Meisenbach, R. J. (2010). Stigma management communication: A theory and Agenda for applied research on how individuals manage moments of stigmatized identity. *Journal of Applied Communication Research*, *38*(3), 268–292. doi:10.10 80/00909882.2010.490841

Monteiro, N. M. (2015). Addressing mental illness in Africa: Global health challenges and local opportunities. *Community Psychology in Global Perspective*, *1*(2), 78–95.

Onwuegbuzie, A. J., Dickinson, W. B., Leech, N. L., Annmarie, G., & Zoran, P. (2009). A qualitative framework for collecting and analyzing: Data in focus group research. *International Journal of Qualitative Methods*, *8*(3), 87–111. doi:10.1177/160940690900800301

Smith, R. (2007). Language of the lost: An explication of stigma Ccmmunication. *Communication Theory, 17*(4), 462–485. doi:10.1111/j.1468-2885.2007.00307.x

Smith, R. A. (2012). An experimental test of stigma communication content with a hypothetical infectious disease alert. *Communication Monographs, 79*(4), 522–538. doi:10.1080/03637751.2012.723811

Thoits, P. A. (2011). Resisting the stigma of mental illness. *Social Psychology Quarterly, 74*(1), 6–28. doi:10.1177/0190272511398019

Van Brakel, W. H. (2006). Measuring health-related stigma—a literature review. *Psychology Health and Medicine, 11*(3), 307–334. doi:10.1080/13548500600595160 PMID:17130068

Wakanyi-Kahindi, L. (2012). *The Agikuyu concept of THAHU and its bearing on the biblical concept of sin* (Doctoral dissertation).

World Health Organization. (2001). *Mental health: new understanding, new hope.* World Health Organization.

KEY TERMS AND DEFINITIONS

Cultural Beliefs: Are systems of knowledge shared by a relatively large group of people.

Cultural Misdemeanor: Refers to committing a 'cultural sin' according to the respondents. It is a form of gross violation of the norms of the communities.

Culture: Is people's way of life which encompasses the knowledge, experiences, beliefs, values, attitudes, meanings, language, religion, and material wealth accumulated by a social group.

Labels: Are terms used to reference the members of the society with mental illness. Such terms are called labels. The label promotes the cognitive process of entitativity, or perceiving a collection of people as a distinct, actual group, and highlights intergroup differences.

Mark: Refers to a cue that allows someone to identify another person as a member of a stigmatized group.

Responsibility: Refers to the implied blame, which is carried by the information entailed in messages. Put differently, responsibility points to the argument that those in the stigmatized group are to blame for the choices they made and such choices put the community at risk.

Stereotypes: Are overgeneralized set of ideas that people have about what someone or something is like, but often incorrect.

Stigma: Refers to the loss of status that arises from being in possession of an attribute, for example a health condition that has been culturally defined as "undesirably different" and so as "deeply discrediting."

Stigma Communication: Refer to the processes through which stigma messages are communicated within a community to allow for group categorization, recognition, stereotyping, discrimination, and exclusionist behaviors to occur.

Taboos: Are defined as cultural prohibitions by the community.

Chapter 3
Media, Social Media, and the Securitization of Mental Health Problems in Nepal:
Yama Buddha's Case Study

Sudeep Uprety
Tribhuvan University, Nepal

Rajesh Ghimire
Tribhuvan University, Nepal

ABSTRACT

This chapter attempts to unfold the trend and nature of mainstream and social media coverage on mental health issues in Nepal through suicide case of Yama Buddha, a popular musician. Using the securitization theory and concepts of threat construction and threat neutralization, major findings through content analysis and key informant interviews reveal reputed mainstream media following cautious route towards threat neutralization and therefore, maintaining a level of journalistic professionalism. However, especially in the other online media, blogs, and other social media, there were sensationalist words and tone used to attract the audience, triggering various sorts of emotional responses, thereby fulfilling the act of securitization. Major recommendations from this chapter include more awareness and understanding about the nature and type of mental health problems; capacity building of journalists and media professionals to better understand and report on mental health problems; development and proper implementation of media guidelines on reporting mental health issues.

DOI: 10.4018/978-1-5225-3808-0.ch003

INTRODUCTION

Anil Adhikari, popularly known as Yama Buddha, a celebrated Nepali rapper reportedly died of suicide at his residence in Ruislip, United Kingdom on January 14, 2017, leaving scores of his fans and followers in shock. This tragic incident triggered a wide attention about celebrity suicides, especially linking to the dreaded late twenty's club of global celebrities such as Jimi Hendrix, Janis Joplin, Jim Morrison and Amy Winehouse. Extensive mainstream and social media coverage of Yama Buddha's suicide also led to the ongoing debates and thereby public discourses on rising cases of suicides and mental health problems in Nepal.

About 90 percent people living in Nepal are suffering from psychiatric problems and there is 'insignificant attention' given to this sector (Uprety & Lamichhane, 2016). Furthermore, the lack of proper knowledge and understanding about the subject matter, lack of mental health specialists; poor implementation of policies and guidelines and lack of adequate resource allocation for mental health sector has aggravated the stigma surrounding mental health in Nepal (Luitel, et al., 2015). This stigmatization has led to under-reporting of many mental health cases and lack of proper care and attention towards the issue.

This chapter attempts to unfold the trend and the nature of stories reported in mainstream and social media on mental health and suicides in Nepal, meticulously unfolding the media reporting about Yama Buddha's case and how different discourses on mental health, suicides and stigma have been developed as a result of the attention the celebrity's death gathered.

Events occurred in this world including suicides are a 'shared reality' held not only by individuals, but also institutionalized in everyday practices and public artifacts such as media coverage (Uchida et al, 2015). While communicating a certain message through media, stories present socio-cultural attitudes and values apart from presenting objective facts, consequently generating a collective perception. However, the story teller or the journalist brings in his/her individuality making stories more interesting. In that sense, media coverage is not just a collective or macro phenomenon, but also comprises of individual psychological facts.

Social media has added a new dimension in the era of communication. Social media sites such as Facebook and Twitter provide that space of inter-linkage where 'weak links' or connections could be established with another person or group without having any previous interaction or good understanding about such people and groups. The power of digital media is as such today that a celebrity suicide case could go viral in no time that such news can have both effects – positive in terms of building a discourse and bringing mental health issues into the mainstream of national health debates on one hand while on the other hand, the lack of understanding about mental health and suicide, in the lure for 'dying to be famous' thus promoting more number of suicides. The fact that the number of Facebook users in Nepal rose from 0.85 million to 4 million in the space of 4 years (2011 to 2014) goes to show the escalating figures of social media usage amongst Nepalese and the impact as well as vulnerabilities it brings along with growing number of users (Anil, 2014).

In that regard, the authors would like to analyze in depth about the type and nature of media reporting on mental health/suicide issues and whether and how the Nepalese media is 'securitizing' such issues. Furthermore, with the social media analysis, it would also be useful in drawing the nature of discourses on mental health issues carried out at the public level and how that is contributing to the construction or deconstruction of stigma surrounding mental health issues in Nepal.

For the purpose of this chapter, the authors collected primary data about Yama Buddha death stories from various mainstream electronic and print media published from January 14, 2017 until end of April, 2017. Ten Key Informant Interviews (KIIs) were also taken with mental health professionals, mainstream media and social media researchers to understand the broader context. Furthermore, relevant literature reviews were undertaken to gather more global and local evidence to gain an in-depth insight and understanding on the issue.

BACKGROUND

Some studies have attempted to analyze the media reports on suicide – in terms of sensationalizing them in a way to solve problems.

Instances of Securitization by Media

A fact sheet by Media Frame (Pirkis & Blood, 2010) illustrates how media reporting and framing leads to imitation or 'copycat' suicide: when there is repeated and prominent coverage (across multiple media sources and on front page); when the reader or viewer identifies with the person as either someone that is similar to themselves or someone they look up to such as a celebrity; when certain subgroups in the population (e.g. young people; people experiencing a mental illness) may be more vulnerable; and when there are explicit descriptions of the method or location.

Interestingly, there are evidences to illustrate that celebrity suicides had more of imitation/copycat effect than non-celebrity suicides. A comprehensive study covering meta-analysis of 419 findings from 55 studies revealed that studies based on celebrity suicides were 5.27 times more likely to report a copycat effect than studies based on non-celebrity suicides (Stack, 2005).

Of 13 studies of television news reports of suicides on at least two of three national TV networks in the USA, an increase in suicide rates was found after the reports in 10 of the studies. Five of these 'positive' studies were of teenage suicide rates and one was of suicide rates in elderly people. Of 10 further studies of news coverage of suicides in more than one news medium, an increase in suicide rates was found in six (Programme, 2003). In some there was clear evidence of the direct impact of the reports on subsequent suicides (e.g. following the suicide of a very popular Japanese pop singer and of Miss Hungary).

Celebrity suicides are clearly newsworthy, and reporting them is often regarded as being in the public interest. Reports of suicides by famous entertainers and political figures are particularly likely to influence the behavior of vulnerable individuals, because they are revered by the community. Glorifying a celebrity's death may suggest that society honors suicidal behavior (WHO, 2008).

A particular incidence of securitization of a celebrity suicide case using Twitter can be understood from a tweet by the Academy of Motion Pictures and Arts (Dewey, 2014) which tweeted an image of Robin William's death with the phrase, 'Genie, you are free'. The impact of this tweet was as such that almost 340,000 retweets were made, violating the ethical norms of talking about suicide using social media.

Likewise, a review about media reporting on mental health issues (Ma, How the media cover mental illnesses: a review, 2017) of more than four decades of published studies revealed that media portrayals of mental illness were consistently inaccurate and unfavorable; people with mental illness were labeled as inadequate, unlikable, and dangerous. The review further indicated that media portrayals of mental illness influenced people's knowledge and attitudes toward mental illness and that negative depictions could have an unfavorable impact on people's attitudes toward people with mental illness.

Similarly, some of the studies provided evidence that reporting of the graphic and disturbing details of suicides might act as a deterrent, putting people off suicide as a solution to their problems, and that in fact 'sanitizing' the reporting of suicides might encourage suicidal behavior. Although there is evidence to suggest that features which include graphic or disturbing images of suicide methods may inform the majority of the audience about the dangers of a particular method, those individuals who are most at risk may actually be attracted to or encouraged by the same graphic details (Programme, 2003).

Furthermore, there have been numerous other empirical studies showing media's influence in negative portrayal of mental health problems. A study in 2005 found almost 40 percent of newspaper stories portrayed mental illness as dangerous and violent, and the stories often appeared in the front section. Likewise, reviews of the US media found rates of dangerousness of 85 percent in representations and particularly controversial reporting of schizophrenia. Similar trends have been identified in New Zealand and Australian studies, where identified dangerousness in 62 percent of 600 articles drawn from a four-week timeframe. In a particular review of representations in various media over a one-month period, using content analysis, themes of violence and dangerousness were identified in more than 60 percent of the 562 articles. Likewise, another study found significant negative reporting in 1035 articles over a one-year period, and 50 percent of reports depicting danger (Knifton & Quinn, 2008).

Instances of Desecuritization by Media

Although majority of media stories tend towards sensationalizing the mental health issues, especially celebrity suicide cases owing to various socio-political and economic context, there have also been some instances of media encouraging desecuritization or normalizing such suicide cases.

There have been instances of desecuritization through media to discourage such acts such as an Australian study of reporting of Kurt Cobain's suicide in a range of media found that rates of suicide among 15-24 year olds fell during the month following the reporting of Cobain's death as the media was highly critical of the musician's act (Pirkis & Blood, 2010).

A review of 41 empirical studies conducted in 12 years shows that although negative portrayals of mental illness still account for a large portion of the research findings, researchers also found the number of such stories is decreasing (Ma, 2017). In that review, a study revealed recovery about mental illness and advocacy action was beginning to be discussed in the media, and more stories focused on biological or environmental causes instead of personal or parental blame. The researchers claimed that this finding was good news because previous research suggested people tended to view people with mental illness as more responsible for their condition than those with other health disorders. Likewise, another study found a large proportion of articles on autism sampled from The New York Times and The Washington Post provided more solutions for autism than causes and more often used medical experts as the news sources, which could help normalize this disorder.

There have also been efforts to desecuritize mental health issues using various social platforms. One such is PatientsLikeMe.com where people suffering from an illness exchange information with others with the same condition, e.g. to find alternative treatment opportunities. Forums such as these promote a patient centered approach to discuss and share problems, experiences in disease control initiatives – including mental health.

Due to the greater influence of media to influence policies, there have also been some instances of mental health policy influence through media with the help of strong evidence. In Australia (Meurk, Whiteford, & Head, 2015), media have contributed to making mental health a national issue. This has been possible with the global attention towards mental health with the combined with the global reach of media to promote inter-cultural dialogue and bringing stakeholders together for required policy uptake.

The 'shock' and 'celebrity' factor appears to count higher in rating the newsworthiness of a suicidal event than broader issues (debt, depression, despair) that may have a greater resonance with readers/audiences lives (Trust, 2007). At the same time it is evident that media coverage of suicide and suicidal behavior can and does highlight important social and societal issues, especially where time and space is given to examining context and considering policy implications.

Media Ethics on Reporting Mental Health Issues

BBC Editorial Guidelines (BBC, 2017) also provides various tips for journalists in reporting suicide cases such as: avoiding language which sensationalizes or normalizes suicide, or presents it as a solution to problems; avoiding prominent placement and undue repetition of stories about suicide; avoiding explicit description of the method used in a completed or attempted suicide; avoiding detailed information about the site of a completed or attempted suicide; wording headlines carefully; exercising caution in using photographs or video footage; taking particular care in reporting celebrity suicides; showing due consideration for people bereaved by suicide; providing information about where to seek help and recognizing that media professionals themselves may be affected by stories about suicide.

In specific country contexts, Media Guidelines prepared by Ministry of Health of New South Wales, Australia (Health, 2014) suggests the following considerations for reporting suicide:

1. **Volume and Prominence:** Positioning the story on the inside pages of a paper or magazines, or further down in the order of reports in TV and radio news
2. **Context:** Reporting the underlying causes of suicide (e.g. mental illness, drug-related illness or other familial or social risk factors) can help dispel myths and increase community understanding
3. **Method and Location:** Detailed descriptions of suicide methods can prompt some vulnerable people to copy the act. If it is important to the story, discuss the method in general terms only. Particular care should be taken not to promote locations as 'suicide spots' or 'hotspots'.
4. **Add Crisis Support Contacts:** Including phone numbers for 24 hour crisis support services to provide immediate support to those who may have been distressed, or prompted to act, by the story

5. **Language:** If the story is about a death, use the term 'suicide' sparingly and check the language you're using does not glamourize, sensationalize, or present suicide as a solution to problems.
6. **Celebrity Suicide:** Celebrity suicide is often reported where it is considered to be in the public interest. To minimize risk, ensure the story does not glamourize suicide or provide specific details about method or location of death.
7. **Interviewing the Bereaved:** The bereaved are often at risk of suicide themselves. Follow media codes of practice on privacy, grief and trauma when reporting personal tragedy.

Likewise, in early 2009 the Canadian Psychiatric Association issued a position paper on safe media reporting (Medicine P., 2009). The paper urges reporters to avoid the following: giving details of the suicide method; using the term 'suicide' in the headline; including photos or admiration of the deceased; repetitive, excessive, or front page coverage; 'exciting' reporting; romanticized or simplistic reasons for the suicide; the idea that suicide is unexplainable; and approval of the suicide.

Theoretical Framework

Authors, through this chapter have used the Theory of Securitization (Buzan, Waever, & Wilde, 1997) first conceptualized in the mid-1990s. The basic notion of securitization is the positioning through speech acts of a particular issue as a threat to survival, which in turn enables emergency measures and the suspension of 'normal politics' in dealing with that issue. The notion of securitization has also been closely linked with linguistics through scholars like Jacques Derrida. Derrida's theory of deconstruction, where his famous quote that "a text matters more for what it does than for what it says".

Authors have also aligned their analysis of the stories covered in mainstream and social media through the lens of Copenhagen School of Security Studies (Sulovic, 2010), conceptualizing security as a process of social construction of threats which includes securitizing actor, who declares certain matter as urgent and a posing threat for the survival of the referent object, that, once accepted with the audience, legitimizes the use of extraordinary measures for neutralization of the threat.

This sort of analysis is very important in the current context of the use of social media for developing and spreading fake news about suicides of certain celebrities that create a lot of fear, shock, anxiety and confusion among the public, thus contributing to the stigma surrounding mental health/suicide issues.

Therefore, for the sake of analysis of this case study, the term securitization has been defined as the process of sensationalizing the celebrity's death and his act of killing with the deliberate use of certain words and terminologies – thereby contributing to threat building with regards to suicidal tendencies. Likewise, the process of desecuritization has been linked with efforts by media to normalize the act of suicide and rather promote better education and awareness of mental health problems.

In a figurative presentation, the theoretical analysis of this chapter rests on analyzing the elements of securitization and desecuritization prevalent in reporting mental health issues by Nepalese mainstream and social media (see Figure 1).

FINDINGS

Mainstream and Online Media Coverage

Republica (Sharma, 2017), covered this event of Yama Buddha's death with the title, 'Famous rapper Yama Buddha no more'. The choice of words in the title is mild with no negative connotations hinting at suicide or any mental health problem, therefore no direct association of securitization can be drawn directly from the title. The phrase 'no more' just suggest the rapper's death and the readers need to read through the content to get more details of the content.

Figure 1. Securitization and Desecuritization of Mental Health Issues

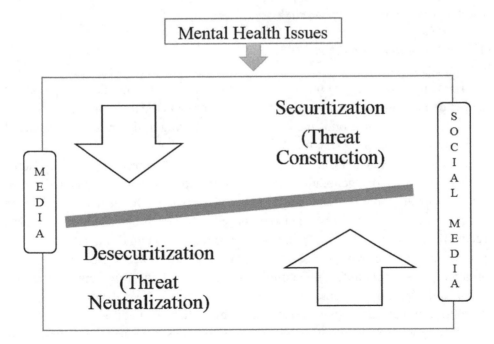

As in the title, the content of the news also avoids any terminologies that securitizes the mental health issues or suicide incidents. The news agency attempts to put forward its event based reporting. Excerpts from the media story:

In an apparent suicide, famous Nepali rapper Anil Adhikari, widely known as Yama Buddha, has been found dead here on Saturday morning.

Quoting the family sources, journalist Bhagirath Yogi of BBC reported that the singer committed suicide in his residence in northern London.

Marhatta added that the cause for the death will be known only after the postmortem is conducted.

With lack of detailed information, the news agency does not give any suggestion or indication about the cause of his death. Professional ethics also seems to be maintained while the source of the death has been quoted (BBC) as well as mentioning the death of the rapper ('in an apparent suicide').

Some of the interesting reactions to the online version of the story are:

It is more important to not lose hope than winning. I am having a nightmare before sleep.

Damn, goose bumps as I read this!

My soul is dead hearing this.

These reactions suggest that shocking news that too of a suicide of a celebrated rapper could trigger grave responses from their fans and the reactions could be very pessimistic such as the ones mentioned above ('having a nightmare before sleep' and 'my soul is dead hearing this').

Daily Mail (Summers, 2017) chose a very long and provoking title: 'Nepal mourns its 'voice of a generation' after the mysterious death of the country's most famous rapper who was found hanged at his wife's parents' home in a west London suburb' of the event. The choice of words used by the news agency definitely has a securitization angle with description of the cause of death (found hanged at his wife's parents' home). Likewise, the phrase 'Nepal mourns its 'voice of a generation' also an attempt to trigger an overwhelming response especially from youth and music fraternity. The story is mentioned as 'exclusive' news in block letters, specifically highlighting that Yama Buddha had hanged himself in the bathroom.

The major content of the story provides a detailed description of the event such as:

When his father-in-law went to use the bathroom at 6am he found he was unable to open the door and could not get an answer.

Eventually he forced his way in and found his son-in-law hanging from his belt in the bathroom.

The rapper had not left a note and friends and relatives are mystified why he would want to end his life.

Providing as detailed information as possible to the readers could be the motive behind publishing such content by the media agencies. However, these sorts of explicit descriptions may also lead to securitization and result in negative connotation of the news agency.

Some of the interesting reactions to the online version of the story are:

The disillusionment of many people in this world is reaching epidemic proportions. So sad to see this happen.

I am a Nepali and I am baffled by his suicide. He could get any sort of help from his fans if he had appealed or gave some signals. It feels so bad. Why?

Nepal is one of the poorest countries in the world and has spent several decades in severe political turmoil. After what they've been through I very much doubt if the country has been "thrown into mourning" by the death of a rapper.

Why would he kill himself when he got the world? There is more to it.

There have been mixed reactions to this story. While the fans of Yama Buddha were in despair, there was also desire to know more about the cause of his death. Likewise, the reactions also suggest the worry about the increasing trend of mental health problems. One of the interesting comment was also related to the title of the story – with the inclusion of the term 'thrown into mourning', clearly having the securitization element to gather attention to the readers while the situation might not have been so extreme.

The Himalayan Times (Times, 2017), a mainstream English news daily chooses a shorter self-explanatory title, 'Yama Buddha commits suicide' to cover the event. The title provides an enough detail for the readers regarding the cause of the rapper's death and moreover as debated by various mental health experts, deems the act as an offense with the term 'commits suicide'.

The Himalayan Times presents an event based reporting of the incident as per the available information, also quoting the source of information:

Famous rapper Yama Buddha has reportedly committed suicide. Anil Adhikari, popular as Yama Buddha, reportedly took his life at his residence in northern London on January 14, according to BBC Nepali Service. He was 29 years old. Quoting his family sources, BBC Nepali Service confirmed that his dead body was found in the bathroom.

There were no apparent reactions to this coverage by the news agency in the comments section.

A popular online website among non-resident Nepalese, Canada Nepal (Baral, 2017) also chooses a similar shorter self-explanatory title, 'Rapper Yama Buddha committed suicide'. Similar to the choice of words for the title by The Himalayan Times, Canada Nepal opts for usage of the term 'committed suicide' linking it as an act of offense.

Canada Nepal chooses to provide a rather detailed account of the event – not just informing about the death of the rapper but also additional detail of his death, stating that he was found dead in his bathroom. However, the tone of the story does not have an explicit securitization angle as it obtains its information from trusted sources (such as BBC and family members) and mentions that additional details about the cause of the death would be revealed after the post mortem report.

In an apparent suicide, famous Nepali rapper Anil Adhikari, widely known as Yama Buddha, has been found dead here on Saturday morning. Adhikari's brother-in-law Resh Marhatta confirmed the death talking to Republica Online. BBC Nepali Service said that the rapper is no more. Quoting the family sources, journalist Bhagirath Yogi of BBC reported that the singer committed suicide in his residence in northern London.

According to family sources, the singer was found dead in his bathroom at around 3 am. Adhikari, 29, had been living in London with his wife. The dead body has been kept at Northwick Park Hospital, Harrow. Source added that police have told the family members to contact them only on Monday. It is learnt that the postmortem will be conducted on Wednesday. Marhatta added that the cause for the death will be known only after the postmortem is conducted.

Another online Nepali portal XNepali.net (2017) does have a securitization component in its coverage. The title itself is attracting the audience when it says,

'Why Yama Buddha committed suicide?' for the audience to be interested to know the cause of its death.

The news agency put forward its arguments to its readers questioning the official report of the rapper's death that it was a suicide case.

This story also has many horrific pictures about the dead body of the rapper further securitizing the act of suicide.

An online portal, Habamoment.com (2017) explicitly mentions about the cause of the rapper's death and also associated with other celebrity suicides with the title, 'Yama Buddha and Three Other Nepali Celebrities Who Committed Suicide'.

The online portal discusses about how Yama Buddha's death 'has made all Nepali think about all high-profile suicides in Nepal'. The article has a negative tone filled with shock with the choice of words such as: "he had name, fame, money, and most importantly the love from his family, wife, and fans but who knew that he too had the courage to kill himself!"

The title of the story by another online portal Update Medicine (2017) attracts the audience in terms of asking the audience one pertinent question: 'The Case of Death: Suicide or Murder?' Through this title, the story gathers attention of the readers to unfold the mystery surrounding the rapper's death.

The story follows a negative tone, inclined towards a fan/follower's reaction towards his death. The story provides additional detail about the death of the rapper and some of the suspicions surrounding Yama Buddha's death:

His near ones say he had not been under any ongoing personal conflict with anybody. After hearing the news, some people in Nepal had some kind of suspicion (correlating to Rap & Hip Hop Culture) that Rapper abused some form of drug before it all had happened but it is said the post mortem examination did not find evidence of drugs over his body. Rather it's been said that they found some traces of alcohol regarding which it said that he had drunk few sips of wine with his wife after returning from his work at Royal Mail that night.

The Guardian published an article the next day stating that rapper's father in law found him after his second attempt to open bathroom door with the next set of keys they had inside the house. On the other hand, other media sources state that it was another person living in the next floor of the same house who on an attempt to enter into bathroom that morning found the door locked from inside. He then opened the door with the next keys and found him hanging dead. The same question gives rise to next suspicion that how can a door be opened with the next key from outside when it was locked with the original set of key from inside.

It has also been reported that torn pieces of passport was found on the scene but the reason behind and its relation with his death still remains a mystery. There seems no other way to assume why Yama Buddha had done so. The absence of any reports regarding the footprints investigation has also become the matter of suspicion. Another mystery regarding this case is relevance of fractured lower molars (some sources report lower jaw) with hanging. It is still unclear if those got fractured before it all took place (due to some other incident) or the knot simply broke off after his death leading to that fracture.

The story had plenty of securitization elements especially with the big bold sub-headings such as 'Who saw the dead body first?' and 'The torn pieces of passport and the torn pieces of molars/jaw'.

Barun Ghimire, a Nepali blogger pays an emotional tribute through his blog (Ghimire, 2017) to the rapper as reflected in the title, 'Rest in Beats Yama Buddha'. Ghimire attempts to desecuritize the event with suggestions on more awareness about suicide and mental health issues.

We need to connect, communicate and care if we are to combat suicide. Let us work together towards suicide prevention and let people know them that they matter more than they think they do. We need to talk about suicide and create awareness in the underlying cause or at least we need to explain to everyone that suicide is not the ANSWER.

To those who want to express respect and tribute to Yama Buddha, I urge them to work towards suicide awareness and suicide prevention so we'd deal with actual killer. Let's talk about suicide and spread awareness. It is high time we do something about it.

Ghimire also expresses a strong message that 'suicide doesn't end the chances of life getting worse, it eliminates the possibility of it ever getting any better'.

Another attempt of desecuritization to this story was made by a blogger Shiva Neupane from Melbourne in his letter to The Himalayan Times (Neupane, 2017) emphasizing on more diffusion of academic knowledge and awareness on psychological studies especially to the younger generation as he writes:

We all have different level of capacities to resist suicidal tendencies. The capacities come from our deeper understanding of life, and the way we look at what it means to live. As long as we are mindful in what it takes to know the internal locus of control, then nothing would happen to us. However, it is our independent mindset to contemplate the entwined fabric of our likes and dislikes about our own boundary of our personal life.

Surprisingly enough, we can see the national and international examples that even the celebrities who have name, fame and money commit suicide just because of their pseudo-views that may be logical for what they do in the first place. The society is the sole- reason why they commit suicide. Directly or indirectly society is culpable for blanketing the individual's framework of understanding about how they view life in which they are encapsulated.

What I personally perceive is the material gains may not fulfill our life. The singer lived in the sophisticated city of London. However, he committed suicide. This reflects the fact that it is not a conscientious decision to readily accept the fact that the people's class and status may not be the only yardstick to measure that they are living in harmony with peace of mind. When there is no peace of mind it doesn't matter how rich you are or how popular you are, death will steal you away in a matter of few minutes. We need psychological studies about mitigating and finding the root causes of this kind of incident.

Social Media Coverage

YouTube

A YouTube video by a channel, Efact TV (2017) has uploaded a video on January 15, 2017 explaining the reason why Yama Buddha committed suicide. The video as of April 11, 2017, 6 am Nepal time has reached 267,573 views with 1220 likes and 145 dislikes.

The title itself has a lot of securitization element with the choice of words, 'Why Yama Buddha hanged himself using belt?' drawing curiosity among readers in terms of not just the cause of the suicide but also the method used by the rapper to kill himself.

The video mentions that the rapper killed himself by hanging in his bathroom. The video also provides details of his hanging mentioning why he chose belt as the rod to hang clothes was located at some height and using belt was easier. The video also mentions that the reason behind his act of killing himself mainly was the gradual erosion of his popularity which sore in 2002/03 and then there was downfall which led him to prolonged depression.

Some of the viewers of the video have commented suspecting the details provided by the media that the rapper woke up from his bed at around 3:30 am and was inside the bathroom for more than 3 hours without his wife even noticing that while she was just sleeping beside him.

Another YouTube video by Thuloparda TV channel (2017) uploaded on January 28, 2017 shows the pathetic emotional condition of a father while his son's corpse was brought for cremation to Kathmandu. This video with images of his corpse surrounded by his family members and relatives along with scores of his fans and other commoners interested to take his photograph triggered a lot of rage amongst its readers. Some of the readers' comments were:

How insensitive people have become? In such a tragic moment, some people are finding it interesting to take photographs using mobiles while the poor parents are in such a shock.

So sad to see that most people are concerned taking pictures only instead of offering prayers and condolences.

Likewise, this video also triggered some of the extreme reactions from the rapper's fans, thus fulfilling the securitization motive of the media agency:

Why is media all the time trying to prove that Yama Buddha committed suicide by assuming that he went into depression after being revealed publicly that the celebrated rapper was earning money by being a postman in the UK?

This life is such a waste! All the time we are worried about what we don't have and what others have. Ultimately, we all will be worthless one day!

Another YouTube channel NK TV goes further extreme in terms of choosing its title for covering the Yama Buddha story. The chosen title is 'True story behind Yama Buddha's death now revealed: the reason you hear will shake your heart'. The choice of words used in the title such as 'true story now revealed' and 'shake your heart' has securitization move. Consequently, this video had a high viewership (422, 307 views with 2161 likes and 243 dislikes as of April 11, 2017, 6:30 am Nepal Time).

This video without citing any source provides an elaborate description on why Yama Buddha killed himself mentioning that the rapper was in a state of worry with him residing in his in-law's house in the UK. Furthermore, the media states that he went into a state of depression having lost all his pride as a celebrated rapper in Nepal and having to work as a postman, delivering letters in the UK. He went into contemplating how could he earn his living just by singing rap songs? According to this channel, one incident really triggered Yama Buddha in killing himself. Once while he was delivering letter in one of the residences in UK, he met one of his fans.

She was so excited to meet him. She called all her friends and took photographs with him. This incident went viral on social media and everybody came to know that a celebrated Nepali rapper was doing the 'menial job' of a postman in UK. Furthermore, sympathizing his condition, those people who knew him used to give him tips while delivering letters, which made him feel very uncomfortable. The media concluded that the rapper being fed up with his life, ultimately, committed suicide.

Another YouTube channel Nepal Reviews chooses the title, 'Yama Buddha suicide letter' with the strategic attempt to securitize the story and attract more viewership (Reviews, 2017). There is no mentioning of the suicide letter. Instead the video runs through some of the photographs of the rapper and the audio narration in the background explaining the reason (all based on assumptions and no quoting of the source) why the rapper killed himself. The channel claims that he had already had a fame but deep down he was frustrated. He was not able to make money and was also into drugs occasionally. He was struggling financially to keep up to his name.

With the choice of emotional words, the channel makes an attempt to securitize this story to his followers:

It might be true that good persons go to heaven earlier. He used to rock at live performances. The Almighty might also be interested in his live performances – so the God also might have been interested in his live performance.

Naya Naya News Nepal – another YouTube channel chooses to desecuritize the Yama Buddha case (2017). Published on January 30, 2017 (with 102, 069 views – 367 likes and 66 dislikes as of April 7, 2017 6:30 am Nepali time), with the title, 'Who is this Person who is revealing death secret of Yama Buddha?'

Rather than providing any first-hand detailed account of the rapper and its audience, this video is more of a commentary about the social, psychological and economic factors leading to the rapper's death:

Why competent youth go abroad? This trend needs to stop. This death teaches us a lesson how to manage our life effectively. There is a trend of Burger nationalism where competent youth go abroad and preach about how Nepal should develop. Yama Buddha wasted his time and competence by engaging in menial jobs such as that of a postman. Some people assumed that he was embarrassed and depressed after it was revealed in social media that he was working as a postman. Yama Buddha's weakness is not to feel proud about the work that he was doing. We should not do activities that embarrass us. Recently, another youngster committed suicide after his piracy scandal of Chakka Panja movie was revealed. Life is not synonymous to sadness and failures. Life should be spent with joy and happiness. He/She should do justice to the talent/skills he/she bears. There is an increasing trend of going abroad to earn money. Student visa has been misutilized not to study abroad but to work as laborers. Greater attention needs to be paid in terms of stopping from going abroad in the lure of earning dollars, getting depressed and committing suicide. There is no point of toiling hard in the abroad. Rather than that, it would have been worthwhile to work hard in own homeland and do something for the country.

Furthermore, the video also talks of various pertinent questions raised in the social media about his suicide such as:

In Britain, there wouldn't be appropriate place to hang oneself inside the bathroom.

Yama Buddha's wife who had slept with him – how could she not notice that her husband was in the bathroom for over 3 and half hours and the dead body was noticed by another member in the family only in the morning?

Yama Buddha's jaw was also broken. How did that happen?

How was the door of the bathroom unlocked?

Overall, the video makes a good effort to desecuritize the story and give a positive message to its viewers with these closing remarks:

These [assumptions made in the media] are all just unproven doubts and until they are proven, we should not be highlighting these issues in the media. We should not be assuming that this could have happened and that could have happened.

Rather we should support the family of the deceased at this time of need.

A talented Yama Buddha – how he spent his life was a wrong message. Nepali youth should take a lesson from this tragic event.

Twitter

There has also been mixed reactions from Yama Buddha's fans and other general public reacting to his death. Some of the interesting tweets collected by the authors are as follows:

I feel ashamed to see the fake cheap videos on YouTube regarding Yama Buddha' death and people accusing his wife who isn't in right state of mind

And the irony is that it took the death of a celebrity for many Nepalese to understand that depression is deadly.

Let the poor soul, loved by everyone rest in peace. Dammit, don't use his death as earning source. Truth will find its way.

Please, stop putting up Yama Buddha's picture as you DP, it's unpleasant, the reminder of his mode of death.

We can't judge anyone as a coward unless we dun know the pain behind the suicide as their last way out.

With curiosity searched about Yama Buddha, ended up with Kurt Cobain's' suicide note

Couldn't tear out a single page of life, so decided to throw the whole book into the fire.

I wish all my books to do suicide like Yama Buddha

The demise of Anil Adhikari (Yama Buddha) Yama Buddha resembles Swiss cheese, lots and lots of holes. Does not sounds suicide to me.

I wish I could actively get involved in case of Yama Buddha's death/suicide conspiracy. I had few question to ask to his acquaintances.

Yama Buddha, you had the guts to commit suicide. There are several people who have no desire to live longer but are not able to kill themselves. You are great.

Yama Buddha is a legend in his own right. His death (reportedly suicide) bursts the bubble our newsrooms & society in general dwells in.

I also have an excuse to kill myself, but I these days I also seek to find excuses to live every day and defeat the death.

People say that suicide is a permanent answer to a temporary problem, but sometimes that problem isn't so temporary.

If Yama Buddha had really committed suicide, then he must be a coward.

Thus, these reactions are filled with extreme love and support and at the same time hatred for the rapper as well as disappointment in his act. Some of the tweets do have desecuritization elements – with appeals to leave this case aside and not to blow this story out of proportion but rather analyze the contexts that lead to such acts and hopefully control such incidents in the future.

Facebook

Similar reactions were received on Facebook and with no word limitations as in Twitter, there have been elaborate discussions about the causes of his death and in general why people, especially celebrities end up killing themselves.

Anil Adhikari's (Yama Buddha) death by suicide is a sad news indeed as is hundreds of Nepalese who commit suicide every year. Mental illness is still such a stigmatized subject. It's about time we speak out about it and encourage people in need to seek support!

Am I the only one who wants to find out the actual reason behind the so called 'suicide' of Yama Buddha? What is written in Nepali news sites is so unclear. Hope to find out the reason soon. I still can't believe that he did suicide and he is with us no more) I am so confused.

I read somewhere, suicide is a temporary solution of a permanent problem. I don't know if you ever read that, but I'm sad to let you know that the problem that you thought you got rid of just got amplified by a larger scale. You thought that you had a valid reason to decide for yourself, but, do we really get to decide for ourselves?

If he had committed suicide there's no space for him on heaven.

Yama Buddha did not commit suicide because he was weak or out of options or in pain. He was just too fed up with these human structured unemotional machines. He only tried to escape them.

As illustrated above, some were in total shock and disbelief about the incident and blamed Nepali media for not providing clear information about his suicide. On the other hand, there were also attempts made to understand the real context that led him to such circumstances as well as appeals to discourage such acts by being sensible and attempting to address our problems rather than taking an escapist route.

Findings From Key Informant Interviews (KIIs)

Few mental health and media experts were also consulted through Key Informant Interviews to gather their perception and opinion about the media coverage of mental health issues in Nepal, particularly linking with celebrity suicides.

Limited Understanding of Mental Health Issues

Both mental health and media experts have pointed towards limited understanding of mental health issues in Nepal.

Mental health as a discipline is very broad subject in itself. However, due to very less proportion of mental health experts, wide misconceptions regarding mental health exists. It is therefore imperative that wider awareness, knowledge and understanding regarding mental health needs to be spread to the public. – Consultant Clinical Psychiatrist

As a mental health researcher, sometimes I am surprised that even the 'educated' and 'informed' citizens have very limited understanding of mental health. Major reasons for this could be limited academic orientation on the subject; lack of resources easily accessible about mental health through the media and social media; more focus on urban settlements – linking mental health issues more towards work related stress management, anger management, depression, among others. – Mental health researcher working in an NGO

As a journalist reporting for the past 9 years on health and social sector, as an honest confession, I admit that I have limited understanding of mental health issues. We have very few journalists (equal to none), who have academic background on health reporting in Nepal. – Journalist of a national daily

Capacity of Journalists to Report on Mental Health Issues

It is striking to notice that the media sector itself was skeptical of its capacity to understand and report mental health issues in a proper way.

The reality of media reporting needs to be taken into consideration. Media professionals are educated mostly on the theories and practical approaches to journalism and mass communication. Yes, we do have some academic training on development journalism, but in terms of mainstream media coverage, the principles of development journalism are not applied to a larger extent. Nowadays, as a positive sign, development agencies have started engaging media professionals on different issues such as health and education. Therefore, there are some opportunities for journalists through fellowships to learn and understand more about the health – including mental health sector. However, these efforts and initiatives are miniscule considering the wider network of commercial media and journalism sector. – Sub editor of a national daily

I have been reporting on health issues for the past seven years now and the basis of my reporting is self-exploration and consultation with mental health experts. The problem with us is that with various constraints for us to report on a regular basis – including time and resource factor for an investigative reporting, it should be admitted that our understanding on mental health issues is not adequate. Furthermore, we are not provided with adequate training and orientation on mental health issues for us to report better unless we take the initiative ourselves through self-learning. In simple terms, there is no institutionalized practice for capacity development of the journalists. – Journalist of a national daily

Media's Role in Securitization on Mental Health Issues

There have been mixed reactions by the key informants when it comes to media's role in securitization of mental health issues.

A section of the key informants believed that at least in the Nepalese context, mental health issues have not been securitized to that extent through media, unless there was a major celebrity suicide or mental health disorder incident.

Frankly speaking, Nepali media sector has not matured enough to that extent where there is institutionalized practice or intention to securitize on 'soft issues' such as health and education. Yes, there have been some instances where there has been some 'over-reporting' or 'sensationalism' created over media reporting of celebrity suicides but, still to a great deal as securitization principle envisages of an existential threat. – Media researcher

As a nation, we are still yet to experience that kind of celebrity 'mania' or 'paparazzi' as experienced in the West or even in India. Nepali celebrities are found accessible to the commoners. In a way, this is a good thing as it limits general public to be idolizing or patronizing acts or deeds of celebrities. In real life incidents elsewhere, there have been many instances of 'copy-cat suicides' which hasn't been 'viral' yet in Nepal. – Clinical Psychiatrist

Whereas, some of the key informants also believed that there is increasing trend of securitizing acts on mental health issues in Nepal.

Yes, to some extent, we are heading towards it [securitization of mental health issues] and moreover, with the increasing growth of media agencies and social media use, the tendency to be interested in celebrity incidents such as suicide cases will increase. – Psychologist

As a media researcher and enthusiast, though I am excited about the staggering growth of media outlets and social media platforms, I am also equally cautious about the consequences of growth of this nature. This ultimately brings us to an interesting debate on media freedom and ethical reporting. It is not a hidden thing that the growth of social media has led to securitization of mental health problems, particularly celebrity suicides and Nepal is no exception. – Media researcher

On Securitization of Yama Buddha Suicide Case

As a reader, I was also confused initially with the nature of stories reported in the media about Yama Buddha's suicide story. The act of securitization really began when there were numerous story links posted in online and social media about horrific pictures of the rapper's dead body and his parents crying in shock, symbolic photographs about the rapper's act of hanging using belt, and various assumptions based coverage about why the rapper could have killed himself. This definitely had a negative impact upon the minds of his young followers. – Psychiatrist

As a close observer of the digital media activities in Nepal, I was well aware of the patterns and intentions of the media agencies in reporting Yama Buddha stories. During informal chats with the media agency owners, they have also revealed about the need for the 'masala' or 'spicy' content to increase their views and shares of their stories. Yama Buddha was a big name and an inspiration for the youth, with his followership growing. His most recent tweet, four days before his death declaring that his latest album was soon to be released had also contributed to his greater fan following. In other words, this is click bait journalism in simple sense. – Media researcher

On developing an interface between media and mental health professionals to improve reporting on mental health issues

Both media and mental health professionals appreciate that there has been a positive response towards improving the practice of media reporting on mental health issues in Nepal. However, they admit that it is more of a 'reactive' rather than a 'proactive' response:

Yes, there has been greater realization that mental health issues are sensitive to have a significant impact upon wider public due to media reporting and we have had discussions at the policy level to address this issue. However, no substantial steps have been taken to institutionalize this practice. – Mental health professional

What strikes me, at this point of time, as media professionals, is that, we do realize that an intermediary is required to strike a balance between a 'journalistic reporting' and policy uptake, may be more in the line of principles of development journalism. This realization has been there at all levels from a novice journalist to a seasoned editor. However, we haven't taken this to the next level, which I suppose is a strategic policy engagement by a civil society organization, a critical media group or similar structures.

Overall, the key informants have shared that the current journalistic practice and lack of adequate information and underlying misconceptions about mental health in Nepal definitely leads to securitization of mental health issues in the long run if the concerned agencies working in the field of media ethics and media education are not cautious enough at an early stage.

CONCLUSION AND RECOMMENDATIONS

This study attempted to understand the nature of media reporting on mental health issues in Nepal, particularly investigating the Yama Buddha suicide case and the extent of securitization applied by the mainstream and social media channels, while covering the story.

Though the Yama Buddha case might not be entirely sufficient to make a comprehensive conclusion, given the high mainstream media and social media attention the story gathered, certain conclusions can certainly be drawn.

Reputed mainstream media outlets in general have chosen a cautious route towards threat neutralization. From the choice of words used for the title to the content, there was an attempt made to ensure that the followers/fans of the celebrity do not follow the path of 'copycat suicide'. In this regard, it can be deduced that a level of understanding and journalistic professionalism is maintained at least by mainstream media outlets.

However, especially in the other online media, blogs and other social media, there were sensationalist words and tone used to attract the audience. This definitely drew the audiences towards such stories and triggered various sorts of emotional responses – thereby fulfilling the act of securitization. The suicide case of Yama Buddha, as a famous celebrity and his songs being widely popular, became a perfect story for click bait journalism for Nepali online media sites. This nature of click bait journalism, knowingly or unknowingly has resulted in mental health issues being 'over-reported' in the media as compared to, previously, even though through an individual case like that of Yama Buddha. Particularly, in the Youtube videos, the securitization element was prominent with titles suggesting explicit details of the rapper's suicide including the cause as well as method of killing himself while the content of such videos barely described such minute details. Some of those videos receiving almost half million views shows the extent of reach among his fans/followers.

Through the key information interviews, it was also revealed that the mushrooming of online and social media globally and in Nepal with increased competition and trend of click bait journalism, the securitization on sensitive issues such as celebrity suicides have also been justified in some occasions. However, this doesn't negate the fact that the capacity of journalists to report on mental health issues, especially suicide cases sensibly needs to be improved to a great extent. The context of story production – the tight deadlines, limited resources and the interest of media houses to capitalize on the celebrity coverage could also have triggered on the nature and extent of media reporting on such issues. Furthermore, with some level of realization and advocacy for the need for an 'intermediary' to take the initiative forward for evidence informed policy development exercise following the media reporting, some efforts have already been made such as a collaboration between Primary Health Care Revitalization Division (PHCRD) under the Ministry of Health and Health Research and Social Development Forum (HERD), a non-government organization to improve media reporting on urban health issues in Nepal (Uprety, McGrath, McNerney, Ghimire, & Baral, 2016).

More often, the triggers resulting in a response become more important than the response itself. When the mental health issues in Nepal are over-reported and in most cases, without substantial details or readers/viewers being misled, three major recommendations can be drawn from this study:

1. More awareness and understanding about the nature and type of mental health problems as well as the existing myths and misconceptions at the public level.
2. Capacity building of journalists and media professionals to better understand and report on mental health problems and consequences of securitization at the public level with over-reporting on suicide cases. This could be done in collaboration with organizations working on mental health.

Figure 2. Multi-sectoral coordination between policy makers, media agencies and mental health organizations

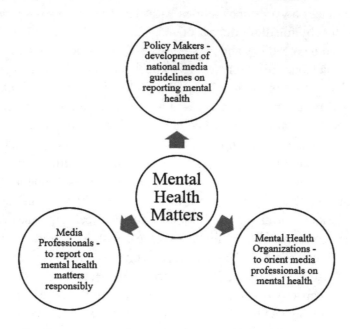

3.   Development and proper implementation of media guidelines on reporting suicide and other mental health issues.

Thus, these recommendations form a multi-sectoral coordination between policy makers, media agencies and mental health organizations promoting better reporting on mental health matters, as presented in Figure 2.

The authors, through this chapter, thus, advocate for the desecuritization of mental health issues in order to deconstruct the stigma and myth surrounding mental health in Nepal.

REFERENCES

Anil, A. (2014, August 20). *Facebook Users in Nepal*. Retrieved April 12, 2017, from Aakarpost: http://tech.aakarpost.com/2014/08/facebook-users-in-nepal.html

Baral, A. (2017, January 14). *Canada Nepal*. Retrieved April 8, 2017, from Rapper Yama Buddha committed suicide: http://www.ecanadanepal.com/2017/01/rapper-yama-buddha-committed-suicide.html

BBC. (2017, April 26). *Editorial Guidelines*. Retrieved April 26, 2017, from BBC: http://www.bbc.co.uk/editorialguidelines/guidelines/harm-and-offence/suicide

Buzan, B., Waever, O., & Wilde, J. d. (1997). *Security: A New Framework for Analysis*. London: Lynne Rienner Publishers.

Dewey, C. (2014, August 12). *Suicide contagion and social media: The dangers of sharing 'Genie, you're free'*. Retrieved April 20, 2017, from The Washington Post: https://www.washingtonpost.com/news/the-intersect/wp/2014/08/12/suicide-contagion-and-social-media-the-dangers-of-sharing-genie-youre-free/?utm_term=.c20fcac2338f

Ghimire, B. (2017, January 16). *Rest in beats Yama Buddha*. Retrieved April 8, 2017, from Sharing my opinion with the world: http://barunghimire.blogspot.com/2017/01/rest-in-beats-yama-buddha.html

Habamoment.com. (2017, January 20). *Yama Buddha and three other Nepali celebrities who committed suicide*. Retrieved March 26, 2017, from Habamoment.com: http://habamoment.com/yama-buddha-and-three-other-nepali-celebrities-who-suicided/

Health, N. M. (2014). *Supporting Fact Sheet: Suicide and the Media*. Retrieved March 26, 2017, from Conversations Matter: http://www.conversationsmatter.com.au/LiteratureRetrieve.aspx?ID=4631

Knifton, L., & Quinn, N. (2008, February). Media, Mental Health and Discrimination: A Frame for Reference for Understanding Reporting Trends. *International Journal of Mental Health Promotion*, *10*(1), 23–31. doi:10.1080/14623730.2008.9721754

Luitel, N. P., Jordans, M. J., & Adhikari, A., Upadhyay, Nawaraj, Hanlon, C., . . . Komproe, I. H. (2015). Mental health care in Nepal: Current situation and challenges for development of a district mental health care plan. *Conflict and Health*, *9*(3), 1–11. doi:10.118613031-014-0030-5 PMID:25694792

Ma, Z. (2017). How the media cover mental illnesses: A review. *Health Education*, *117*(1), 90–109. doi:10.1108/HE-01-2016-0004

Medicine, P. (2009). Media Portrayals of Suicide. *PLoS Medicine*, *1-2*. doi:10.1371/journal.pmed.1000051 PMID:19296719

Medicine, U. (2017, January 29). *Update Medicine*. Retrieved March 26, 2017, from Unanswered Questions on Yama Buddha's death: http://updatemedicine.com/yama-buddha-death-mystery/

Meurk, C., Whiteford, H., Head, B., Hall, W., & Carah, N. (2015, June). Media and evidence-informed policy development: The case of mental health in Australia. *Contemporary Social Science: Journal of the Academy of Social Sciences, 10*(2), 160–170. doi:10.1080/21582041.2015.1053970

Nepal, A. (2017, January 29). *XNepali.net*. Retrieved March 18, 2017, from Why did Yama Buddha committed suicide, Anil is cremated at Pashupati Aryaghat: http://xnepali.net/why-did-yama-buddha-committed-suicide-anil-is-cremated-at-pashupati-aryaghat/

Nepal, N. N. (2017, January 30). *Yama Buddha Death Secret*. Retrieved April 7, 2017, from Youtube: https://www.youtube.com/watch?v=EHaUdfcdvds

Neupane, S. (2017, January 17). *Letters: Causes of Suicide*. Retrieved March 25, 2017, from The Himalayan Times: https://thehimalayantimes.com/opinion/letters-causes-of-suicide/

Pirkis, J., & Blood, W. (2010). *Suicide and the news information media*. Mindframe National Media Initiative. Retrieved April 6, 2017, from http://www.mindframe-media.info/__data/assets/pdf_file/0016/5164/Pirkis-and-Blood-2010,-Suicide-and-the-news-and-information-media.pdf

Programme, R. F. (2003). *Suicide and the Media: Pitfalls and Prevention*. Reuters Foundation Programme; University of Oxford Centre for Suicide Research. Retrieved February 26, 2017, from http://cebmh.warne.ox.ac.uk/csr/Suicide%20&%20the%20Media%20seminar.pdf

Reviews, N. (2017, January 14). *Yama Buddha suicide letter*. Retrieved April 11, 2017, from Youtube: https://www.youtube.com/watch?v=GTuL4Evrbcc

Sharma, C. (2017, January 15). *Famous rapper Yama Buddha no more*. Retrieved March 14, 2017, from My Republica: http://www.myrepublica.com/news/13100/

Stack, S. (2005). Suicide in the media: A quantitative review of studies based on non-fictional stories. *Suicide & Life-Threatening Behavior, 35*(2), 121–133. doi:10.1521uli.35.2.121.62877 PMID:15843330

Sulovic, V. (2010, October 5). Meaning of Security and Theory of Securitization. *Belgrade Centre for Security Policy*. Retrieved April 15, 2017, from http://www.bezbednost.org/upload/document/sulovic_(2010)_meaning_of_secu.pdf

Summers, C. (2017, January 22). *Nepal mourns its 'voice of a generation' after the mysterious death of the country's most famous rapper who was found hanged at his wife's parents' home in a west London suburb*. Retrieved March 8, 2017, from MailOnline: http://www.dailymail.co.uk/news/article-4145452/Nepal-mourns-death-country-s-famous-rapper.html

Times, T. H. (2017, January 15). *Yama Buddha commits suicide*. Retrieved March 6, 2017, from The Himalayan Times: https://thehimalayantimes.com/entertainment/anil-adhikari-yama-buddha-commits-suicide/

Trust, M. (2007). *Sensitive Coverage Saves Lives*. Leeds, UK: MediaWise Trust. Retrieved March 3, 2017, from http://www.mediawise.org.uk/wp-content/uploads/2011/03/Sensitive-Coverage-Saves-Lives.pdf

TV, T. (2017, January 28). *Yama Buddha bakasma auda pitako halat yesto, Kathmanduma ruwabasi*. Retrieved April 13, 2017, from Youtube: https://www.youtube.com/watch?v=1zWxxaBiifk

TV, E. (2017, January 15). *Kina Beltma Jhundiyeka Thiye Ta Yama Buddha? Rahasya Yesto*. Retrieved April 11, 2017, from Youtube: https://www.youtube.com/watch?v=KVEIMVcO_w4

Uprety, S., & Lamichhane, B. (2016). *Mental Health in Nepal - A Backgrounder*. Kathmandu: HERD. Retrieved April 21, 2017, from http://www.herd.org.np/publications/27

Uprety, S., McGrath, N. A., McNerney, S., Ghimire, R., & Baral, S. (2016). *Media mentoring in Nepal: helping journalists write better stories on urban health issues*. HERD; COMDIS-HSD. Retrieved March 23, 2017, from http://comdis-hsd.leeds.ac.uk/resource/media-mentoring-nepal-helping-journalists-write-better-stories-urban-health-issues/

WHO. (2008). *Preventing Suicide: A Resource for Media Professionals*. Geneva: WHO. Retrieved March 25, 2017, from http://www.who.int/mental_health/prevention/suicide/resource_media.pdf

Chapter 4

Understanding and Addressing the Stigma in Mental Health Within the Asian and Asian-American Culture

Ben Tran
Alliant International University, USA

ABSTRACT

Mental health stigma can be defined as the display of negative attitudes, based on prejudice and misinformation, in response to a marker of illness. Stigma creates mental distress for individuals, which furthers stigmatizing attitudes, thereby making it a relentless force and as incompetent in achieving life goals such as living independently or having a good job. Over the years, researchers have consistently highlighted the problem of mental health service underutilization within the Asians and Asian-Americans communities. As such, understanding the cultural contexts that facilitate good outcomes may offer a lever or stigma reduction. Thus, the purpose of this chapter is to understand and address the sociocultural and psychological paradigms of the stigma in mental health within Asians and Asian-Americans. This chapter will cover the history of stigma within the Asian culture, Asian's mental health, mental health services utilization within the Asian culture, and methods of addressing the stigma within the Asian culture to promote the utilization of mental health services.

DOI: 10.4018/978-1-5225-3808-0.ch004

INTRODUCTION

Mental health stigma can be defined as the display of negative attitudes, based on prejudice and misinformation, in response to a marker of illness (Sartorius, 2007). Link and Phelan (2001) describe four characteristics that distinguishes mental health stigma from other social phenomena: (1) it is fundamentally a label of an out-group; (2) the labelled differences are negative; (3) the differences separate the 'normal' from the out-group, and (4) label and separation leads to discrimination. Stigma creates mental distress for individuals, which furthers stigmatize attitudes, thereby making it a relentless force (Seeman, Tang, Brown, & Ing, 2016). Nevertheless, it is widely acknowledged that psychiatric diagnoses are stigmatized, and associated with negative public attitudes (Angermeyer & Matschinger, 2003). Hence, social cognitive models pin point stigma as a relationship between stigma signals (cues), stereotypes (attitudes), and behaviors (discrimination) (Corrigan, 2000), stemming from socialization (Abdullah & Brown, 2011). People with mental illness are perceived as dangerous and unpredictable, incompetent at achieving life goals such as living independently or having a good job (Angermeyer & Dietrich, 2006), and often blamed for their own illllnesses. Prejudice arises when people endorse such stereotypes and discrimination is the behavioral result of prejudice (Corrigan, Druss, & Perlick, 2014; Jenks, 2011).

On a macrosocial level, institutional policies endorse mental health stigma by restricting opportunities for people with mental illness (Corrigan, Markowitz, & Watson, 2004). According to the Global Burden of Disease Study (Murry & Lopez, 1996), stigma lies in the world-wide impact of mental illness on overall health and productivity. Profoundly under-recognized, mental illness constitutes 11% of the global burden of disease, with major depression alone currently ranking fourth and expected to rise to second by 2020. In some regions of the world, mental disorders already represent the largest contributor to the total disease burden, and there is great concern with the *morality crisis* related to mental illness in Eastern Europe (Rutz, 2001). In the face of these concerns, the World Health Organization's (WHO) International Pilot Study of Schizophrenia (IPSoS), the International Study of Schizophrenia (ISoS), and the Study of the Determinants of Outcomes of Severe Mental Disorders (DOSMD), have all documented enormous heterogeneity in the outcomes of mental illness within and across countries (Hopper & Wanderling, 2000; Kulhara & Chakrabarti, 2001; Sartorius, Gulbinat, Harrison, Laska, & Siegel, 1996; Sartorius, Jabensky, & Shapiro, 1978). While it is generally agreed that the reasons for these differences are "far from clear" (Kulhara & Chakrabarti, 2001), one predominant explanation revolves around culturally defined processes.

Scholars and policymakers suggest that stigma may be the reason behind such findings and lies at the root of recovery from mental illness (Remschmidt, Nurcombe, Belfer, Sartorius, & Okasha, 2007). As such, understanding the cultural contexts that facilitate positive outcomes may offer stigma reduction. In particular, whether individuals and others around them recognize mental illness, stigmatize these conditions and support seeking care is critical, since each represent key aspects of culture that can influence the outcome of mental illness (Pescosolido, 1991; 2006). The purpose of this chapter is to understand and address the sociocultural and psychological paradigms of stigma in mental health within Asian culture. For the purpose of this chapter, within the focus of Asians, emphasis will be on Chinese and Chinese Americans. This chapter will cover the history of stigma within the Asian culture, Asian's mental health, mental health services utilization within the Asian culture, and methods of addressing the stigma within the Asian culture to promote the utilization of mental health services.

ASIANS: THE CHINESE

Based on U.S. Census information from 2011, according to Ali (2014), it is estimated that 18.2 million persons of Asian descent living in the United States, and that Asians comprise approximately 5.8% of the total population (Pew Research, 2012; United States Census, 2013a) and growing. Of the 50 states in the United States, California and New York have the largest numbers of Asians in 2010 (United States Census, 2013a). Asians were the fastest growing racial group with the largest proportional population increase between the 2000 and 2010 census, even compared to Hispanic and Latinos, which was one of the largest increase in population (United States Census, 2013a; United States Census, 2013b). Among Asians of Chinese descent, followed by Filipino Americans, Indian Americans, Vietnamese Americans, Korean Americans, and then by Japanese Americans (United States Census, 2013a). Not surprisingly, after English and Spanish, Chinese is the third most widely spoken language in homes in the United States. While Asians are making tremendous strides in acculturation since the first Chinese and Japanese immigrants came to the United States in the mid 1800's, Asians are still largely a population made up of immigrants, with 74% of Asian adults having been in another country (Pew Research, 2012).

Among Asians, 28% live in a multigenerational family, defined by having at least two adult generations in the same household, which is higher than Whites, Blacks, and Hispanic Americans (Pew Research, 2012). On the whole, Asians have a relatively high educational status, with approximately 85% of adults over age 25 having attained a high school diploma, 49% of Asian adults over age 25 are college graduates, compared to 28% of the general population. However, there is a disparity in the percentage of college graduates in different Asians ethnic groups. For example, according to Ali (2014), only 26% of Vietnamese Americans over age 25 are college graduates, which is lower than the general population. Approximately half of Korean, Chinese, Japanese, and Filipino Americans over age 25 are college graduates. Indian Americans have a much higher percentage of college graduates over age 25 (70%). These interethnic differences may reflect different immigration patterns from the countries of origin. While the median income of an Asian household is $66,000, and higher than the national median, 12.5% of Asians lived in poverty in 2009 and 17.2% were without health insurance (United States Census, 2013a). Additionally, Asians households are often larger than those of other ethnic groups. While these facts and figures do not reflect the diversity of the Asians population, they help to provide a broad characterization of the group (Ali, 2014).

Brief Immigration History: The Chinese

The first Asian category of immigrant to the United States arrived from Japan in 1843 and were soon followed by Chinese men who came in 1850s and 1860s to work on the trans-continental railroad, gold mines, and in agriculture (Takaki, 1998, pp. 80-98; United States Census, 2013a). The Chinese Exclusion Act of 1882, which put an end to all immigration from China, was a reflection of the opposition to Asians immigrating to the United States and becoming permanent residents. The Asian Exclusion Act of 1924 was a continued response to concern about Asian immigration, which limited the new immigrants per year from East Asia, Southeast Asia, and South Asia (Pew Research, 2012). Asian immigrants were thought to be unable to assimilate into the U.S. population due to phenotypic differences in appearance, unlike European immigrants. A Supreme Court case in 1923 of U.S. vs. Bhagat Singh Third denied an Indian immigrant the ability to apply for citizenship citing this concern in the official decision (Takaki, 1998, pp. 80-98). The doubt about the allegiance of those of Asian origin to the United States lasted well into the middle of the twentieth century. During World War II, over 80,000 U.S.-born citizens of Japanese origins were held in concentration camps by the government (Takaki, 1998, pp. 80-98).

Immigration from Asia radically changed over the course of the twentieth century with different ethnic subgroups greatly increasing as a response to the loosening of governmental restrictions and quotas. For example, according to Ali (2014), in the middle of the 20th century, naturalization and immigration of the war brides of U.S. soldiers from Japan, Korea, and Vietnam became permissible (Cottrell, 1990; Lopez & Yamazato, 2003; Takaki, 1998, pp. 80-98). In 1965, the Immigration and

Nationality Act ended quotas with regard to Asian immigrants from Asia. This act also changed the ethnic landscape of Asian immigrants, who until that time had largely been from Japan, China, and the Philippines. In the 1970s, there was an influx of refugees from war-torn Laos and Cambodia (Tseng & Strelzer, 2001). Currently, Asian immigrants are most likely to come to the United States with work visas, but also come through student visas, temporary visas, and unauthorized status (Pew Research, 2012).

Moving forward, as a result of the varied historical waves of immigration, there is tremendous diversity among the immigration and acculturation experiences among Asians. The term Asian captures the breadth of experience of an elderly Japanese American man whose family has been in the United States for many generations and the 18-year-old female refugee from Myanmar who recently arrived to the United States. Despite their age gap, the Japanese American man whose grandparents immigrated in one of the early waves of immigration will likely be more acculturated than the 18-year-old who arrives to resettle in a very foreign culture. As the chapter's focus turns toward mental health in Asians, specifically the Chinese, it will be important to continue to consider each patient or family's immigration history as it informs aspects of who they are and what issues may arise when they present themselves to mental health professionals.

Brief History of the Prevalence of Mental Health Disorders in Asians and the Utilization of Mental Health Services

According to Ali (2014), the Surgeon General's Report on Mental Health in 2001, now well over 15 years old, there was little adequate data about the prevalence of mental health disorders in Asians. One of the larger studies mentioned in this report, the CAPES study, demonstrated that Chinese Americans in the Los Angeles area had a moderate rate of depression, with 7% of the studied participants endorsing having experienced depression in their lifetime and 3% in the prior year (U.S. Center for Mental Health Services, 2001; U.S. National Institute of Mental Health, 2001; U.S. Office of the Surgeon General, 2001; United States Substance Abuse and Mental Health Services Administration, 2001). Studies in the 1980s and early 1990s that assessed symptoms of depression rather than the diagnosis of depression in the Asian population found higher rates of depressive symptoms in Japanese American, Korean Americans, Filipino Americans, and Chinese Americans in various major cities in the United States (U.S. Center for Mental Health Services, 2001; U.S. National Institute of Mental Health, 2001; U.S. Office of the Surgeon General, 2001; United States Substance Abuse and Mental Health Services Administration, 2001). One of the concerns underscored in the Surgeon General's report is the lack of adequate data about DSM diagnoses in the Asian population and the report questioned whether or not Asians truly have lower rates of psychiatric disorders compared to other populations. Due to the potential cultural bias in the reporting of and asking about symptoms, it was unclear whether or not accurate data about mental health conditions in Asians were captured by numerous studies. Culturally informed ways of expressing symptoms, prevalence of somatization, and culture-bound syndromes were all raised as possible confounding factors. The report clearly states that there were inadequate data about the prevalence of disorders in Asians who did not report mental health concerns and did not see mental health professionals. Rather than demonstrating that Asians were a resilient model minority group (Tran, 2016, 2017), the report showed that the scope of mental health problems of Asians were not adequately detected. Without perceiving a realistic mental health need, treatment could not occur, except for high-acuity populations, like Southeast Asian refugees with post-traumatic stress disorder, whose need was more evident (U.S. Center for Mental Health Services, 2001; U.S. National Institute of Mental Health, 2001; U.S. Office of the Surgeon General, 2001; United States Substance Abuse and Mental Health Services Administration, 2001).

Moving forward, large-scale studies have yielded more useful data about the prevalence of mental health diagnoses in Asian Americans and utilization of mental health services. However, diagnosis-specific studies have focused only on ethnic subgroups of Asians and there is no reliable data on the prevalence of psychiatric diagnoses in Asians as a whole. One of the large-scale studies is the National Latino and Asian American Study (NLAA) that reflects the prevalence of psychiatric diagnoses to be 0.8%. This study was designed to assess the 12-month prevalence of mental health disorders from 2002 to 2003 among Asians and Latinos, to assess the psychosocial context of the emergence of the disorders, and to determine how often mental health services were sought, in comparison with White, Hispanic, and Black populations (Alegría, Takeuchi, Canino, Duan, Shrout, Meng, Vega, Zane, Vila, Woo, Vera, Guarnaccia, Aguilar-Gaxiola, Sue, Escobar, Lin, & Gong, 2004). In one analysis by Dr. Jennifer Abe-Kim of the NLAAS data, 8.6% of the population surveyed sought mental health treatment compared to 17.9% of the general population when assessed in other large-scale studies (Abe-Kim, Takeuchi, Hong, Zane, Sue, Spencer, Appel, Nicdao, & Alegría, 2007). In the general population, 41.1% of persons with a probable DSM-IV diagnosis sought psychiatric treatment compared to 34.1% of Asians. Additionally, the propensity to use mental health services was inversely correlated to generation of immigration, such that second generation immigrants were more likely to use mental health services than immigrants, and third generation immigrants were more likely to use mental health services than second generation immigrants at a rate more similar to the general population (Abe-Kim et al., 2007).

In the NLAAS study, the prevalence of lifetime suicidal ideation in Asian populations were found to be 8.8% and the prevalence of suicide attempts were found to be 2.5%. Factors that were positively correlated with suicidal ideation and attempts include being female, conflict with family, a history of depression or anxiety, and perception of discrimination. Stronger identification and sense of belonging with one's ethnic group was negatively correlated with suicidal ideation and attempts (Cheng, Fancher, Ratanasen, Conner, Duberstein, Sue, & Takeuchi, 2010). The 2010 National Drug Use Survey on Health by the Substance Abuse and Mental Health Services Administration (SAMHSA), a large-scale survey on mental health and alcohol, tobacco and drug use patterns among over 60,000 responders over 12 years old, showered that the rate of illicit drug use was 3.5% in the month prior, lower than Whites, Native Americans, Blacks, or Hispanics. Among the 38.4% of Asian Americans who endorsed alcohol use in the month prior, 8.8% were binge drinkers and 2.4% were heavy drinkers of alcohol (The 2010 National Drug Use and Survey on Health, 2012). Rates of substance abuse or dependence were lower among Asians at 4.1% compared to other ethnic groups, which is consistent with what others studies have found (The 2010 National Drug Use and Survey on Health, 2012).

Smaller scale studies in specific ethnic populations of Asians have identified prevalence rates in these subgroups, but conclusions from these studies do not necessarily generalize to the heterogeneous group of Asians. For example, according to Ali (2014), Yeung, Chan, Mischoulon, Sonawalla, Wong, Nierenberg, and Fava (2004) found the prevalence of major depressive disorder among Chinese Americans in a primary care setting in Boston to be 19.6%, much higher than the estimate from the CAPES study in Los Angeles described earlier (Yeung et al., 2004). Another study from 2000 found that the prevalence of panic disorder in Cambodian refugees being treated at a psychiatric clinic disorders in Asians based on data from NLAAS study and found overall low prevalence of eating disorders in Asians, less than 1% for anorexia and bulimia. Women had a higher lifetime prevalence of binge eating disorder than men, 2.67% compared to 1.35% (Nicadao, Hong, & Takeuchi, 2007). The author believes that it is difficult to draw conclusions about a particular individual based on these heterogeneous data. One interpretation of these data is that mental health professional should expect that refugees from Asia will likely exhibit symptoms of anxiety disorders. However, with less high-acuity populations, the mental health professional should be more vigilant for mental health symptoms, which may be underrepresented or may manifest in different ways.

The Surgeon General's Report in 2001, according to Ali (2014), in addition to emphasizing the need for better epidemiological data on mental health conditions, also highlighted the low utilization of mental health services by Asians compared to other minority groups, which has continued to be true when compared to Whites, Blacks, and Hispanics (Sue, Yan-Cheng, Saad, & Chu, 2012; U.S. Center for Mental Health Services, 2001; U.S. National Institute of Mental Health, 2001; U.S. Office of the Surgeon General, 2001; United States Substance Abuse and Mental Health Services Administration, 2001). Since that time, many studies have examined this question with differing results, because barriers for the individual Asian patient may include any of the following: cultural bias in how the patient describes his symptoms, bias in how the clinician or researcher assesses the symptoms, decreased perception of need for treatment, stigma, foreign-born status, wishing to save face, initial use of family support and traditional healing methods, focus on somatic symptoms, length of time in the United States, lack of culturally appropriate services, lack of language appropriate services, and lack of health insurance (Abe-Kim et al., 2007; Lu, 2010; Sue, et al., 2012; U.S. Center for Mental Health Services, 2001; U.S. National Institute of Mental Health, 2001; U.S. Office of the Surgeon General, 2001; United States Substance Abuse and Mental Health Services Administration, 2001). According to Ali (2014), for every 100,000 Asian and Pacific Islanders, there are 70 Asian and Pacific Islander mental health care providers, which is less than half of the number of providers for Whites. Also, Asians may have difficulty accessing the U.S. health care system in general, as suggested by the fact that Asians who are Medicaid eligible are much less likely to have Medicaid than their White counterpart (Lu, 2010). While it is not possible to review all of the nuances of the methodological difficulties in assessing the prevalence of mental health disorders in Asians and the disparity in their treatment, excellent reviews are provided elsewhere (Lu, 2010; Sue et al., 2012).

There have been calls for systematic, comparable studies of stigma within and across social and cultural contexts in order to understand its origins, meanings and consequences (Aggarwal, Cedeño, Guarnaccia, Kleinman, & Lewis-Fernández, 2016; Caracci & Mezzich, 2001; Hopper & Wanderling, 2000; Ng, 1997; Rutz, 2001; Slu, 1989). Despite these calls and findings that document the pervasive existence and impact of stigma in different countries (Crisp, Gelder, Rix, Meltzer, & Rowlands, 2000; Fabrega, 1991; Pescosolido, Martin, Link, Kikuzawa, Burgos, & Swindle, 2000; Stuart & Arboleda-Flórez, 2001; Wahl, 1999), relatively little about the cross-cultural distribution of stigma. Researchers across the global have collected data on stigma, but differences in samples and instrumentation make it difficult, if not impossible, to compare findings. Thus, questions about whether and how the social reaction to mental illness varies across countries, whether the underlying operative processes are similar, and whether it maps onto the distribution of outcome heterogeneity remain unanswered. Thus, the important question of whether these differences can offer a wedge into decreasing stigma's negative impacts, also remains unanswered. In sum, while the influence of cultural context on health and well-being is widely acknowledged, the empirical literature on the cross cultural nature of stigma remains underdeveloped (Aggarwal et al., 2016; National Research Council and Institute of Medicine, 2000). The World Psychiatric Association's (WPA) Global Programme Against Stigma and Discrimination because of Schizophrenia (Sartorius, 1997) has encouraged the developed the development of a comparative catalogue of information and, to date there have been only a few large-scale studies. Even recent cross-national effort, while springing from and being influenced by the WPA initiative, have not been linked in practice, making inference about comparative influence difficult. Moreover, according to Pescosolido, Olafsdottir, Martin, and Long (2008), there has never been a methodologically coordinated attempt to understand the extent to which mental illness is understood and stigmatized across countries (Townsend, 1975).

Mental Health Disorders and Stigma: Asians

The concepts of stigma and shame play an important role in Asians' low services use (Chu & Sue, 2011). According to Chu and Sue (2011), *Haji* among Japanese, *Hiya* among Filipinos, *Mianzi* among Chinese, and *Chaemyun* among Koreans are terms that reveal concerns over the process of shame or the *loss of face* (Sue, 1994). Many Asians tend to avoid the juvenile justice or legal system, mental health agencies, health services, and welfare agencies, because the utilization of services for certain problems is a tacit admission of the existence of these problems and may result in public knowledge of these familial difficulties. Older adult Korean Americans, for example, report greater misconceptions and stigmatizations about mental health as a weakness that would bring shame to a family if one were to reveal their mental illness by seeking treatment (Jan, Chiriboga, & Okazaki, 2009). Other studies have confirmed that greater personal stigma and lower stigma tolerance predicts a lower likelihood to seek help among Asian students, and that stigma about mental illness is higher among Asians (Eisenberg, Downs, Golberstein, & Zivin, 2009; Ting & Hwang, 2009).

System-level and care process factors also contribute to the considerable problem of mental health care disparities in Asians. Higher rates of poverty and rates of being uninsured or underinsured, particularly among Southeast Asians like the Cambodians, Hmong, or Laotians, can prevent access to needed mental health services (Reeves & Bennett, 2204). Compounding this problem of financial resources is the dearth of available language-appropriate and culturally-appropriate services for many Asian individuals. Beyond the need to increase the availability of Asian-language clinicians, research has pointed to the need for culturally-competent providers who are able to understand and deliver mental health treatments with similar worldviews and cognitive styles to that of Asian clients (Aggarwal et al., 2016; Zane, Sue, Chang, Huang, Huang, Lowe, Srinivasan, Chun, Kurasaki, & Lee, 2005). Asians who make the difficult decision to initiate contact with mental health providers may be more likely to stay in treatment if they encounter these culturally-congruent aspects of the care process (Aggarwal et al., 2016; Ivey, Ivey, & Simek-Morgan, 1997; Sue & Sue, 1999).

ASIANS: MENTAL HEALTH

Asians in the United States are comprised of many subgroups including Cambodians, Chinese, Japanese, Filipinos, Koreans, Laotians, Asian Indians, Vietnamese, etc. who speak over thirty languages. Asian comprise 58% of the U.S. population but 60% of the world's population (Chu & Sue, 2011). Despite the fact that Asian groups are heterogeneous, researchers have often studied the subpopulations as an aggregate group because Asians often show similar cultural values that are in contrast to Westerners (Chu & Sue, 2011). Despite the high prevalence of mental health-related problems, mental health is commonly overlooked in Asian communities, and cultural barriers have been identified as the most imperative factor (Aggarwal et al., 2016; Lee, Juon, Martinez, Hsu, Robinson, Bawa, & Ma, 2009). Nguyen and Anderson (2005) stated that some Asians hold the belief that individuals who have mental illness may be possessed by supernatural entities such as demons or spirits. Therefore, mental illness is highly stigmatized in many Asian cultures, and the root of mental illness stigma can be found in Asians' cultural beliefs toward mental health (Kung, 2004; Lee et al., 2009; Masuda, Anderson, Twohig, Feinstein, Chou, Wendell, Stormo, 2009; Nguyen & Anderson, 2005). Indeed, among Asian immigrants, extra-familial intervention is often considered shameful, as it indicates the inadequacy of family members and causes them to *lose face* within their community (Chu & Sue, 2011).

Consequently, instead of seeking professional help, Asians may try to change this behavior through self-control and willpower or may try to keep out bad thoughts by keeping busy (Zhang, Snowden, & Sue, 1998). When these attempts fail, they may choose to address problems and needs first, within the family system (Hsu, Davies, & Hansen, 2004). External help is sought only after all other resources are exhausted or when legal or social services force the issue. Even when seeking mental health services, many Asians might first seek medical services or traditional resources such as herbalists, acupuncturists, fortunetellers, or religious/spiritual leaders for help, which are less stigmatized sources of help (Nguyen & Anderson, 2005). Depending on the severity of their illness, they may then seek a mental health professional (Kung, 2004). If the Asian culture and stigma play a significant role in help-seeking behaviors, given the interconnected nature of culture, stigma, and the acculturation process among ethnic minorities (Hsu, Davies, & Hansen, 2004), it follows that acculturation might predict help-seeking behaviors.

MENTAL HEALTH SERVICES UTILIZATION WITHIN THE ASIAN CULTURE: ACCULTURATION, PREFERENCE FOR COUNSELORS, AND HELP-SEEKING BEHAVIORS

In the Asian culture, empirical studies have shown that the identification, express and acknowledgement of psychiatric problems are influenced by culture. According to Han and Pong (2015), studies show that many Asians believe that emotional anguish is seen as the consequence of bad thoughts, a lack of will power and self-control, and personality weakness, and therefore disclosing that one has mental illness is considered to be shameful (Kung, 2004; Lee et al., 2009). These beliefs may deter individuals from seeking help for their symptoms. Furthermore, in Asian cultures, mental illness often is not considered as an individual problem. Rather, mental illness potentially represents a negative reflection on the immediate family as well as their ancestors. For Asian immigrants, stigma attached to mental illness is a multifaceted phenomenon which is related to loss of face and status that us beyond the individual level (Chu & Sue, 2011). It is likely that such an intense and complex stigma attached to mental health issues further exacerbates disparities in mental health service utilization. Indeed, among Asian immigrants, extra-familial intervention is often considered shameful, as it indicates the inadequacy of family members and causes them to *lose face* with their community (Chu & Sue, 2011). Consequently, instead of seeking professional help, Asians may try to change this behavior through self-control and willpower or may try to keep out bad thoughts by keeping busy (Zhang, Snowden, & Suc, 1998). When these attempts fail, they may choose to address problems and needs first within the family system, such as immediate nuclear family, then extended family (Hsu, Davies, & Hansen, 2004). External help is sought only after all other resources are exhausted or when legal or social services force the issue.

Another cultural-bound contributor to low mental health service utilization is one's level of acculturation. Acculturation is a process of changing one's culture by incorporating elements of another culture and entails a mutual blending of culture, both psychologically and behaviorally (Berry, 1997). Thus, acculturation reflects the extent to which individuals learn the psychological and behavioral aspects of the dominant culture (Zane & Mak, 2002). Thus, Asians' reluctance to seek professional help and their lack of acceptance of Western psychotherapy, based on their level of acculturation, is known as a contributor to barriers in seeking mental health services (Wong, Marshall, Schell, Elliott, Hambarsoomians, Berthold, & Chun, 2006). Furthermore, studies also show that many Asians, in addition to the cultural factors such as stigma and acculturation, do not feel comfortable speaking to a mental health professional who does not share their same ethnic background, primarily due to cultural/language difference (Lee et al., 2009).

Mental Health Services Utilization Within the Asian Culture: Characteristics and Professional Mental Health Help-Seeking Behavior

Most existing studies have emphasized the cultural contextual factors in Asians' professional mental-health-seeking behavior. Previous research has shown that demographic characteristics seem to play a role in the willingness to seek professional help among Asians (Takayama, 2010). According to Han and Pong (2015), Asian females tend to have more positive attitudes toward seeking help than do Asian males (Leong & Zachar, 1999; Yoo, Goh, & Yoon, 2005). Also, while some studies have not found any relationship between age and seeking formal psychological help (Abe-Kim, Takeuchi, & Hwang, 2002; Abe-Kim et al., 2007; Shea & Yeh, 2008), some argue that younger Asians, especially those who ae male, may be less traditional, which results in a positive view of psychological help-seeking behavior (Solberg Ritsma, Davism Tata, & Jolly, 1994).

Cultural-Bound Syndromes

Culture-bound syndromes are repeated clusters of symptoms and behaviors specific to a geographic region which can cause both physical and mental distress in an individual and may result in impairment of functioning and help seeking behavior. The symptoms may include somatic symptoms as well as symptoms that may or may not overlap with a psychiatric disorder classified in the DSM (Task Force on DSM-IV, 2000). Various culture-bound syndromes are associated with particular Asian populations and are a continued area of study as psychiatric researchers and clinicians alike determine how best to approach their diagnosis and treatment. Identification and management of culture-bound syndromes is a continued controversial area of inquiry. A recent review challenged the notion of this being only a culture-bound syndromes given the more frequent episodes of violence and aggressive behavior in Western countries as well as Asian countries, by people of Asian descent and non-Asian descent (Saint Martin, 1999). The prevalence of culture-bound syndromes may also continue shift. In Lee and Kleinman's study (2007), reviewing the history and prevalence of neurasthenia in China, Lee and Kleinman (2007) postulate that the worldwide impact of the DSM has made it less likely that Chinese psychiatrists use the diagnosis of neurasthenia in China (Lee & Kleinman, 2007). Culture-bound syndromes continue to evolve over time, particularly as technology and communication continue to impact cross-cultural exchange of information and ways of understanding illness.

Shame and Stigma

According to Wynaden, Chapman, Orb, McGowan, Zeeman, and Yeak (2005), Asians reported that their communities stigmatized people who had a mental illness and that the ill person experienced feelings of shame. Several Chinese elaborated that for the community, the meaning of *shame* had a very intense and profound meaning. Wynaden et al. (2005, p. 90) found it difficult to describe in English the intensity of the expression of the feeling of *shame* that a person with a mental illness would feel: "The [Chinese] feel shame, the meaning of shame is [non-Chinese people] can't understand the meaning of shame. For Chinese people shame is very deep meaning. It means that you can't go out and face other people (p. 3)". Thus, shame and stigma prevented people from seeking help from mainstream mental health services. According to Wynaden et al., (2005, p. 91), the family tried to manage the problem and isolated themselves from the community to prevent knowledge of the family member's illness from becoming public: "They [family] don't want to accept it and those that do [they feel that they] will be stigmatized and bring bad onto the family...migrants that live in Australia still often live in their own culture...They know that there is a problem but they do not want to accept it (p. 5)". A person with a mental illness, according to Wynaden et al., (2005, p. 91), and his/her family isolated themselves because they believed that they would be labelled as different by their community and viewed negatively: "I think that they [people who are ill] are very sensitive to being labelled being seen as different. You know they are very sensitive to people looking at you in a strange way that you have a mental problem. In Chinese it [a mental problem] is mad! (p. 3)".

Causes of Mental Illness

Asians stated that knowledge about the cause of mental illness depended on the person's: (1) level of education; (2) country of origin; and (3) age According to Wynaden et al. (2005). People who had migrated from countries such as Singapore, with a western lifestyle, were more open to the western concepts of education and scientific information regarding the causes of mental illness. Educated people were also better informed and viewed mental illness as having a genetic/hereditary link.

They understood disorder such as depression and schizophrenia. In contrast, migrants from more remote villages who were less educated and elderly migrants held more traditional beliefs. Hence, religion, and in particular Buddhism and Taoism, was reported to be important in determining the health beliefs of community members. According to Wynaden et al. (2005, p. 91), Buddhists believed in reincarnation and, inherent in this belief is, the philosophy of karma. Karma, the law of cause and effect in eastern spirituality, emphasizes that there is a consequence for every action. Therefore, positive actions result in positive reactions and negative actions result in negative reactions in a later reincarnation. Subsequently, people who produced a child who had a mental illness were perceived as being punished for their conduct in their past lives: "Traditionally they [parent] feel they may have done something wrong for this [mental illness] to happen. What you did in your past lives reincarnation [(前 世) the previous life]. You have not done anything right in your previous life. It is a sin very simply (p. 3)".

Other beliefs, according to Wynaden et al. (2005, p. 91), about the cause of mental illness are linked to the person being possessed by evil spirits: "When you are unwell, people will try to treat you with a witch doctor or spiritual leader...They relate psychiatric problems to spiritual causes (p. 10)". Traditional beliefs were also reported to have a sociological base. This belief was associated with the concept of *bad blood*: "In the old times they thought it was some bad blood in your family that caused it [mental illness]. Sometimes if the child has this problem [mental illness] then it must be the mother's fault, not the father. The mother brought all this to the family. It has a lot to do with the sociological thinking at that time society how they see women and men's roles (p. 6)". Furthermore, refugees from China were identified as an extremely vulnerable population because of the traditional beliefs they held. Many of the customs among this group did not facilitate resolution of problems associated with mental illness. According to Wynaden (2005, p. 91), the family may not attend funerals of a member who had committed suicide: "The refugee group from China...this is the group of people that are really very isolated and have nobody and no support at all...They don't know how to deal with it...Language is a problem culture is another major problem in fact I came across quite a few refugee families and they have a huge problem to adjust to the way of life (p. 6)".

Family and Reputation

According to Wynaden et al. (2005, p. 91), the need to maintain family reputation was reported by all Asians and Asian Americans and were not dependent on people's level of education or country of origin: "They are reluctant to talk about it [mental illness] even if you [a general practitioner] ask them questions. It is something to be ashamed of it is a weakness and there is a stigma attached to it. You will be branded (p. 9)". Maintaining family reputation was particularly important if the problem was viewed as having a hereditary cause. It was reported that many Asian migrants have high expectations for their children. If these children succeeded it gave a good impression for the family. However, if the child developed a mental illness the family's reputation was disgraced (Wynaden et al., 2005, p. 91).

Hiding Up

According to Wynaden et al. (2005, p. 92), hiding up involved keeping the mental illness hidden from the community and/or not doing anything about the ill person's behavior: "There is still a large group of people who hide their [mentally ill] children away. They refuse to believe that they have a history of mental illness…They hide them [the child] they let them stay in the house and they do not let them leave the house (p. 2)". Hiding up meant that the family would not actively look for treatment and they would hide the ill person away hiding that as the child matured the problem would go away. The family would not bring people into their home, they would keep to themselves: "A lot of Chinese families [with a family member with a mental illness] hide up, they do not come out and they do not feel comfortable n going out…If you get an illness like a mental illness you do not understand and it has connotations and there is a lot of pressure to keep it hidden. If a family has mental illness they never want to talk to it. Only the family people know about the illness (p. 3)".

Seeking Help

Seeking help was a difficult process and it was usually left until the ill person's behavior was so bad that it could not be managed any longer within the family: "People who get treatment do it as the last resort (p. 5)". Generally, Asians do not voluntarily seek help from mainstream health services. Instead, they prefer to use prayer and visit temples and churches. Taoism was an important religion as it provided direction about the cause and treatment of mental illness. The family sought help when they were not able to manage the ill person. Some accessed help from a general practitioners (GP) from their country of origin because they believed that the GP would be more likely to understand. Other went to a non-Asian GP to maintain family confidentiality and prevent the risk of information being leaked to their community. Furthermore, language barriers were experienced by people accessing non-Asian doctors, and the use of interpreters was costly.

Lack of Collaboration

Asians explained that health professional had to reach into the community to access people if they wanted to demystify mental illness. According to Wynaden et al. (2005, p. 92), one way was to make contact with spiritual/religious leaders as places of worship played a very important role in determining the health belief of these communities. Health professionals need to understand the impact of mental illness on the family: "[Health professionals need to] develop more understanding of how Asian people feel about having a family member with a mental illness. If they can understand the traditional thinking, how people think about it. Health professionals can support them and let them know that they are not different... You need to make them feel that they are not disrespected (p. 3)". Health professional have to act with compassion, establish rapport and maintain confidentiality (p. 8)".

FUTURE RESEARCH AND RECOMMENDATIONS

Asians may have needs for certain resources that are not reflected in lower service utilization patterns. Experts have criticized the mental health services currently available within the US mental health system as disjointed, culturally mismatched with the treatment preferences of ethnic minority clients, and non-representative of cultural ideas about illness and health (Aggarwal et al., 2016; President's New Freedom Commission on Mental Health, 2003; United States Department of Health and Human Services, 2001). In recent years, culturally-specific service options have emerged to improved fit with the mental health needs of Asians. Cultural treatment adaptations, for example, refer to the process by which evidence-based practices (EBPs) validated in mainstream populations are tested and modified for the specific cultural needs of ethnic minorities like Asians. Culturally-adapted EBPs systematically consider language, culture, and contextual issues consistent with client's cultural values, beliefs, and practices, and have demonstrated beneficial outcomes in diverse populations (Bernal, Jiménez-Chafey, & Rodríguez, 2009; Griner & Smith, 2006; Pan, Huey, & Hernandez, 2011; Sue, Zane, Hall, & Berger, 2009). Several of these culturally-adapted treatment options have emerged as viable options for Asian individuals, including Problem Solving Therapy for depressed Chinese older adults (Chu, Huynh, & Arean, 2012), a culturally-adapted one-session treatment for Asians with phobia (Pan et al., 2011), a culturally-adapted cognitive behavioral intervention to accommodate the somatic symptoms that accompany PTSD in Cambodian refugees (Hinton, Pich, Chhean, Safren, & Pollack, 2006), and a Cantonese language CBT for depressed Hong Kong immigrants in Vancouver Canada (Shen, Alden, Söchting, & Tsang, 2006).

As a relatively new field of study, the science of cultural adaptation has shown recent advances with strides in guideline for when, how, and to what extent treatments should be adapted for a cultural population without significantly compromising fidelity to essential treatment components (Castro Barrera, & Holleran-Steiker, 2010). In fact, several models for the cultural adaptation process have been offered, such as the ecological validity framework (Bernal, Bonilla, & Bellido, 1995), cultural accommodation model (Leong & Lee, 2006). Most of these models recommend variations around four basic adaptation phases: information gathering, developing of initial adaptation design, pilot testing, and additional refinement (Barrera & Castro, 2006). These culturally-adapted treatments show considerable promise to provide treatment options that are congruent with the cultural preferences, coping and interpersonal styles, and psychopathology expressions of Asian clients. Continued work is needed to further develop and refine culturally-adapted treatments, and translational implementation efforts are sorely needed to transport such treatments from research to applied community settings. Unique challenges for the validity of mental disorder research arise from the heterogeneity of Asians populations, cultural biases in reporting style, and cultural idioms of distress. First, the nature of the Asian population is that it is small, diverse, and ever-changing. Second, cultural variations in response style, particularly on self-report rating scales, present important challenges for researchers and mental health professionals in the interpretation and cross-cultural validity of questionnaires. Third, Asians choose to express their distress is that of language terms utilized on research instruments (Chu & Sue, 2011).

CONCLUSION

Over the years, researchers have consistently highlighted the problem of mental health service underutilization within the Asians communities (Abe-Kim, Takeuchi, Hong, Zane, Sue, Spencer, Appel, Nicdao, & Alegría, 2007; Cheung & Snowden, 1990; Sue, Yan-Cheng, Saad, & Chu, 2012; Sue & McKinney, 1975). This mental health disparity manifests in a multifaceted manner, such as lower services utilization rates relatives to Whites (Matsuoka, Breaux, & Ryujin, 1997), presenting for professional help with more severe symptoms compared to other races (Chen, Sullivan, Lu, & Shibusawa, 2003), and a preference for receiving help from sources outside of professional mental health services (Ruzek, Nguyen, & Herzog, 2011). What is especially troubling is the recent evidence based on national data indicating that Asians continue to lag behind other groups (African Americans, Hispanics, and non-Hispanic Whites) in mental health service utilization, even while factoring in rates of distress (Sue, Cheng, Saad, & Chu, 2012). Therefore, a continued effort among researchers to unpack the contributing factors behind this mental health disparity is needed. That said, Kim and Kendall's (2015) study confirmed the recent and powerful data presented by Sue et al. (2012), indicating that the Asians underutilization trend still holds, even after taking into account psychopathology, only serve to further underscore the need for more research addressing this mental health disparity. Such that, the nuanced understanding of when an explanatory mechanism of help-seeking [Asian values → help-seeking attitudes → willingness to see a counselor] is attenuated, is when spiritual and biological etiology beliefs are strongly endorsed

Religion, Philosophy, and Health Beliefs

Many values and beliefs common among Asian populations have underpinnings in Asian religions and philosophy. These value systems are comprehensive, describing the integration of the body and the mind as well and an approach to managing both one's internal and external world. Asians and Asian Americans are an extremely diverse group, and while all Asians and Asian Americans will not uphold these beliefs, it is useful to briefly review them here as they inform the conceptualization of mental health and illness as well as general cultural values in many Asian cultures. That being said, much of Eastern philosophy is based on principles in Confucianism, Taoism, Hinduism, and Buddhism. Confucian thought brought order to Chinese civilization by emphasizing concepts such as interpersonal harmony, acceptance of a person's place in society, hierarchy within the family with older adults and males in higher positions, unconditional obligation toward the family, and orientation toward the group rather than the individual (Uba, 1994; Yang, Narayanasamy, & & Chang, 2011). Taoism emphasizes the importance of maintaining balance and harmony both internally and with the larger world, respecting nature, and maintain personal qualities of humility and receptivity (Stevenson, 1996; Yang, Narayanasamy, & Chang, 2011).

In Buddhism, the individual cultivates compassion for the suffering of others, acceptance of one's fate, or karma as a result of acts in a past life, and an acceptance of the ephemeral nature of life, as well as emphasis on non-attachment to aspects of the self (Hinton, Tran, Tran, & Hinton, 2008; Plakum, 2008). Elements of animism, belief in the existence of spirits, gods, and ghosts and the belief in a larger spirit would infused in natural inanimate and animate objects, has informed elements of Asian philosophy from Taoism, Confucianism, and Buddhism that include respect or worship for ancestors as a virtue (Hinton, Tran, Tran, & Hinton, 2008). Hinduism and Islam are the most common religions in South Asian nations. Aspects of Hindu beliefs have overlap with Buddhism such as the values of knowledge of life, emotional regulation, control-over-desire, the value of humility, and the importance of societal duty (Jeste & Vahia, 2008). Muslims also have a strong belief in destiny or fate, similar to karma, in that events occur because of the will of God, and similar ideas of sin to Judeo Christian religions. Many Muslims also believe in the spirit world of the jinn and some may have supernatural beliefs about the evil eye (Walpole, McMillan, House, Cottrell, & Ghazala, 2013). Hence, for example, a Chinese patient may believe that his low energy and mood are the result of an imbalance of yin and yang and may wish to take traditional herbs from a root doctor along with the antidepressant recommended by his psychiatrist (Castillo, 2002). Understanding traditional beliefs may also help mental health clinicians, researchers, and educators gain insight into a family's approach to managing a particular condition in a family member and the challenges that may arise. The breadth of religious and philosophies upheld by Asians was briefly reviewed here, but the mental health clinician can improve their understanding of the individual Asian patient's approach to his/her mental health by learning more about his/her particular belief systems.

Asian American Family Culture

Based on the deeply ingrained idea of filial piety in the vast majority of Asian cultures, the family is the unit on which society is based. Filial piety is a core value based on Confucian principles. It emphasizes the importance of family throughout the life cycle of the individual. The interdependence of family, members among Asians manifests itself in various ways, one of which is when Asians contemplate making major life decisions. In surveys of Asian adults with children over age 18, 68% felt that parents should have some influence in determining what career their child pursues, and in the same group, approximately 66% felt that parents should have at least some influence in their child's choice of spouse (Pew Research, 2012). On the other hand, behavior against the family or cultural values, such as delinquent behavior, a suicide attempt, being gay or lesbian, or taking a partner from a different religion or ethnic background, may be viewed as bringing shame to the family, or causing the family to *lose face*, and lead to conflict within the family (Rho & Rho, 2009; Walpole et al., 2013). Cultural values of displaying more tempered emotions, and family harmony may lead to more indirect or restrained communication between family members than in non-Asian families (Rho & Rho, 2009; Uba, 1994). Additionally, the emphasis placed on respect and obedience to parental authority can also decrease the likelihood of open communication between different generations as detailed in immigrant families. Acculturation and enculturation are related concepts. Both reflect aspects of the process of change an individual undergoes when one moves to a new culture.

Acculturation and Families

Connections among family members undergo transition as immigrants move to a new culture and attempt to adapt to the culture. In a process known as acculturation, the individual adapts with regard to identity, beliefs, and values in relation to the new dominant culture (Kim, Ahn, & Lam, 2009). Enculturation, a related concept, functions in the opposite manner and is a process in which a person strengthens their ties to social norms and values of their culture of origin (Kim, Ahn, & Lam, 2009). Hwang (2007) has referred to the term as acculturation family distancing (AFD) to combine the parent and child generation in immigrant households may acculturate at different rates, leading to a difference in values and also difficulties in communication (Hwang, 2007; Uba, 1994). Other researchers have referred to this phenomenon as dissonant acculturation and suspect that this is particularly relevant in conflict between parents who may struggle to maintain ties to the older culture and children who because of their age and desire to connect with peers may have greater exposure to the new culture (Kim, Ahn, & Lam, 2009). According to Ali (2014), this acculturation gap can also occur between elderly relatives that are coming from the country of origin, to live in the United States with their children. Grandparents may be brought to the United States with the idea that they can benefit from better health care or provide childcare for the family. Immigration is often alienating for older immigrants, who likely face greater functional limitations and language limitations than younger generations (Baker & Takshita, 2002; Uba, 1994). It is also more challenging for the elderly to establish a peer group and a grandparent new to the United States may experience an acculturation gap with their children and an even greater one with their grandchildren. Acculturation is part of the process of making a cultural and geographic transition and can lead to significant intergenerational conflict in Asian families.

Hence, in previous section, existing evidence of the breadth and depth of stigma across countries and provocative cross-national findings in what empirical work exists. Thus, while stigma is seen as *cross culturally ubiquitous* (Dovidio, Major, & Crocker, 2000; Neuberg, Smith, & Asher, 2000), the earliest work (Goffman, 1963) to the most recent (Dovidio, Major, & Crocker, 2000; Fabrega, 1991) conceptualizes stigma as a phenomenon shaped by cultural and historical forces. Early on, anthropologists described the different ways that cultures shape how individuals with mental illness are viewed and treated (Benedict, 1934; Townsend, 1975). Lefley (1990) contends that chronicity, itself, is a cultural artifact based, at least in part, on differing worldviews, religious traditions, the role of alternative healing systems, and difference in the cultural value of interdependence. Even studies that have documented differences in outcomes for persons with mental illness across countries point to and call for further investigations across cultural contexts (Dovidio, Major, & Crocker, 2000; Ng, 1997). These studies suggest that future research must identify the collective properties of social, cultural, economic and physical environments that influence health and disease outcomes. For example, according to Pescosolido et al. (2008), Sartorius (1998) reports that the ratio of psychiatrists to the population ranges from 1:1,000-5,000 in the more developed societies to 1:50,000-100,000 in the developing world to only 1:5,000,000 in some African countries. Of course, this is not independent of the availability of economic capital in a society which needs to be considered as well, because the World Health Organization (WHO) reports that countries in Western Pacific Region devote less than 5% of their small health budgets to mental health and neurological disorders (World Health Organization, 2005, p. 121). Thus, existing research suggests that researchers and practitioners in the field of mental health need to examine cross-cultural issues directly, rather than making assumptions about their correlation with broad categories.

ACKNOWLEDGMENT

I would like to dedicate this chapter to William Marc Weisman, M.S. (Marc Weisman), at the State of California, Department of Rehabilitation (DOR), in San Francisco, California. Marc is a team manager that I have the pleasure to work under and an opportunity to being mentored by, who demonstrates the behavior and definition of servant leadership, and practices the act of servant leadership. Marc continuously demonstrates the behavior of servant leadership, and practices the act of servant leadership, through the implementation of his knowledge, skills, abilities, wisdom, charm, humor, and charism. Marc exemplifies his managerial skills and (servant) leadership qualities through his actions with how efficiently he is able to handle and resolve situations at hand.

I am a certified bilingual [Cantonese and English (and not certified Mandarin)] Senior Vocational Rehabilitation Counselor, Qualified Rehabilitation Professional (SVRC-QRP) with DOR. I am currently the top performing SVRC-QRP, among 36 counselors in 6 teams in the San Francisco District with the State of California, Department of Rehabilitation. I single-handedly manage the RAMS/Hire-Ability mental health contract, and achieved a 97% successful rate (66/68). The first time since the contract tenure with DOR (approximately 20 years). I am also the only bilingual liaison with the Disabled Students Programs and Services (DSPS) Department for Chinatown North Beach Campus at City College of San Francisco (CCSF) for DOR.

Hire-Ability is non-profit vocational services program partnered with San Francisco Department of Public Health and California State Department of Rehabilitation which serves the San Francisco Bay Area community by connecting employers with trained, assessed and pre-qualified employees. Hire-Ability specializes in providing employers with a pool of employees that reflect the diverse and multicultural population of the region. Specifically, Hire-Ability assists employers in achieving their diversity goals by matching them with qualified individuals with disabilities. Hire-Ability Vocational Services is a division of RAMS, Inc. (Richmond Area Multi-Services, Inc.), which was established in 1974 and has over 30 different community programs that operate in the San Francisco Area. RAMS, Inc. is a private, non-profit mental health agency that is committed to advocating for and providing community based, culturally-competent, and consumer-guided comprehensive services, with an emphasis on serving Asian & Pacific Islander Americans. Founded in San Francisco's Richmond District in 1974, our agency offers comprehensive services that aim to meet the behavioral health, social, vocational, and educational needs of the diverse community of the San Francisco Area with special focus on the Asian & Pacific Islander American and Russian-speaking populations.

REFERENCES

Abdullah, T., & Brown, T. (2011). Mental illness and ethnocultural beliefs, values, and norms: An integrative review. *Clinical Psychology Review*, *31*(6), 934–948. doi:10.1016/j.cpr.2011.05.003 PMID:21683671

Abe-Kim, J., Takeuchi, D., Hong, S., Zane, N., Sue, S., & Alegría, M. (2007). Use of mental health-related services among immigrant and U.S.-born Asian Americans: Results from the national Latino and Asian American study. *American Journal of Public Health*, *97*(1), 91–98. doi:10.2105/AJPH.2006.098541 PMID:17138905

Abe-Kim, J., Takeuchi, D., & Hwang, W. C. (2002). Predictors of help seeking for emotional distress among Chinese Americans: Family matters. *Journal of Counseling and Clinical Psychology*, *70*(5), 1186–1190. doi:10.1037/0022-006X.70.5.1186 PMID:12362969

Abe-Kim, J., Takeuchi, D. T., Hong, S., Zane, N., Sue, S., Spencer, M. S., ... Alegría, M. (2007). Use of mental health-related services among immigrant and US-born Asian Americans: Results from the National Latino and Asian American Study. *American Journal of Public Health*, *97*(1), 91–98. doi:10.2105/AJPH.2006.098541 PMID:17138905

Aggarwal, N. K., Cedeño, K., Guarnaccia, P., Kleinman, A., & Lewis-Fernández, R. (2016). The meanings of cultural competence in mental health: An exploratory focus group study with patients, clinicians, and administrators. *SpringerPlus, 5*(1), 384. doi:10.118640064-016-2037-4 PMID:27065092

Alegría, M., Takeuchi, D., Canino, G., Duan, N., Shrout, P., Meng, X. L., ... Gong, F. (2004). Considering context, place and culture: The National Latino and Asian American Study. *International Journal of Methods in Psychiatric Research, 13*(4), 208–222. doi:10.1002/mpr.178 PMID:15719529

Ali, S. (2014). Identification and approach t treatment of mental health disorders in A0.sian American population. In R. Parekh (Ed.), The Massachusetts general hospital textbook on diversity and cultural sensitivity in mental health (pp. 31-59). Humana Press.

Angermeyer, M., & Dietrich, S. (2006). Public beliefs about and attitudes towards people with mental illness: A review of population studies. *Acta Psychiatrica Scandinavica, 113*(3), 163–179. doi:10.1111/j.1600-0447.2005.00699.x PMID:16466402

Baker, F. M., & Takeshita, J. (2002). The ethnic minority elderly. In W. S. Tseng & J. Streltzer (Eds.), *Culture and psychotherapy: A guide to clinical practice* (pp. 209–222). Washington, DC: American Psychiatric Press.

Barrera, M., & Castro, F. G. (2006). A heuristic framework for the cultural adaptation of interventions. *Clinical Psychology: Science and Practice, 13*(4), 311–316. doi:10.1111/j.1468-2850.2006.00043.x

Benedict, R. (1934). Anthropology and the abnormal. *Journal of General Psychiatry, 10*(1), 59–80. doi:10.1080/00221309.1934.9917714

Bernal, G., Bonilla, J., & Bellido, C. (1995). Ecological validity and cultural sensitivity for outcome research: Issues for the cultural adaptation and development o psychosocial treatments wit Hispanics. *Journal of Abnormal Child Psychology, 23*(1), 67–82. doi:10.1007/BF01447045 PMID:7759675

Bernal, G., Jiménez Chafey, M. I., & Rodríguez, M. M. D. (2009). Culturally adaptations of treatments: A resource for considering culture in evidence-based practice. *Professional Psychology, Research and Practice, 40*(4), 361–368. doi:10.1037/a0016401

Berry, J. (1997). Immigration, acculturation and adaption. *Applied Psychology, 46*(1), 5–34.

Caracci, G., & Mezzich, J. E. (2001). Culture and urban mental health. *The Psychiatric Clinics of North America, 24*(3), 581–593. doi:10.1016/S0193-953X(05)70249-5 PMID:11593865

Castillo, R. J. (2002). *Lessons from Folk healing practices.* Washington, DC: American Psychiatric Press.

Castro, F. P., Barrera, M. Jr, & Holleran-Steiker, L. K. (2010). Issues and challenges in the design of culturally adapted evidence-based interventions. *Annual Review of Clinical Psychology, 6*(1), 213–239. doi:10.1146/annurev-clinpsy-033109-132032 PMID:20192800

Chen, S., Sullivan, N. Y., Lu, Y. E., & Shibusawa, T. (2003). Asian Americans and mental health services: A study of utilization patterns in the 1990s. *Journal of Ethnic & Cultural Diversity in Social Work, 12*(2), 19–42. doi:10.1300/J051v12n02_02

Cheng, J. K. Y., Fancher, T. L., Ratanasen, M., Conner, K. R., Duberstein, P. R., Sue, S., & Takeuchi, D. (2010). Lifetime suicidal ideation and suicide attempts in Asian Americans. *Asian American Journal of Psychology, 1*(1), 8–30. doi:10.1037/a0018799 PMID:20953306

Cheung, F. K., & Snowden, L. R. (1990). Community mental health and ethnic minority populations. *Community Mental Health Journal, 26*(3), 277–291. doi:10.1007/BF00752778 PMID:2354624

Chu, J. P., Huynh, L., & Arean, P. A. (2012). Cultural adaptation of evidence-based practice utilizing an iterative stakeholder process and theoretical framework: Problem solving therapy for Chinese older adults. *International Journal of Geriatric Psychiatry, 27*(1), 97–106. doi:10.1002/gps.2698 PMID:21500283

Chu, J. P., & Sue, S. (2011). Asian American mental health: What we know and what we don't know. *Online Readings in Psychology and Culture, 3*(1). doi:10.9707/2307-0919.1026

Corrigan, P. (2000). Mental health stigma as social attribution: Implications for research methods and attitude change. *Clinical Psychology: Science and Practice, 7*(1), 48–67. doi:10.1093/clipsy.7.1.48

Corrigan, P., Druss, B., & Perlick, D. (2014). The impact of mental illness stigma on seeking and participating in mental health care. *Psychological Science in the Public Interest, 15*(2), 37–70. doi:10.1177/1529100614531398 PMID:26171956

Corrigan, P., Markowitz, F., & Watson, A. (2004). Structural levels of mental illness stigma and discrimination. *Schizophrenia Bulletin*, *30*(3), 481–491. doi:10.1093/oxfordjournals.schbul.a007096 PMID:15631241

Cottrell, A. B. (1990). Cross-national marriages: A review of the literature. *Journal of Comparative Family Studies*, *21*(2), 151–169.

Crisp, A. H., Gelder, M. G., Rix, S., Meltzer, H. I., & Rowlands, O. J. (2000). Stigmatization of people with mental illness. *The British Journal of Psychiatry*, *177*(1), 4–7. doi:10.1192/bjp.177.1.4 PMID:10945080

Dovidio, J. F., Major, B., & Crocker, J. (2000). *The social psychology of stigma*. New York: Guilford Press.

Eisenberg, D., Downs, M. F., Golberstein, E., & Zivin, K. (2009). Stigma and help seeking for mental health among college students. *Medical Care Research and Review: MCRR*, *66*(5), 522–541. doi:10.1177/1077558709335173 PMID:19454625

Fabrega, H. Jr. (1991). The culture and history of psychiatric stigma in early modern and modern western societies: A review of recent literature. *Comprehensive Psychiatry*, *32*(2), 97–119. doi:10.1016/0010-440X(91)90002-T PMID:2022119

Goffman, E. (1963). *Stigma: Notes on the management of spoiled identity*. Englewood Cliffs, NJ: Prentice-Hall.

Griner, D., & Smith, T. B. (2006). Culturally adapted mental health intervention: A meta-analytic review. *Psychotherapy (Chicago, Ill.)*, *43*(4), 531–548. doi:10.1037/0033-3204.43.4.531 PMID:22122142

Han, M., & Pong, H. (2015). Mental health help-seeking behaviors among Asian American community college students: The effect of stigma, cultural barriers, and acculturation. *Journal of College Student Development*, *56*(1), 1–14. doi:10.1353/csd.2015.0001

Hinton, D. E., Pich, V., Chhean, D., Hofmann, S. G., & Pollack, M. H. (2006). Somatic-focused therapy for traumatized refugees: Treating posttraumatic stress disorder and comorbid neck-focused panic attacks among Cambodian refugees. *Psychotherapy (Chicago, Ill.)*, *43*(4), 491–505. doi:10.1037/0033-3204.43.4.491 PMID:22122139

Hinton, L., Tran, J. N., Tran, C., & Hinton, D. (2008). Religious and spiritual dimensions of the Vietnamese dementia caregiving experience. *Hallym International Journal of Aging*, *10*(2), 139–160. doi:10.2190/HA.10.2.e PMID:20930949

Hopper, K., & Wanderling, J. (2000). Revisiting the developed versus developing distinction in course and outcome in schizophrenia: Results from ISoS, the WHO collaborative follow-up project. International Study of Schizophrenia. *Schizophrenia Bulletin*, *26*(4), 835–846. doi:10.1093/oxfordjournals.schbul.a033498 PMID:11087016

Hsu, E., Dabies, C. A., & Hansen, D. J. (2011). *Understanding mental health needs of Southeast Asian refugees: Historical, cultural, and contextual challenges*. Lincoln, NE: University of Nebraska. Available at http://digitalcommons.unl.edu/psychfacpub/86

Hsu, E., Davies, C. A., & Hansen, D. J. (2004). *Understanding mental health needs of Southeast Asian refugees: Historical, cultural, and contextual challenges*. Lincoln, NE: University of Nebraska.

Hwang, W. (2007). Acculturative family distancing: Theory research and clinical practice. *Psychotherapy (Chicago, Ill.)*, *43*(4), 397–409. doi:10.1037/0033-3204.43.4.397 PMID:22122132

Ivey, A. E., Ivey, M. B., & Simek-Morgan, L. (1997). *Counseling and psychotherapy: A multicultural perspective*. Needham Heights, MA: Allyn & Bacon.

Jang, Y., Chiriboga, D. A., & Okazaki, S. (2009). Attitudes toward mental health services: Age group differences in Korean American adults. *Aging & Mental Health*, *13*(1), 127–134. doi:10.1080/13607860802591070 PMID:19197698

Jenks, A. C. (2011). From 'lists of traits' to 'openmindedness": Emerging issues in cultural competence education. *Culture, Medicine, and Psychiatry. An International Journal of Cross-Cultural Health Research*, *35*, 209–235. doi:10.100711013-011-9212-4 PMID:21560030

Jeste, D., & Vahia, I. (2008). Comparison of the conceptualization of wisdom in ancient Indian literature with modern views: Focus on the Bhagavad Gita. *Psychiatry*, *71*(3), 197–208. doi:10.1521/psyc.2008.71.3.197 PMID:18834271

Kim, B. S. K., Ahn, A. J., & Lam, N. A. (2009). Theories and research on acculturation and enculturation experiences among Asian American families. In N. H. Trinh, Y. C. Rho, F. G. Lu, & K. M. Sanders (Ed.), Handbook of mental health and acculturation in Asian American families (pp. 25-43). Humana Press. doi:10.1007/978-1-60327-437-1_2

Kim, P. Y., & Kendall, D. L. (2015). Etiology beliefs moderate the influence of emotional self-control on willingness to see a counselor through help-seeking attitudes among Asian American students. *Journal of Counseling Psychology, 62*(2), 148–158. doi:10.1037/cou0000015 PMID:24635590

Kulhara, P., & Chakrabarti, S. (2001). Culture and schizophrenia and other psychotic disorders. *The Psychiatric Clinics of North America, 24*(3), 449–464. doi:10.1016/S0193-953X(05)70240-9 PMID:11593856

Kung, W. (2004). Cultural and practical barriers to seeking mental health treatment for Chinese Americans. *Journal of Community Psychology, 32*(1), 27–43. doi:10.1002/jcop.10077

Lee, S., Juon, H., Martinez, G., Hsu, C., Robinson, E., Bawa, J., & Ma, G. X. (2009). Model minority at risk: Expressed needs of mental health by Asian American young adults. *Journal of Community Health: The Publications for Health Promotion and Disease Prevention, 34*(2), 144–152. doi:10.100710900-008-9137-1 PMID:18931893

Lee, S., & Kleinman, A. (2007). Are somatoform disorders changing over time? The case of neurasthenia in China. *Psychosomatic Medicine, 69*(9), 846–849. doi:10.1097/PSY.0b013e31815b0092 PMID:18040092

Lefley, H. P. (1990). Culture and chronic mental illness. *Hospital & Community Psychiatry, 41*(3), 277–286. PMID:2179100

Leong, F. T. L., & Zachar, P. (1999). Gender and opinions about mental illness as predictors of attitudes toward seeking professional psychological help. *British Journal of Guidance & Counselling, 27*(1), 123–132. doi:10.1080/03069889908259720

Link, B., & Phelan, J. (2001). Conceptualizing stigma. *Annual Review of Sociology, 27*(1), 363–385. doi:10.1146/annurev.soc.27.1.363

Long, F. T. L., & Lee, S. H. (2006). A cultural accommodation model for cross-cultural psychotherapy: Illustrated with the case of Asian Americans. *Psychotherapy (Chicago, Ill.), 43*(4), 410–423. doi:10.1037/0033-3204.43.4.410 PMID:22122133

Lopez, R. A., & Yamazato, M. (2003). On growing old in America: Perceptions of an Okinawan War Bride. *Journal of Women & Aging, 4*(2/3), 17–31. doi:10.1300/J074v15n04_03 PMID:14750587

Lu, F. G. (2010). Asian Americans and Pacific Islanders. In P. Ruiz & A. Primm (Ed.), Disparities in psychiatric care: Clinical and cross cultural perspectives (pp. 40-51). Baltimore, MD: Lippincott Williams & Wilkins.

Masuda, A., Anderson, P., Twohig, M., Feinstein, A., Chou, Y., Wendell, J., & Stormo, A. (2009). Help-seeking experiences and attitudes among African American, Asian American, and European American college students. *International Journal for the Advancement of Counseling, 31*(3), 168–180. doi:10.100710447-009-9076-2

Matsuoka, J. K., Breaux, C., & Ryujin, D. H. (1997). National utilization of mental health services by Asian Americans/Pacific Islanders. *Journal of Community Psychology, 25*(2), 141–145. doi:

Murray, C. J. L., & Lopez, A. D. (1996). *Global burden of disease: A comprehensive assessment of morality and disability from diseases, injuries, and risk factors 4 in 1990 and projected to 2020.* Cambridge, MA: Harvard School of Public Health.

National Research Council and Institute of Medicine. (2000). From neurons to neighborhoods: The science of early childhood development. Committee on integrating the science of early childhood development. In J. P. Shonkoff & D. A. Phillips (Eds.), *Board on children, youth, and families, commission on behavioral and social sciences and education.* Washington, DC: National Academy Press.

Neuberg, S. L., Smith, D. M., & Asher, T. (2000). Why people stigmatize: Toward a biocultural framework. In T. F. Heatherton, R. E. Kleck, M. R. Hebl, & J. G. Hull (Eds.), *The social psychology of stigma* (pp. 31–61). New York: Guilford Press.

Ng, C. H. (1997). The stigma of mental illness in Asian cultures. *Australian and New Zealand Journal of Psychology, 31*(3), 382–390. doi:10.3109/00048679709073848 PMID:9226084

Nguyen, Q. C., & Anderson, L. P. (2005). Vietnamese Americans' attitudes toward seeking mental health services: Relation to cultural variables. *Journal of Community Psychology, 33*(2), 213–231. doi:10.1002/jcop.20039

Nicadao, E. G., Hong, S., & Takeuchi, D. T. (2007). Prevalence and correlates of eating disorders from Asian Americans: Results from the national Latino and Asian American study. *International Journal of Eating Disorders, 11*(4), 22–26. doi:10.1002/eat.20450 PMID:17879986

Pan, D., Huey, S. J., & Hernandez, D. (2011). Culturally adapted versus standard exposure treatment for phobic Asian Americans: Treatment efficacy, moderators, and predictors. *Cultural Diversity & Ethnic Minority Psychology, 17*(1), 11–22. doi:10.1037/a0022534 PMID:21341893

Pescosolido, B. A. (1991). Illness careers and network ties: A conceptual model of utilization and compliance. In G. L. Albrecht & J. A. Levy (Eds.), *Advances in medical sociology* (pp. 161–184). Greenwich, CT: JAI Press.

Pescosolido, B. A. (2006). Of pride and prejudice: The role of sociology and social networks in integrating the health sciences. *Journal of Health and Social Behavior*, *47*(3), 189–208. doi:10.1177/002214650604700301 PMID:17066772

Pescosolido, B. A., Martin, J. K., Link, B. G., Kikuzawa, S., Burgos, G., & Swindle, R. (2000). *Americans' view of mental illness and health at century's end: Continuity and change. Public report on the MacArthur Mental health module, 1996 general social survey*. Bloomington, IN: Indiana Consortium for Mental Health Services Research.

Pescosolido, B. A., Olafsdottir, S., Martin, J. K., & Long, J. S. (2008). Cross-cultural aspects of the stigma of mental illness. In J. Arboleda-Flórez & N. Sartorius (Eds.), *Understanding the Stigma of Mental Illness: Theory and Interventions* (pp. 19–35). John Wiley & Sons. doi:10.1002/9780470997642.ch2

Pew Research. (2012). *The rise of Asian Americans*. Retrieved on April 9, 2017, available at http://www.pewsocialtrends.org/2012/06/19/the-rise--of-asian-americans/3

Plakum, E. M. (2008). Psychiatry in Tibetan Buddhism: Madness and its cure seen through the lens of religious and national history. *The American Academy of Psychoanalysis and Dynamic Psychiatry*, *36*(3), 415–430. doi:10.1521/jaap.2008.36.3.415 PMID:18834281

President's New Freedom Commission on Mental Health. (2003). *Achieving the promise: Transforming mental health care in America. Final Report. Department of Health and Human Services Publication No. SMA-03-3831*. Rockville, MD: DHHS.

Reeves, T. J., & Bennett, C. E. (2004). *We the people: Asians in the United States, Census 2000 Special Reports*. Washington, DC: U.S. Census Bureau.

Remschmidt, H., Nurcombe, B., Belfer, M. L., Sartorius, N., & Okasha, A. (2007). *The mental health of children and adolescents: An area of global neglect*. Chichester, UK: Wiley. doi:10.1002/9780470512555

Rho, Y., & Rho, K. (2009). Clinical considerations in working with Asian American children and adolescents. In N. Trinh, Y. Rho, F. Lu, & K. M. Sanders (Eds.), *Handbook of mental health and acculturation in Asian American families* (pp. 143–166). New York, NY: Humana Press. doi:10.1007/978-1-60327-437-1_8

Rutz, W. (2001). Mental health in Europe: Problems, advances and challenges. *Acta Psychiatrica Scandinavica. Supplementum, 410*(s410), 15–20. doi:10.1034/j.1600-0447.2001.1040s2015.x PMID:11863046

Ruzek, N. A., Nguyen, D. Q., & Herzog, D. C. (2011). Acculturation, enculturation, psychological distress and help-seeking preferences among Asian American college students. *Asian American Journal of Psychology, 2*(3), 181–196. doi:10.1037/a0024302

Saint Martin, M. L. (1999). Running Amok: A modern perspective on a culture-bound syndrome. *Primary Care Companion to the Journal of Clinical Psychiatry, 1*(3), 66–70. doi:10.4088/PCC.v01n0302 PMID:15014687

Sartorius, N. (1997). Fighting schizophrenia and its stigma. A new world psychiatric association educational programme. *The British Journal of Psychiatry, 170*(4), 297. doi:10.1192/bjp.170.4.297 PMID:9246243

Sartorius, N. (1998). Stigma: What can psychiatrists do about it? *Lancet, 352*(9133), 1058–1059. doi:10.1016/S0140-6736(98)08008-8 PMID:9759771

Sartorius, N. (2007). Stigma and mental health. *Lancet, 370*(9590), 810–811. doi:10.1016/S0140-6736(07)61245-8 PMID:17804064

Sartorius, N., Gulbinat, W., Harrison, G., Laska, E., & Siegel, C. (1996). Long-term follow-up of schizophrenia in 16 countries. A description of the international study of schizophrenia conducted by the world health organization. *Social Psychiatry and Psychiatric Epidemiology, 31*(5), 249–258. PMID:8909114

Sartorius, N., Jablensky, A., & Shapiro, R. (1978). Cross-cultural differences in the short-term prognosis of schizophrenic psychoses. *Schizophrenia Bulletin, 4*(1), 102–113. doi:10.1093chbul/4.1.102 PMID:746359

Seeman, N., Tang, S., Brown, A., & Ing, A. (2016). World survey of mental illness stigma. *Journal of Affective Disorders, 190*(15), 115–121. doi:10.1016/j.jad.2015.10.011 PMID:26496017

Shea, M., & Yeh, C. (2008). Asian American students' cultural values, stigma, and relational self-construal: Correlates and attitudes toward professional help seeking. *Journal of Mental Health Counseling, 30*(2), 157–172. doi:10.17744/mehc.30.2.g662g5l2r1352198

Shen, E. K., Alden, L. E., Söchting, I., & Tsang, P. (2006). Clinical observations of a Cantonese cognitive-behavioral treatment program for Chinese immigrants. *Psychotherapy (Chicago, Ill.)*, *43*(4), 518–530. doi:10.1037/0033-3204.43.4.518 PMID:22122141

Slu, T. (1989). Short-term prognosis of schizophrenia in developed and developing countries. WHO international study program. *Zhurnal Nevropatologii i Psikhiatrii Imeni S. S. Korsakova*, *89*(5), 66–72. PMID:2781923

Solberg, V. S., Ritsma, S., Davis, B. L., Tata, S. P., & Jolly, A. (1994). Asian American students' severity of problems and willingness to seek help from university counseling centers: Role of previous counseling experience, gender, and ethnicity. *Journal of Counseling Psychology*, *41*(3), 275–279. doi:10.1037/0022-0167.41.3.275

Stevenson, C. (1996). The Tao, social constructionism and psychiatric nursing practice and research. *Journal of Psychiatric and Mental Health Nursing*, *3*(4), 217–224. doi:10.1111/j.1365-2850.1996.tb00115.x PMID:8997982

Stuart, H., & Arboleda-Flórez, J. (2001). Community attitudes toward persons with schizophrenia. *Canadian Journal of Psychiatry*, *46*(3), 245–252. doi:10.1177/070674370104600304 PMID:11320678

Sue, D. W., & Sue, D. (1999). *Counseling the culturally different: Theory and practice* (3rd ed.). New York: Wiley and Sons.

Sue, S. (1994). Mental health. In N. Zane, D. T. Takeuchi, & K. Young (Eds.), *Confronting critical health issues of Asian and Pacific Islander Americans* (pp. 266–288). Newbury Park, CA: Sage.

Sue, S., & McKinney, H. (1975). Asian Americans in the community mental health care system. *The American Journal of Orthopsychiatry*, *45*(1), 111–118. doi:10.1111/j.1939-0025.1975.tb01172.x PMID:1167437

Sue, S., Yan-Cheng, J. K., Saad, C. S., & Chu, J. P. (2012). Asian American mental health: A call to action. *The American Psychologist*, *67*(7), 532–544. doi:10.1037/a0028900 PMID:23046304

Sue, S., Zane, N., Hall, G. C. N., & Berger, L. K. (2009). The case for cultural competency in psychotherapeutic interventions. *Annual Review of Psychology*, *60*(1), 525–548. doi:10.1146/annurev.psych.60.110707.163651 PMID:18729724

Takaki, R. (1998). *Strangers from a different shore*. Boston, MA: Little, Brown, and Company.

Takayama, J. (2010). *Ecological systems theory of Asian American mental health service seeking* (School of Professional Psychology, paper 121). Retrieved on April 8, 2017, available at http://commons.pacificu.edu/spp/121

Task Force on DSM-IV. (2000). *Diagnostic and statistical manual of mental disorders: DSM-IV TR* (4th ed.). Washington, DC: American Psychiatric Publishing.

The 2010 National Drug Use and Survey on Health. (2012). *SAMHSA*. Retrieved on April 9, 2017, available at http://www.samhsa.gov/data/nsduh/2k10nsduh/2k10results. html

Ting, J., & Hwang, W. C. (2009). Cultural influences on help-seeking attitudes in Asian American students. *American Journal of Public Health*, *79*(1), 125–132. PMID:19290732

Townsend, J. M. (1975). Cultural conceptions, mental disorders, and social roles: A comparison of Germany and America. *American Sociological Review*, *40*(6), 739–752. doi:10.2307/2094177 PMID:1211687

Tran, B. (2016). The impact of the model minority culture in higher education institutions: The cause of Asian Americans' psychological and mental health. In N. P. Ololube (Ed.), *Handbook of research on organizational justice and culture in higher education institutions* (pp. 282–323). Hersey, PA: IGI Global. doi:10.4018/978-1-4666-9850-5.ch012

Tran, B. (2017). *The impact of the model minority culture in higher education institutions: The cause of Asian Americans' psychological and mental health (Reprint Collection). In Gaming and technology addiction: Breakthroughs in research and practice* (Vol. 1, pp. 404–445). Hersey, PA: IGI Global.

Tseng, W., & Strelzer, J. (2001). *Culture and psychotherapy: A guide to clinical practice* (pp. 173–191). Washington, DC: American Psychiatric Press.

Uba, L. (1994). *Asian American personality patterns, identity, and mental health*. New York: The Guilford Press.

United States Census. (2013a). *Facts for features: Asian /Pacific American heritage month*. Retrieved on April 9, 2017, available at http://www.census.gov/newsroom/releases/archives/facts_for_features_special_editins/cb13-ff09.html

United States Census. (2013b). *The Hispanic population: 2010 brief.* Retrieved on April 9, 2017, available at http://www.census.gov/prod/cen2010/briefs/c2010br-04.pdf

United States Department of Health & Human Services. (2000). *Healthy People 2010: Understanding and Improving Health* (2nd ed.). Washington, DC: U.S. Government Printing Office.

United States Department of Health and Human Services. (2001). *Mental health: Culture, race and ethnicity: A supplement to mental health: A report of the surgeon general.* Rockville, MD: Author.

United States National Institutes of Mental Health. (2001). *Mental health: Culture, race, and ethnicity. A supplement to mental health: A report of the surgeon general.* Rockville, MD: Author.

United States Office of the Surgeon General. (2001). *Mental health: Culture, race, and ethnicity. A supplement to mental health: A report of the surgeon general.* Rockville, MD: Author.

United States Substance Abuse and Mental Health Services Administration. (2001). *Mental health: Culture, race, and ethnicity. A supplement to mental health: A report of the surgeon general.* Rockville, MD: Author.

Wahl, O. F. (1999). Mental health consumers' experience of stigma. *Schizophrenia Bulletin, 25*(3), 467–478. doi:10.1093/oxfordjournals.schbul.a033394 PMID:10478782

Walpole, S. C., McMillan, D., House, A., Cottrell, D., & Ghazala, M. (2013). Interventions for treating depression in Muslim patients: A systematic review. *Journal of Affective Disorders, 145*(1), 11–20. doi:10.1016/j.jad.2012.06.035 PMID:22854098

Wong, E., Marshall, G., Schell, T., Elliott, M., Hambarsoomians, K., Berthold, S. M., & Chun, C. (2006). Barriers to mental health are utilization for U.S. Cambodian refugees. *Journal of Counseling and Clinical Psychology, 74*(6), 1116–1120. doi:10.1037/0022-006X.74.6.1116 PMID:17154740

World Health Organization. (2005). *Mental health atlas.* Geneva: World Health Organization.

Wynaden, D., Chapman, R., Orb, A., McGowan, S., Zeeman, Z., & Yeak, S. H. (2005). Factors that influence Asian communities' access to mental health care. *International Journal of Mental Health Nursing, 14*(2), 88–95. doi:10.1111/j.1440-0979.2005.00364.x PMID:15896255

Yang, C., Narayanasamy, A., & Chang, S. (2011). Transcultural spirituality: The spiritual journey of hospitalized patients with schizophrenia in Taiwan. *Journal of Advanced Nursing, 68*(2), 358–367. doi:10.1111/j.1365-2648.2011.05747.x PMID:21707724

Yeung, A., Chan, R., Mischoulon, D., Sonawalla, S., Wong, E., Nierenberg, A. A., & Fava, M. (2004). Prevalence of major depressive disorder among Chinese-Americans in primary care. *General Hospital Psychiatry, 26*(1), 24–30. doi:10.1016/j.genhosppsych.2003.08.006 PMID:14757299

Yoo, S. K., Goh, M., & Yoon, E. (2005). Psychological and cultural influences on Koreans' help-seeking attitudes. *Journal of Mental Health Counseling, 27*(3), 266–281. doi:10.17744/mehc.27.3.9kh5v6rec36egxlv

Zane, N., & Mak, W. (2002). Major approaches to the measurement of acculturation among ethnic minority populations: A content analysis and an alternative empirical strategy. In K. M. Chun, P. B. Organista, & G. Martin (Eds.), *Acculturations: Advances in theory, measurement, and applied research* (pp. 39–60). Baltimore, MD: United Book Press.

Zane, N. W., Sue, S., Chang, J., Huang, L., Huang, J., Lowe, S., ... Lee, E. (2005). Beyond ethnic match: Effects of client-therapist cognitive match in problem perception coping orientation, and therapy goals on treatment outcomes. *Journal of Community Psychology, 33*(5), 569–585. doi:10.1002/jcop.20067

Zhang, A. Y., Snowden, L. R., & Sue, S. (1998). Differences between Asian and White Americans' help-seeking and utilization patterns in the Los Angeles area. *Journal of Community Psychology, 26*(4), 317–326. doi:

ADDITIONAL READING

Aggarwal, N. K., DeSilva, R., Nicasio, A. V., Boiler, M., & Lewis-Fernández, R. (2015). Does the cultural formulation interview for the fifth revision of the diagnostic and statistical manual of mental disorders (DSM-5) affect medical communication? A qualitative exploratory study from the New York site. *Ethnicity & Health, 20*(1), 1–28. doi:10.1080/13557858.2013.857762 PMID:25372242

Aggarwal, N. K., Nicasio, A. V., DeSilva, R., Boiler, M., & Lewis-Fernández, R. (2013). Barriers to implementing the DSM-5 Cultural Formulation Interview: A qualitative study. *Culture, Medicine, and Psychiatry. An International Journal of Cross-Cultural Health Research, 37,* 505–533. doi:10.100711013-013-9325-z PMID:23836098

Brown, L. A., Gaudiano, B. A., & Miller, I. W. (2001). Investing the similarities and differences between practitioners of second- and third wave cognitive-behavioral therapies. *Behavior Modification, 35*(2), 187–200. doi:10.1177/0145445510393730 PMID:21324946

Chou, K. L., & Mak, K. Y. (1998). Attitudes to mental patients among Hong Kong Chinese: A trend study over two years. *The International Journal of Social Psychiatry, 44*(3), 215–224. doi:10.1177/002076409804400307

Chu, J. P., Hsieh, K., & Tokars, D. (2011). Help-seeking tendencies in Asian Americans with suicidal ideation and attempts. *Asian American Journal of Psychology, 2*(1), 25–38. doi:10.1037/a0023326

Cumming, E., & Cumming, J. (1957). *Closed ranks: An experiment in mental health education.* Cambridge, MA: Harvard University Press. doi:10.4159/harvard.9780674491779

Dain, N. (1994). Reflections on antipsychiatry and stigma in the history of American psychiatry. *Hospital & Community Psychiatry, 45*(10), 1010–1014. PMID:7829037

Lai, Y. M., Hong, C., & Chee, C. Y. (2001). Stigma and mental illness. *Singapore Medical Journal, 42*(3), 111–114. PMID:11405561

Lin, K. M., & Cheung, F. (1999). Mental health issues in Asian Americans. *Psychiatric Services (Washington, D.C.), 50*(6), 774–780. doi:10.1176/ps.50.6.774 PMID:10375146

Lin, K. M., & Kleinman, A. M. (1988). Psychopathology an clinical course of schizophrenia: A cross-cultural perspective. *Schizophrenia Bulletin, 14*(4), 555–567. doi:10.1093chbul/14.4.555 PMID:3064282

Link, B. G., & Phelan, J. C. (2001). Conceptualizing stigma. *Annual Review of Sociology, 27*(1), 363–385. doi:10.1146/annurev.soc.27.1.363

Link, B. G., Phelan, J. C., Bresnahan, M., Stueve, A., & Pescoslido, B. A. (1999). Public conceptions of mental illness: Labels, causes, dangerous and social distance. *American Journal of Public Health, 89*(9), 1328–1333. doi:10.2105/AJPH.89.9.1328 PMID:10474548

Link, B. G., Yang, L., Phelan, J. C., & Collins, P. (2004). Measuring mental illness stigma. *Schizophrenia Bulletin, 30*(3), 511–541. doi:10.1093/oxfordjournals.schbul. a007098 PMID:15631243

Mak, K. Y., & Gow, L. (1991). The living conditions of psychiatric patients discharged from half-way houses in Hong Kong. *The International Journal of Social Psychiatry, 37*(2), 107–112. doi:10.1177/002076409103700205 PMID:1655669

Masuda, A., Wendell, J. W., Chou, Y., & Feinstein, A. B. (2010). Relationships among self-concealment, mindfulness and negative psychological outcomes in Asian American and European American college students. *International Journal for the Advancement of Counseling, 32*(3), 165–177. doi:10.100710447-010-9097-x

Napier, A. D., Ancarno, C., Butler, B., Calabrese, J., Chater, A., Chatterjee, H., ... Woolf, K. (2014). Culture and health. *Lancet, 384*(9954), 1607–1639. doi:10.1016/S0140-6736(14)61603-2 PMID:25443490

Pan, D., Huey, S. J., & Hernandez, D. (2011). Culturally adapted versus standard exposure treatment for phobic Asian Americans: Treatment efficacy, moderators, and predictors. *Cultural Diversity & Ethnic Minority Psychology, 17*(1), 11–22. doi:10.1037/a0022534 PMID:21341893

Rabkin, J. (1974). Public attitudes toward mental illness: A review of the literature. *Schizophrenia Bulletin, 10*(Fall), 9–33. doi:10.1093chbul/1.10.9 PMID:4619493

Renzaho, A. M. N., Romios, P., Crock, C., & Sønderlund, A. L. (2013). The effectiveness of cultural competence programs in ethnic minority patient-centered health care—a systematic review of the literature. *International Journal for Quality in Health Care, 25*(3), 261–269. doi:10.1093/intqhc/mzt006 PMID:23343990

Roman, P. M., & Floyd, H. H. Jr. (1981). Social acceptance of psychiatric illness and psychiatric treatment. *Social Psychiatry. Sozialpsychiatrie. Psychiatrie Sociale, 16*(1), 21–29. doi:10.1007/BF00578066

Sartorius, N., & Schulze, H. (2005). *Reducing the stigma of mental illness: A report from a global association*. New York: Cambridge University Press. doi:10.1017/CBO9780511544255

Swindle, R., Heller, K., Pescosolido, B. A., & Kikuzawa, S. (2000). Responses to nervous break-downs in American over a 40-year period: Mental health policy implications. *The American Psychologist, 55*(7), 740–749. doi:10.1037/0003-066X.55.7.740 PMID:10916863

Takeuchi, D. T., Chung, R. C. Y., Lin, K. M., Shen, H., Kurasaki, K., Chun, C. A., & Sue, S. (1998). Lifetime and twelve-month prevalence rates of major depressive episodes and dysthymia among Chinese Americans in Los Angeles. *The American Journal of Psychiatry, 155*(10), 1407–1414. doi:10.1176/ajp.155.10.1407 PMID:9766773

Vargas, S. M., Cabassa, L. J., Nicasio, A. V., De La Cruz, A. A., Jackson, E., Rosario, M., ... Lewis-Fernández, R. (2015). Toward a cultural adaptation of pharmacotherapy: Latino views of depression and antidepressant therapy. *Transcultural Psychiatry, 52*(2), 244–273. doi:10.1177/1363461515574159 PMID:25736422

Villareal-Armas, G. (2010). Cultural competence in the trauma treatment of Thai survivors of modern-day theory slavery: The relevance of Buddhist mindfulness practices and healing rituals to transform shame and guilt of forced prostitution. In A. Kalaykian & D. Eugene (Eds.), *Mass trauma and emotional healing around the world: Rituals and practices for resilience and meaning-making* (pp. 269–285). Santa Barbara, CA: Praeger.

Yeung, A., Shyu, I., Fisher, L., Wu, S., Yang, H., & Fava, M. (2010). Culturally sensitive collaborative treatment for depressed Chinese Americans in primary care. *American Journal of Public Health, 100*(12), 2397–2402. doi:10.2105/AJPH.2009.184911 PMID:20966373

KEY TERMS AND DEFINITIONS

Asian Americans (Americans of Asian Descent): The term refers to a panethnic group that includes diverse populations who have ancestral origins in East Asia, Southeast Asia, or South Asia, as defined by the U.S. Census Bureau. This includes people who indicate their race(s) on the census as Asian or reported entries such as Asian Indian, Chinese, Filipino, Korean, Japanese, Vietnamese, and Other Asian.

Asian Exclusion Act of 1924: A continued response to concern about Asian immigration, which limited the new immigrants per year from East Asia, Southeast Asia, and South Asia.

Diagnostic and Statistical Manual of Mental Disorders (DSM-5): Used by clinicians and researchers to Diagnose and classify mental disorders.

Hiding Up: Involved keeping the mental illness hidden from the community and/or not doing anything about the ill person's behavior.

Karma: The law of cause and effect in eastern spirituality, emphasizes that there is a consequence for every action.

Mianzi: Refers to one's own sense of dignity or prestige in social contexts. It is a strategy that protects self-respect and individual identity.

Multigenerational Family: Having at least two adult generations in the same household.

Stigma: Stigma can be defined as the display of negative attitudes, based on prejudice and misinformation, in response to a marker of illness.

Chapter 5
Barriers to Practitioners' Endorsement of a Recovery Perspective:
Considering Attitudes Through a Schema Lens

Debra Kram-Fernandez
Empire State College (SUNY), USA

ABSTRACT

This chapter is concerned with the impact of practitioner biases on the experience of a meaningful life for individuals who live with serious mental illness (SMI). Professional biases, systemic biases that originate in societal fear and lack of knowledge, and internalized stigma taken on by the consumer affect life decisions. Following a history of treatment initiatives experienced by consumers as abusive, it is important to understand how a system envisioned to protect and treat was often experienced as harmful. In the 1980s a movement emerged to transform the nature of mental health treatment to a client-centered, recovery-oriented model. In 1999, the Surgeon General proclaimed that all agencies serving this population should be recovery oriented. Yet, the shift to this approach to understanding people with SMI has not been complete. While there are many explanations why practitioners may not fully embrace this perspective, this chapter introduces the concept of "schemas" from cognitive behavioral theory as a way of examining professional biases in the field of SMI.

DOI: 10.4018/978-1-5225-3808-0.ch005

INTRODUCTION

This chapter concerns the impact of professional biases on the ability of individuals with Serious Mental Illness (SMI) to experience a life of meaning and purpose in the same way as those who do not live with SMI. Due to the inherent power differential between patient and therapist, client and coach, or consumer and guide, professional biases can devastate the dreams of individuals who turn to the mental-health system, voluntarily or involuntarily, for the purpose of learning strategies to manage life with SMI. Most studied is the impact on help-seeking behaviors of people with SMI due to public and professional stigmas (Hailamariam et al., 2017; Henderson et al., 2013). When professionals are not able to reflect on their own schemas, there is potential for a cyclical and damaging dynamic. This dynamic is one based on personal biases of the professional, systemic biases originating in societal fear and lack of knowledge, and subsequently the internalized stigma taken on by the consumer, can prevail (Beretta et al., 2005; Orbell & Henderson, 2016). In the face of obvious reservations on the part of their treating professional, rare is the individual who will have the courage to move forward in pursuit of a life course of their choosing (Mead & Copeland, 2000; Deegan, 1996).

The mental health system has a long history of offering interventions that were ineffective and sometimes barbaric. However, when professionals act on the science and data of the time, interventions are usually reasonable and calculated risks. Bloodletting, ice baths, and even frontal lobotomies most likely emerged in a genuine effort to effect healing. Yet, these treatments often continue long past the acquisition of evidence that they are ineffective and in fact harmful, and the realization of their effects. One explanation of how this happens might be the impact of professional stigma. At what point does the practitioner embrace an "us and them" attitude toward his or her charges? At what point is it easy to detach from empathizing with the other because the other has become somehow less human?

In 1999, the Surgeon General proclaimed that all agencies serving this population should be recovery oriented; yet, the shift to this more client-centered approach to helping people with SMI has not been seamless or complete. Many reasons impede greater embrace of this directive, including but not limited to lack of consistent and widely disseminated data that a Recovery Perspective is more effective; lack of understanding of the practices that make an agency recovery oriented; and misconceptions that suggest this orientation is cost-prohibitive. Thinking critically about the recovery perspective reveals that this "perspective" or "paradigm" is not an evidence-based practice. In fact, it is not so much a "practice" as it is a way of working with people—an ethical focus on an individual's right to self-determination, dignity, and respect. Therefore, failure to fully embrace these principles remains somewhat curious. This chapter will define the cognitive behavioral concept of schemas, and consider how a greater understanding of this psychological mechanism may be a way of examining professional biases and their impact on consumers in the field of SMI.

By the end of this chapter, readers should have a basic understanding of the Recovery Perspective in mental health, and areas of common ground as well as conflict when compared with the more traditional Medical Perspective. We discuss how this perspective offers a client/consumer-centered approach to services for people with SMI, and how attention to professional schemas may be a vehicle for understanding the perpetuation of stigma against the people with SMI by professionals in the field of mental health. In closing, the chapter will offer some possible directions for mitigating the inherent harm that can occur from unchecked schemas among mental-health professionals.

TYPES OF STIGMA AND THE PERSPECTIVES THAT MAY HELP DRIVE THEM

Understanding a number of key concepts can assist the reader in fully appreciating the impact that stigma and bias have had on the lives of adults with SMI. First, this chapter refers to individuals who utilize mental-health services as "consumers." The nomenclatures for this population and the terms by which they are identified have morphed with the emergence of new scholarly and political developments. The term "patient" gave way to "client" as many recognized that the original term promoted a sense of illness and a role or position of dependence upon a person with a title suggesting "expert" status. "Client" gave way to the term "consumer" in the 1990s. This coincided with the emergence of the recovery movement that quickly became a formidable component of the mental-health landscape. The title "consumer" emphasizes a shift in the understanding of the relationship between a person in need of services and a service provider. Rather than a person with a disability being acted upon, "consumer" connotes a sense of the system working for the person in need of service. The battle for adoption of this change has been hard-fought and the term remains in inconsistent usage. Other important concepts include the notion of personal biases among professionals, social and systemic bias among others in the society, and bias that consumers of mental-health services often internalize.

Personal bias among helping professionals is one type of stigma. Numerous factors influence the development of individual perspectives on SMI, and like lay people, professionals are not immune to these factors. Lessons learned from family of origin, school and community experiences, religious organizations and affiliations, the political climate, and everyday experiences impact expectations and assumptions about human beings with SMI. The inclination toward science and/or religion can have an impact on how people understand the world around them, and the influence of the media cannot be overstated. Images of SMI in popular culture, such as sound bites on television or radio news broadcasts, movies, sitcoms, miniseries, and even social media, can have a profound influence on a person's understanding of causes, prognoses, appropriate treatment alternatives, and implications for public safety.

Haller (2010) makes the argument many representations of disability in the media show a tendency toward distortion that betrays the "ableist" values so dear to society. "Ableist" values essentially promote the worth of physical and mental, and intimate that their lack may even be a reasonable excuse for suicide. Haller uses the notion of assisted suicide to make this argument. If it is understandable that under the circumstance of losing a physical or sensory ability, one should have a right to end one's own life, what message does this convey to a person who never had that sense or ability? In her content analysis of media images of disability, although she observes shifts in public consciousness that were promising, the theme of disability represented as weakness remains prevalent. In addition, the theme of disability deserving derision or ridicule continues to be a problem.

Science in and of itself can exhibit bias. While greater learning and science can challenge misconceptions and fallacies, the history of the treatment of people with SMI is plagued by interventions founded in science that ultimately proved ineffective, dangerous, or sometimes even downright barbaric. Azar, Benjet, Fuhrmann, and Cavallero (1995) emphasize that "scientific facts" are laden with personal values.

Personal values of professionals informed by beliefs and perceptions that stigmatize can be profoundly detrimental to life outcomes for individuals with SMI. A professional making a decision based on an unsubstantiated fear can exert tremendous and unfair power over the life choices of a consumer. Not all mental-health professionals are experts on the scholarly literature of mental illness and societal risk; however, all mental-health professionals influence decisions over the lives of others, which their unchecked personal views may govern.

History has played a role in professional bias—perhaps small, but nonetheless a definitive role in the perpetuation of personal biases held by many mental-health professionals and lay people. For instance, Emil Kraepelin was the first to distinguish a separate set of symptoms that could be associated with what is now called schizophrenia. Kraepelin (1919, cited in Warner, 2004) named this separate disorder Dementia Praecox, which translates in essence to an illness that begins in adolescence (praecox) and results in a dementia-like state. He proclaimed that what differentiated dementia praecox from other forms of mental illness was its incurability. Thus, over a hundred years later and in spite of evidence to the contrary, diagnosis of a SMI, particularly a psychotic disorder such as schizophrenia, is often thought incurable. In fact, Kraepelin himself conducted numerous studies and found that a small percentage recovered from SMI (Kraepelin, as cited in Warner, 2004).

Even today, many professionals believe recovery is hopeless with a diagnosis of schizophrenia.

A further historical blow came later in early 1900s when one of the greatest minds in psychiatric and psychological history, considering the diagnosis of schizophrenia, declared that psychotic illness falls on a continuum separate from the mental health of the average person. In his contemplations about varying types and levels of neurosis, Sigmund Freud (1911) in his work on dream interpretation expressed concerns about the ability of a person with damaged ego strength to delve into this material without exacerbating psychotic symptoms. Regardless of Freud's personal reckoning of the implications of that assertion, the message suggests that people with SMI were somehow less than capable of psychological growth and change.

Another factor in professional bias might be the influence of a theoretical framework to which a given professional subscribes. Freud was the father of psychoanalysis, and psychoanalytically oriented mental-health professionals understand the cause of mental-health issues to be rooted in unconscious conflicts, usually traceable from childhood. In other words, symptoms or behaviors for which a consumer might seek help from a professional are a result of these unconscious conflicts. Recovery is thus a cessation of symptoms that results from working through past traumas by putting them into words with affect. Particularly in classical psychoanalytic theory, the roles of analyst and patient were clearly delineated and hierarchical. The treatment was usually quite long term, with a belief in recovery. However, whether this type of treatment is appropriate for people with more serious disorders is still a question, suggesting that there is actually no strong belief in recovery from SMI. Even today, some professionals see psychodynamic treatment of serious mental illness such as schizophrenia as akin to malpractice (Fuller Torrey, 2006). The value in this theory is the idea that motivations and drives made conscious free the consumer to make choices of his or her own free will. Recovery is ultimately the moment when through complex psychodynamic processes, the consumer "internalizes" the therapist and is able to do this kind of detective work on his or her own.

Alternatively, cognitive behavioral theory (CBT) was a bold and radical shift that emerged at a time when the "unconscious" was a household word. Albert Ellis (1994) proposed the idea that perhaps rather than an unconscious that would require long-term detective work with an expert professional, the locus of why people behave and feel as they do lies in how they interpret cues from their environment. In other words, the thoughts that go through a person's head in a given situation will determine how they feel and then act, and then perhaps think, feel, and act again. Thoughts, feelings, and behaviors are cyclically related. However, with just a few sessions with a cognitive behavioral therapist, a person can learn to identify thought distortions and thus interrupt the unhelpful patterns. CBT is an active therapy, particularly for the consumer. While both theories require hard work, CBT requires specific homework assignments and activities. Therapist and consumer roles are more level, and the therapist is more of a coach. Therefore, after just a few sessions, the consumer will have the tools to coach him- or herself. There is once again an expectation that with this work, recovery is a possible outcome.

Sociocultural theory minimizes the impact of internal dialogue and unconscious conflicts on the functioning of an individual or group. On the contrary, this theory suggests that if we resolved societal inequities and injustices, people would not behave in symptomatic ways. This theory sees causality as related to social injustice, and therefore the cure lies in social change. The role of a helping professional might be to stand side by side with a consumer at a march, painting a mural, lobbying legislators, and fighting together for social change.

Dividing theories into separate categories—biological, psychodynamic, cognitive, behavioral, family or systems, and sociocultural theories—is neat and organized. But in practice, varying degrees of each theory have an impact on the individual's emotional health in different and unique ways. Societal biases and systemic bias are crucial issues, and different consumers respond well to different approaches fueled by different theories. In sum, professional bias can be attributed to personal life experiences of the practitioner, to historical inaccuracies perpetuated over a century, and even to the theory that most resonates for the individual helping professional.

Internalized stigma is another level of presupposition that negatively affects the lives of consumers. People with SMI are members of the same social system as everyone else. The images they see of SMI are the same as the rest of the population sees. In addition, many have experienced a medical-model culture where calling an individual "a schizophrenic," "a borderline," or "a depressive" was standard nomenclature. This can be very demoralizing. The problem with this language is that once an identity becomes a label that entails lesser social and professional expectations for a meaningful life, only an extraordinary human being could overcome such expectations and thrive.

Expectations expressed by the professional community have a tremendous impact on people with SMI and greatly affect their expectations for themselves. In an editorial piece in *Schizophrenia Bulletin*, a family member explains that when the disease affects the brain, it is difficult to see where the disease ends and the person begins (Sundstrom, 2004). This difficulty is compounded when professionals in the field cannot make this distinction either.

The Recovery Perspective

Harry Stack Sullivan (1962), a renowned psychoanalytic theorist and practitioner in his own right, was a disciple of Sigmund Freud. Their paths diverged due to professional disagreements. One important difference in their understanding of mental health was that while Freud saw psychosis on a continuum separate from that of the rest of humanity, Sullivan saw humanity in SMI. On many points, he presaged innovations of the late 20th and early 21st centuries. Long before evidence-based practices were a celebrated initiative in mental health, Sullivan made the claim that any treatment offered to a person with a SMI requires study. He also understood that when a person with a SMI believes that the treatment provider considers the illness degenerative, the patient is at great risk of losing hope for the future. He also believed that an illness that affects the life of people as young as adolescents must be curable. Although his contributions were made before the onset of the recovery movement (and subsequently the recovery perspective), crossovers between his humanistic theory and the recovery perspective are noteworthy.

Although a large number of studies throughout the 20th century document recovery from the most serious mental disorders (see Warner, 2004; Calabrese & Corrigan, 2005), in 1987 Courtney Harding published an article on a study that she conducted, which also presaged aspects of the recovery movement. Not too distant history conjures up an image of SMI housed in a mental institution from which many people never were discharged. Images included restraints, screaming, electric-shock treatments, and lack of care such that human adults sat for interminable periods of time in soiled clothing. Harding (1987) wondered what the impact might be of a twofold intervention, the first being inpatient skills training, and the second a coordinated plan for support, from the same team that taught the inpatient skills, for patients reintegrating into the world-at-large. She led a team that provided this intervention, and conducted a longitudinal analysis. Her findings were quite positive and became a turning point in the scholarly discourse around the notion of recovery from SMI. This skills-building and environmental-support model presaged the Psychiatric Rehabilitation Model that, in addition to sharing office space with proponents of the Recovery Perspective, is in many ways the operationalization of the Recovery Perspective.

While standing up for the dignity and appropriate treatment of people with SMI is not a late 20th-century phenomenon, (e.g., Dorothea Dix, Philipe Pinel), in the 1980s this movement developed leadership among consumers, their families, and professionals, which turned it into quite a formidable movement. Some leaders and advocates of this movement include individuals who identify with attributes of both scholars and consumers, including Patricia Deegan, Ph.D. (1988; 1996), Mead & Copeland, (2000), and Anthony (2000), to name a few.

In the 1980s, the recovery movement was born, and it would change the face of mental-health treatment. Two divergent forces were the impetus for this transformation. First, people with SMI began writing in large numbers, not only about their experiences with recovery, but also of abuse that they experienced in the mental-health system.

Second was the development of the Psychiatric Rehabilitation Model, dovetails with the Recovery Perspective in that both are strengths-based models of care that recognize the value of peer support, encourage integration into the community-at-large, and maintain core values in understanding recovery from SMI.

Today's scholarly discourse about the definition of recovery from SMI considers what recovery means to those with serious mental illness. Up until the 1980s, recovery was essentially synonymous with cure, and thus meant a cessation of symptoms, cessation of hospitalizations, and the achievement of a "normal" level of functioning (Warner, 2004). This provided a measurable definition that would satisfy medical practitioners and quantitative researchers alike. This Medical Model perspective sees recovery from SMI as an endpoint that does allow for measuring recovery in a consistent and unbiased manner. On the other hand, recovery-oriented clinicians and consumers tend to view recovery as a nonlinear process. Although from a Recovery Perspective there is variation in the way in which recovery is defined, certain key elements are present in most definitions, including the restoring of a sense of hope, a sense of meaning, and a sense of purpose in life (Noordsy et al., 2002). Other important elements of this newer definition include creating and/or maintaining a peer-support network outside the mental-health system (Davidson, 2006), taking responsibility for one's own recovery journey, and considering one's own understanding of spirituality (Anthony, 2000; Davidson, 2006 Noordsy et al., 2002). Measuring recovery by this definition is a greater challenge than examining the number of hospitalizations, symptoms, and defined levels of functioning, but there is tremendous value in the endeavor. This method of measuring recovery recognizes the identity of a person as more than an illness and a number, and instead as a multidimensional human being.

Mental illness is rarely an event from which recovery is linear. While measures and numbers are clear and concise, mental health is a grey and murky concept best envisioned as multilayered and inexact. All human beings are learning, growing, and changing in different aspects of their lives at any given time. Thus, envisioning recovery from serious mental illness as a process that evolves in stages rather than as an endpoint is compelling (Lieberman & Kopelowicz, 2002). Proponents of the recovery movement invest their energy in changing the way we provide services. Rather than being acted upon by a system of experts, recovery-oriented consumers strive to be equal partners in determining their course of treatment.

Although this philosophy resonates with the social work code of ethics, a code that specifically emphasizes a need to respect client self-determination and the dignity of a person (NASW, 2017), like any organizational change, this paradigmatic transition has experienced some obstacles. In fact, the vast majority of agencies serving those with SMI may not be fully compliant with the Surgeon General's directive.

There is a real and critical need to address myths and assumptions on the part of professional helpers. In general, stigma creates an "us and them" environment that enables people to behave in inhumane ways towards others. This can become routine and acceptable. Germaine to the experience of people with SMI are numerous concrete examples of how stigma against people with SMI has resulted in harmful and inhumane treatment of this population. A right to participate in one's own treatment-plan development is a recent addition to consumer rights. Prior to this, once a person bore the label of SMI, the norm became being acted-upon with little if any of their input. Protections to ensure that people with SMI would be free to live in the least restrictive environment that could allow for both their personal safety and society's is also a new phenomenon. Providers are attempting to review the use of restraints, and further, to recognize the element of retraumatization inherent in many of these routine practices. Only recently have programs begun to examine the risks of abuse of power within programs for people with SMI, and to implement strategies to mitigate this potential. Although the notion of internalized stigma and the knowledge of how institutional care can foster this situation has been documented as far back as 1961 when Erving Goffman published *Asylums*, rigorous efforts to address internalized stigma are still in their infancy.

In many ways, the greatest and perhaps the most critical negative impact of stigma, for people with SMI in particular, has been the impact on the psychological concept of hope (Davidson, 2006). Having lost hope, a person has lost a sense of controlling his or her destiny. Without enabling a sense of hope for the possibility of change, for the possibility of something better, we greatly diminish a person's motivation to find any meaning or purpose in life. Consumers have documented numerous examples of mental-health services that demonstrate how the mental-health system perpetuates this state of hopelessness, due to stigmatization based on lack of understanding, experience, and knowledge about SMI. This undermining of hope for a positive future robs many of years of their lives.

Frequently when treatment does not appear to be yielding positive outcomes, clinicians blame the consumer. Linehan (1994) has argued that if the treatment is not working, it is the treatment at fault, not the person. This perspective can promote compassion and recognition that SMI is not a willful attempt to sabotage treatment interventions.

"Schemas" are semifixed and long-held beliefs that individuals often develop from childhood experiences, which drive how they organize data in their world and make decisions, and how they relate to one another. This concept of schemas may offer a way of looking at professional attitudes influenced by stigma, and an understanding of how providers maintain errant views.

SCHEMAS

A Manner of Understanding Professional Biases From the Cognitive Behavioral Theoreticians

Many initiatives have been geared toward helping people with mental illness find strategies to cope and even fully recover. The historian Gerald Grob (1994) has separated periods in the history of treatment for the mentally ill into four discrete eras. Each period represents a shift in the understanding of the cause of mental-health issues and a new direction for providing treatment.

The first of these periods he called the Asylum Period, which occurred from approximately the mid-1800s through the early 20th century. While members of society with mental illness and without economic privilege found themselves in asylums, others found themselves in "sanctuaries," removed from the stresses of everyday society. These patients received "moral treatment" offered in some of the state hospitals. The rationale was that disorders of the mind were a by-product of the chaos, greed, and sense of meaninglessness in society, and thus the cure was to remove the afflicted person from these social stressors. Providing a sanctuary promotes a peaceful environment designed around a routine of purposeful and structured activities, and healing occurs. In fact, this type of treatment did prove successful. The industrial revolution led to overcrowding in an overwhelmed system that provided custodial care at best, and at worst neglect and abuse.

The Mental Health Hygiene period began in the 1890s with the notion that cure of SMI could be an outcome of proper scientific approaches to treatment. The shift was to small hospitals that were associated with medical schools. The emphases were on early diagnosis and reenvisioning mental-health care as equivalent to medical care, and thus moving into the mainstream. However, this model also met its demise with a loss of funding and an increase in demand for services, which overwhelmed the system.

The shift in the mid-20th century to Community Mental Health Care grew out of a few important developments. First was the discovery in the 1950s of psychotropic medications that could be combined with other medications, resulting in a calming affect that made community reintegration a real possibility. In addition, societal awareness of the conditions in mental hospitals put pressure on government officials to take action. President Kennedy, with a personal interest in human beings with mental disabilities of varying kinds, both emotional and intellectual, was persuaded to sign into legislation the Mental Health Centers Act of 1963 (Community Mental Health Centers Construction Act, public law 88-164) (Clark, 1993). Deinstitutionalization was the outcome of this bill, but the results were not as anticipated. Moneys earmarked for community treatment centers that were unaccustomed to meeting the needs of this challenging population were used to provide treatment to higher-functioning clients, and mass numbers of people discharged from the psychiatric institutions became homeless and in danger.

The Community Support period began around 1975 and continues today. This period represents a shift in the understanding of causes of mental illness, and recognition of the importance of addressing the stigma of SMI. One shift was the emergence of the recovery movement, wherein consumers began disseminating anecdotal data about recovery from SMI. The understanding of what causes SMI shifted from faulty parenting to a neuroscientific perspective. The development of new technology that allowed for neuro-imaging of the brain greatly supported this shift. The shift from bad parents to neuroscience promoted two ideas: that recovery is possible, and that the biggest challenges to societal reintegration for people with SMI were attributable to social stigma, not the illness itself. Social stigma was used to block appropriate housing for people with SMI (ex. group homes, scattered site homes) from receiving permits in safe neighborhoods, as well as funding that could help to integrate people with SMI into the competitive workforce. Social stigma interacts with personal stigmas imposed by professionals, and stigmas internalized by those with SMI.

Studying cognitive behavioral theory requires that a thought, feeling, or behavior that seems intractable or impermeable to change be questioned as to what mechanisms are perpetuating the problem. Similar to the difficulty many people experience when attempting to break a habit or develop a new behavior, professionals and lay people who determine the care that will be provided to people with serious mental illness may be vulnerable to acting on schemas that might be outside of their completely conscious control.

The intractability of stigmatized thinking may be a by-product of the cognitive behavioral concept called "schema." Schemas are a fact of development; human beings develop schemas throughout life in order to help them to make sense of the world around them (Azar et al., 1995). Schemas emerge as children collect a repertoire of life experiences, and familial as well as social relationships and interactions can impact them. They are also developed as we observe images of popular culture including television, movies, books, games, and all sorts of social media. Schemas respond to social norms, cultural beliefs, and experiences from infancy to the present, with families, schools, community centers, religious affiliations, and more. Further, human beings develop role schemas (Azar et al., 1995), which allow them to conceive of expectations or definitions for mental fitness, competence, and essentially mental health. The experiences that enable people to develop these schemas also determine their understanding of how human beings should act when confronted with various social relationships. This can elicit preconceived ideas of how consumers should act in the presence of a mental-health professional. This has crucial implications for professional decision-making. There is an inherent power differential between a provider and a consumer. Providers can determine what services and opportunities are available to a consumer. Thus, providers have an ethical responsibility to make decisions not driven by stigma and bias.

Schemas are not necessarily a negative construct. Like any personal characteristic, schemas can be rigid or flexible, closed or permeable to new data. They can encompass a negative assessment or evaluation, or a positive one. Professionals making decisions guided by fixed and negative schemas have the capacity to detract from client self-determination in a powerful and negative way. For example, how a provider writes a biopsychosocial report for an application for independent housing can be the deciding factor as to whether or not a consumer obtains the housing he or she desires. Like unchecked biases, unchecked schemas can result in professionals taking full responsibility for the life situations of their charges. Every professional possesses his or her own set of schemas, and thus can positively or negatively affect the basic right to self-determination of consumers of mental-health services. Schemas can determine the roles and expectations that practitioners hold for their charges.

Azar et al. (1995) have used the concept of schemas to offer a compelling way of examining bias in child-welfare decisions about termination of parental rights. Likewise, this chapter uses the concept of schemas as a manner of examining bias in decision-making on the part of professionals in the field of mental health. One way of examining schema is to look at expectations of people within role relationships. Often without realizing it, we have predetermined expectations of how individuals should behave in their role as consumers, toward others in the role of practitioners. One dyadic role that might be somewhat commonplace is that of the compliant client. What is a compliant client, and what happens when that role is not satisfied?

The Compliant Client

Although most professionals today would probably agree that the hallmark of a successful treatment is not fostering compliance and dependence, but rather fostering critical thinking, self-advocacy, problem solving, and a wide repertoire of safe coping mechanisms, adherence to this philosophy can be complicated in practice. Reasons for this conundrum may be the history of mental-health professions, and the context of the world in which people today practice.

From an historical perspective on the field of mental health, direct-service providers have struggled to enjoy respect as both professionals and scientists when their area of specialization is studies of the mind and behavior. Although psychiatrists were devalued by other medical doctors, many social workers made the choice to associate with both the medical and the psychiatric professions in an effort to enhance their professional status. This social work profession carries a past haunted by functioning as "friendly visitors" who, while largely pure of heart, practiced by imparting knowledge about what was moral, as keepers of the social order. Therefore, it is not surprising that when the profession arrives at the 1980s, working from a position of more or less "equal" status with patients could be perceived as a threat to the psychiatrist's or social worker's public image of professional and scientist.

In addition, there is no denying that society has become increasingly litigious and blaming. There are very real professional consequences at risk when promoting consumers' right to self-determination and the kind of risk-taking that promotes growth and learning that other citizens can take for granted. Should a consumer voice a desire for independent housing, and a professional assist in exploring wants and desires before making a global assessment of the consumer's overall functioning; and should that housing situation result in a loss of the apartment, and emotional stress and suffering, who would be held accountable? On the other hand, what percentage of the population without a diagnosis of SMI learns in the absence of experience? Is there really another way to learn the skills of living independently?

These tensions trouble a field that values strengths-based and client-centered approaches to treatment, and that honors the right to self-determination for all people and aim to empower all charges.

The Mentally Deranged

Another expectation of the role imposed on persons diagnosed with SMI is that they are a threat and dangerous to society. Until quite recently, film and television stories of individuals with mental illness have consistently portrayed people with mental illness as regressed, dangerous, and irrational. When struggling, stressed, and symptomatic, lack of a clear sense of reality can be a symptom of many with these afflictions, which can be frightening to observe. On the other hand, frightened people are not sufficient to support an assessment of dangerousness. In fact, studies support the idea that the vast majority of people with SMI are at much greater risk of victimization than of ever committing a violent crime.

When a news story begins with a report of a terrifying, distressing, and unconscionable mass shooting, immediately followed by reporting that indicates belief that SMI was a factor, it creates a specific social response. That the gunman unsuccessfully sought treatment twice in the week before the incident due to a shortage of staff would create a different story and result in a different public sentiment. It would be a story less about the danger of the SMI, but rather about the need to provide adequate supports to all citizens to enable them to participate in the world safely and successfully. A story beginning with: "The shooter had never been known by the mental-health system . . . " would communicate a different message. If there were a weekly segment on every news broadcast that showcased the contributions of a different people living in the world with SMI, fully contributing and functioning as valuable members of society, again we would have a different story.

Diagnosis, Stigma and Schema

Diagnosis is a wonderful tool for identifying a set of symptoms that respond well to certain interventions, and for securing funding to help consumers obtain the supports required for growth and development. Diagnoses simply allow consumers access to various programs. Other than these uses, it is always a potentially dangerous practice to put a label on a human that can have far-reaching consequences with respect to how they view themselves, how they are seen by society, and even how the community of helping professionals sees them. Diagnoses result in expectations that can be a detriment to growth and change.

Cognitive behavioral theorists are interested not only in the schemas that drive our actions, but also in the conditions that maintain and perpetuate these thoughts, feelings, and actions. In other words, it is not enough simply to strive to change a behavior; one must understand what maintains that behavior. When individuals look for confirmations of their expectations, they can very often find them. There is an abundance of societal expectations for how someone with SMI will behave in a given situation. Retroactively, people can often find ways to interpret what they see in a manner that supports their expectations. When looking through the lens of one's own schemas, we interpret multiple layers of a situation accordingly. Thus to be mental health professionals who promote recovery rather than stand in its way, the field will need to identify improved methods of helping professionals to better identify, understand, and resist acting on their existing schemas about people with SMI.

There are numerous schemas held by lay people, people with SMI, and professionals in the field of mental health, which are based on feelings rather than facts. These schemas have a tremendous impact on consumers' rights to self- determination, a life of dignity, and living in the least restrictive environment that allows for their care and safety and the safety of others. Identifying ways to ensure that professionals make decisions and recommendations they base on accurate information, and not long-held schemas, is a necessary priority in deconstructing stigma around mental illness.

SOLUTIONS AND RECOMMENDATIONS

Failing to address professional schemas is unethical, and it causes genuine harm in a number of ways. One issue is the notion of a self-fulfilling prophecy. Orbell

121

and Henderson (2016) discuss the findings of a study that suggest that we activate subliminally based on a schematic representation of illness. In other words, the messages that consumers receive might be automatically activating behaviors that we then document as symptoms.

Studies around the word also suggest that social expectations about SMI drive beliefs that this group needs or deserves fewer social comforts to survive. One study (Rayan & Obiadate, 2017) examined the impact of stigma and poverty on people with SMI in Arab countries, and found that they experienced significant differences in overall quality of life.

One consequence that receives considerable attention is the impact due to stigma on help-seeking behavior in people with SMI (Corrigan, Druss, & Perlick, 2014; Clement et al., 2015; and Natan, Drori, & Hochman, 2017). In examining how specifically professional stigma acts as a barrier to help-seeking behavior, Clement et al. (2015) identify fear of disclosure—i.e., of being revealed as a "mental patient"—as a strong factor that keeps people from seeking treatment. Corrigan et al. (2014) concur and note as a deterrent the lack of accurate information possessed by not only the consumer, but also families and communities.

A concerning finding is that consumers in a 2017 study identified power relations in mental-health care as a primary locus of stigmatized behaviors. Sercu & Bracke (2017) found that one in four experiences of stigma occur at mental-health facilities. Professionals communicate these attitudes to consumers when they infantilize consumers and take no interest in aspects of their humanity outside of the diagnosis. The presence of other power attributes such as class and social inequalities compound these effects. Another study found that poor quality of life for people with SMI in India was significantly greater due to poverty. People with SMI were unable to pay for treatment and received unreliable medications, particularly those that could reduce side effects of the primary medications. There was a lack of understanding about the potential long-term nature of the illness, and that made sustaining support and connections a challenge. There was also a lack of education, and therefore a lack of flexibility in methods of engagement when someone was actively delusional, or unwilling or unable to enter treatment options (Hailamariam, Fecadu, Prince, & Hanlon, 2017).

Disclosure of mental illness has been correlated with better outcomes for people in recovery who are reintegrating into society (Pahwah, Brekke, Rice, & Fulginiti, 2017). However, stigma from professionals and people in the society-at-large is a factor in dissuading people from disclosure. The issue here is that many of the professionals who should be providing community education and advocating against stigma are unaware of their own discomfort and tendency to stigmatize consumers. Other studies support this idea and state that the mistrust of mental-health professionals might not be unfounded (Zieger et al., 2017). Many studies are showing that there is little success in most of our initiatives to reduce stigma and its harmful effects (Clark et al., 2013).

Some studies demonstrate that anti stigma campaigns help. Musyimi, et al. (2017) reviewed a study that analyzed results of campaigns at numerous levels. The study looked at how anti stigma efforts affected the attitudes of children, social media, adults, social marketing, and community initiatives. Indications appeared that initial help-seeking among people with SMI increased, and stigma from friends, family, and even community members decreased. Unfortunately, there was no indication that stigma perceived by health professionals decreased, and it is unclear as to why that occurred. This may identify long-held schemas about mental health and mental illness. How do we work to change stigmatizing behaviors, bias, and schema that we are unaware we carry?

Unexpected Consequences

Interesting studies have found that negative cognitive self-schemas increase self-stigma (Shimotsu et al., 2014). Pedersen and Paves (2014) addressed a perplexing question: Since we know that perceived public stigma is a barrier to young adults seeking treatment, how does this relate to personal stigma? In other words, they wondered how people with SMI would view and treat others, and how would this compare with perceived public stigma? Interestingly, the majority of responders would not have thought less of someone who had SMI or sought help; yet they believed others would think less of them. Also perplexing is that for so many people around the world, having a quality life is less important than avoiding the pain of a stigmatizing label. Stigma diminishes self-esteem and robs people of opportunities (Corrigan, Druss & Perlick, 2014).

In the United States and Western European countries, Sontag & Sontag (1990) observes a relationship between campaigns to overcome illness and other psychosocial stressors. As we call for a war on poverty, on homelessness, on AIDS, we communicate that to have an illness or any psychosocial concern is weak, vulnerable, and unacceptable. We communicate this in such a manner that often the person is lost in the war against their illness.

What Is Important to Successful Treatment?

Engagement and ability to connect with a benevolent other is an important element in successful treatment. Beretta et al., 2005 suggest that the therapeutic alliance is associated with the patient's wish to be close, to perceive others as trustworthy and helpful. However, they found that people with low alliance, relates not to a wish to avoid, but to a patient's wish to be close impeded by perceptions of others' responses as negative, with diminished capacity for affiliation. This is further complicated by the reality that many professionals unwittingly communicate the same fears, low expectations, and stigmas to consumers as people in the general population.

For instance, another study found that while most medical doctors, primary-care nurses, psychiatrists, psychiatric nurses, and psychologists self-report respect for the dignity of their patients, follow-up exploration of a vignette reveals that most would not want to hire or be neighbors or friends of people with SMI (Smith, Mittal, Chekuri, Han, & Sullivan, 2017). Likewise, in Sweden a study explored whether professionals would hire, date, or let a person with SMI take care of young people. Responses were quite negative. Like public perceptions of SMI, professionals on some level fear that people with SMI are dangerous, unpredictable, and difficult in relationships. This stigmatizing view does not seem to change in spite of global efforts to challenge stigma (Hansson, Jormfeldt, Svedberg, & Swensson, 2011).

Schemas drive decision-making. If reading an article exposing facts could change practitioner behavior, this would be a simple solution and likely would have been accomplished long ago, eliminating decisions based on negative schemas. Mechanisms that retrigger long-held beliefs make challenging schemas difficult. A practitioner may be privy to reliable, trustworthy data indicating that the majority of people with SMI are not a danger to other people. Nonetheless, this may not be enough to change the deeply wired mindset that drives how the practitioner makes decisions related to his or her work with consumers.

In order to address unconscious schemas that may drive treatment decisions, new and innovative training to identify negative schemas must be sought. Finding ways not only to identify schemas held by mental-health professionals, but also to examine the myths upon which they are built, where they originated, and how they are perpetuated, and to challenge them in a safe environment in which the professionals can do this personal work, will be a challenge. Research utilizing structured conversations to assist mental-health professionals in examining the schemas they may have about individuals with SMI may be a place to begin. Small-group dialogue that surfaces schemas in a safe environment can help identify those that are negative and biased, and find adequate ways of challenging those beliefs in a rigorous, yet safe manner as a means of practitioner training.

What Reduces Stigma and Professional Stigma?

O'Reilly, Bell, and Chen (2012) suggest that fostering empathy is a major factor in decreasing stigma. Others have recommended a need to recognize the culture within which one hopes to campaign against the stigma of SMI (Pawluk & Zolezzi, 2017). For instance, in Qatar, health professionals shared that they supported efforts to decrease stigma but thought efforts should target school-age children to provide education about SMI and appropriate pathways to treatment. Others concur, stating that mental-health literacy may be more effective than challenging stigma once it is entrenched (Greenwood et al., 2016). In another study, strategies such as role-play were not found to be as effective as direct contact with a person with SMI, and indirect contact (e.g., through film). Even educational emails showed short-term positive impact on decreasing stigma (Stubbs, 2014).

There are four accepted paths to changing perceptions. First, people learn from training (Bedregal, O'Connell, & Davidson, 2006). Numerous studies have found that specifically training on the Recovery Perspective and its operational model, Psychiatric Rehabilitation, opens professionals to growth and learning. Second, people learn from meeting and having meaningful connections with real human beings who have SMI (Eack & Newhill, 2008). The implication of this path to change is that as trainings are re-envisioned to improve professionals' ability to monitor their own schemas, it is logical that consumer participation in structured discussions be included. Third, people learn from self-reflection and genuine openness to challenging their own misperceptions (Kadushin & Harkness, 2014). Fourth, people learn from open dialogue (Brown & Isaacs, 2005). A tenet of group therapy is trusting that a group of people can come together to support one another. People can come together for the purpose of solving social problems, particularly when all acknowledge that they do not have the single answer that needs to be imposed on others. When people can demonstrate a willingness to share and contemplate their own thoughts and ideas and those of others, a willingness to work towards learning, growth and consensus building, there is hope for finding ways to end stigma. People come together willing to ask deeper questions and trust that together they may be able to identify innovative and positive solutions to stigma within the field of mental health, even those notions of stigma held by professionals.

CONCLUSION

When reviewing moments and shifts in the history of treatment of people with SMI, one can come away with a sense that people who cared about and empathized with the plight of people with mental illness often initiated efforts to heal, which ultimately went awry. One can look at the role of stigma—in particular stigma emanating from mental-health professionals—and see harmful interventions that required Herculean efforts to eradicate. Cognitive behavioral theory, when a thought, feeling, or behavior is recurrent or difficult to change, may aid in attending to the schemas that drive that behavior, and provide a place to begin. Thoughts, feelings, behaviors, and attitudes can be difficult to change because environmental factors retrigger them. This chapter argues for understanding the concept of schemas and considering training alternatives to help mitigate the harm resulting from stigma on the part of mental-health professionals.

Social workers provide the majority of services to adults with SMI (Kirk, 2005). The Social Work Code of Ethics posits ideas about service provision that are very much in sync with the Recovery Perspective. Therefore, it is curious that this would not be a smooth, timely, and easy transition. Yet there have been barriers to professionals embracing this client-centered perspective.

Recovery-oriented care represents a paradigm shift that not only has implications for clients but also involves a rather formidable shift in the role of the professional and how services are provided. In the litigious and blame-oriented environment that surrounds current practice, social workers who may wish to fully embrace a Recovery Perspective would have considerable concerns. This perspective supports people with SMI taking risks—the same risks that people who are not diagnosed with SMI are able to take for granted. This perspective honors a consumer's expressed desire for an independent apartment, and seeks it without a global assessment of functioning. While this does not mean abdicating responsibility for assessing consumer safety and problem solving around potential skills deficits that can be addressed, its premise is that in the absence of data suggesting the person is not competent, we can assume the ability to budget and/or learn from mistakes, as a person without a diagnosis would. To work from an assumption that people with SMI can learn these lessons, in the same way as their non-SMI counterparts can, is a shift that can be threatening to a professional who may be held accountable by families and/or systems when a worthwhile risk does not work out.

Another challenge is failure to accurately understand definitions of the Recovery Perspective and the Medical Perspective. Some professionals see the Recovery Perspective as an anti-medication movement. While many consumers and professionals do question whether medication is overprescribed, this is not a Recovery Perspective agenda. Similarly, some believe a Medical Perspective is solely about medication. This again is inaccurate, as evidenced by a longstanding and ongoing history of Medical Perspective practitioners diligently working to identify new and progressive methods of helping consumers, which go far beyond medication.

One key difference between the two models can be articulated in terms of the shifting role of the professional. Recovery-oriented professionals see their role more as a coach or guide on the journey of recovery, while the medical model assumes more of an expert stance. Another key difference is the very definition of what it means to recover. In practice, however, this is not always the case. Greater attention to the role of schema in professional decision-making is one recommendation.

REFERENCES

Anthony, W. (2000). A recovery-oriented service system: Setting some system level standards. *Psychiatric Rehabilitation Journal, 24*(2), 159–169. doi:10.1037/h0095104

Azar, S., Benjet, C., Fuhrmann, G., & Cavallero, L. (1995). Child maltreatment and termination of parental rights: Can behavioral research help Solomon? *Behavior Therapy, 26*(4), 599–623. doi:10.1016/S0005-7894(05)80035-8

Bedregal, L., O'Connell, M., & Davidson, L. (2006). The Recovery Knowledge Inventory: Assessment of mental health staff knowledge and attitudes about recovery. *Psychiatric Rehabilitation Journal, 30*(2), 96–103. doi:10.2975/30.2006.96.103 PMID:17076052

Beretta, V., Roten, Y., Stigler, M., Drapeau, M., Fischer, M., & Despland, J. N. (2005). The influence of patients' personal schemas on early alliance building. *Swiss Journal of Psychology, 64*(1), 13–20. doi:10.1024/1421-0185.64.1.13

Brown, J., & Isaacs, D. (2005). *The World Café: Shaping the World Through Conversations that Matter*. Berret-Kohler Publishers Inc.

Calabrese, J., & Corrigan, P. (2005). Beyond dementia praecox: Findings from long-term follow-up studies of schizophrenia. In R. Ralph & P. Corrigan (Eds.), *Recovery in Mental Illness: Broadening Our Understanding of Wellness* (pp. 60–72). Washington, DC: American Psychological Association. doi:10.1037/10848-003

Clark, C. S. (1993). Mental illness. *CQ Researcher, 3,* 673-696. Retrieved April 11, 2009 from http://library.cqpress.com/cqresearcher/cqresrre1993080600

Clark, W., Welch, S., Berry, S., Collentine, A., Collins, R., Lebron, D., & Shearer, A. (2013). Reducing stigma: Self-stigma. California's historic effort to reduce the stigma of mental illness: The Mental Health Services Act. *American Journal of Public Health, 103*(5), 786–794. doi:10.2105/AJPH.2013.301225

Clement, S., Schauman, O., Graham, T., Maggioni, F., Evans-Lacko, S., Bezborodovs, N., ... Thornicroft, G. (2015). What is the impact of mental health related stigma on help-seeking? A systematic review of quantitative and qualitative studies. *Psychological Medicine, 45*(1), 11–27. doi:10.1017/S0033291714000129 PMID:24569086

Corrigan, P., Druss, B., & Perlick, D. (2014). The impact of mental illness stigma on seeking and participating in mental health care. *Psychological Science in the Public Interest, 15*(2), 37–70. doi:10.1177/1529100614531398 PMID:26171956

Davidson, L. (2006). Recovery guides: An emerging model of community-based care for adults with psychiatric disabilities. In A. Lightburn & P. Sessions (Eds.), *Handbook of community-based clinical practice* (pp. 476–502). Oxford, UK: Oxford University Press.

Deegan, P. (1988). Recovery: The lived experience of rehabilitation. *Psychosocial Rehabilitation Journal, 11*(4), 11–19. doi:10.1037/h0099565

Deegan, P. (1996). Recovery as a journey of the heart. *Psychiatric Rehabilitation Journal, 19*(3), 91–98. doi:10.1037/h0101301

Eack, S. M., & Newhill, C. E. (2008). What influences social workers' attitudes toward working with severe mental illness? *The Journal of Contemporary Social Services, 89*(3), 419–428. PMID:24353397

Ellis, A. (1994). *Reason and emotion in psychotherapy. Revised and updated.* Secaucus, NJ: Carol Publishing Group.

Freud, S. (1911). The case of Schreber, papers on technique, and other works. In *The standard edition of the complete psychological works of Sigmund Freud* (Vol. 12). London, UK: The Hogarth Press and the Institute of Psychoanalysis.

Fuller Torrey, W. (2006). *Surviving schizophrenia: A manual for families, patients and providers.* New York, NY: Harper Collins.

Goffman, E. (1961). *Asylums: Essays on the social situation of mental patient and other inmates.* New York, NY: Anchor Books.

Greenwood, K., Carroll, C., Crowter, L., Jamieson, K., Ferraresi, L., Jones, A. M., & Brown, R. (2016). Early intervention for stigma towards mental illness? Promoting positive attitudes towards severe mental illness in primary school children. *Journal of Public Mental Health, 15*(4), 188–199. doi:10.1108/JPMH-02-2016-0008

Grob, G. (1994). *The mad among us: A history of the care of America's mentally ill.* New York, NY: The Free Press.

Hailamariam, M., Fecadu, A., Prince, M., & Hanlon, C. (2017). Engaging and staying engaged: A phenomenological study of barriers to equitable access to mental health care for people with severe mental disorders in a rural African setting. *International Journal for Equity in Health, 16*(1), 156. doi:10.118612939-017-0657-0 PMID:28851421

Haller, B. (2010). *Representing disability in an ableist world.* Louisville, KY: The Advocado Press.

Hansson, L., Jormfeldt, H., Svedberg, P., & Swensson, B. (2011). Mental health professionals' attitudes towards people with mental illness: Do they differ from attitudes held by people with mental illness? *International Journal of Social Psychology, 59*(1), 48–54. doi:10.1177/0020764011423176 PMID:21954319

Harding, C. M., Brooks, G., Ashikaga, T., Stauss, J., & Breier, A. (1987). The Vermont longitudinal study of persons with severe mental illness. *The American Journal of Psychiatry, 144*(6), 718–735. doi:10.1176/ajp.144.6.718 PMID:3591991

Kadushin, A., & Harkness, D. (2014). *Supervision in social work.* New York, NY: Columbia University Press. doi:10.7312/kadu15176

Kirk, S. (2005). *Mental disorders in the social environment.* New York, NY: Columbia University Press.

Leiberman, R., & Kopelowicz, A. (2002). Recovery from schizophrenia: A challenge for the 21ˢᵗ century. *International Review of Psychiatry (Abingdon, England), 14*(4), 245–255. doi:10.1080/0954026021000016897

Linehan, M. (1994). *Cognitive behavioral treatment of borderline personality disorder.* New York, NY: Guilford Press.

Mead, S., & Copeland, M. (2000). What recovery means to us: Consumer's perspectives. *Community Mental Health Journal, 36*(3), 315–328. doi:10.1023/A:1001917516869 PMID:10933247

Natan, M., Drori, T., & Hochman, O. (2017). The impact of mental health reform on mental illness stigmas in Israel. *Archives of Psychiatric Nursing, 31*(6), 610–613. doi:10.1016/j.apnu.2017.09.001 PMID:29179829

National Association of Social Workers. (n.d.). *Code of Ethics.* Retrieved from http://www.naswdc.org/pubs/code/code.asp

Noordsy, D., Torrey, W., Mueser, K., Mead, S., O'Keefe, C., & Fox, L. (2002). Recovery from severe mental illness: An intrapersonal and functional outcome definition. *International Review of Psychiatry (Abingdon, England), 14*(4), 318–326. doi:10.1080/0954026021000016969

O'Reilly, C., Bell, J. S., & Chen, T. (2012). Mental health consumers and caregivers as instructors for health professional students: A qualitative study. *Social Psychiatry and Psychiatric Epidemiology*, *47*(4), 607–613. doi:10.100700127-011-0364-x PMID:21384120

Orbell, S., & Henderson, C. J. (2016). Automatic effects of illness schema activation on behavioral manifestations of illness. *Health Psychology*, *35*(10), 1144–1153. doi:10.1037/hea0000375 PMID:27253428

Pahwah, R., Brekke, J., Rice, E., & Fulginiti, J. (2017). Mental illness disclosure decision making. *The American Journal of Orthopsychiatry*, *87*(5), 575–584. doi:10.1037/ort0000250 PMID:28394157

Pawluk, S., & Zolezzi, M. (2017). Health care professionals perspectives on a mental health educational campaign for the public. *Health Education Journal*, *76*(4), 479–491. doi:10.1177/0017896917696121

Pedersen, E., & Paves, A. (2014). Comparing perceived public stigma and personal stigma of mental health treatment seeking in a young adult sample. *Psychiatry Research*, *219*(1), 143–150. doi:10.1016/j.psychres.2014.05.017 PMID:24889842

Rayan, A., & Obiadate, K. (2017). The correlates of quality of life among Jordanian patients with schizophrenia. *Journal of the American Psychiatric Nurses Association*, *23*(6), 404–413. doi:10.1177/1078390317710498 PMID:28569084

Sercu, C., & Bracke, P. (2017). Stigma, social structure and the biomedical framework: Exploring the stigma experiences of in-patient service users in two different psychiatric hospitals. *Qualitative Health Research*, *27*(8), 1249–1261. doi:10.1177/1049732316648112 PMID:27251609

Shimotsu, S., Horikawa, N., Emora, R., Ishikawa, S. I., Nagao, A., Hiejima, S., & Hosomi, J. (2014). Effectiveness of Cognitive Behavioral Therapy in reducing self-stigma in Japanese Psychiatric Patients. *Asian Journal of Psychiatry*, *10*, 39–44. doi:10.1016/j.ajp.2014.02.006 PMID:25042950

Smith, J., Mittal, D., Chekuri, L., Han, X., & Sullivan, G. (2017). A comparison of provider attitudes towards SMI across different health care disciplines. *Stigma and Health*, *4*(2), 327–337. doi:10.1037ah0000064

Sontag, S. (1989). *AIDS and its metaphors*. New York, NY: Picadur.

Stubbs, A. (2014). Reducing mental illness stigma in health care students and professionals: A review of the literature. *Australasian Psychiatry*, *22*(6), 579–584. doi:10.1177/1039856214556324 PMID:25371444

Sullivan, H. S. (1962). *Schizophrenia as a human process*. New York, NY: WW Norton.

Sundstrom, E. (2004). The Clogs. *Schizophrenia Bulletin*, *30*(1), 191–192. doi:10.1093/oxfordjournals.schbul.a007063 PMID:15176773

Warner, R. (2004). *Recovery from schizophrenia: Psychiatry and political economy*. New York, NY: Brunner-Routledge.

Zieger, A., Mungee, A., Schomerus, G., Ta, T. M. T., Weyers, A., Boge, K., ... Hahn, E. (2017). Attitude towards psychiatrists and psychiatric medication: A survey from five metropolitan cities in India. *Indian Journal of Psychiatry*, *59*(3), 341. doi:10.4103/psychiatry.IndianJPsychiatry_190_17 PMID:29085094

KEY TERMS AND DEFINITIONS

Cognitive Behavioral Theory: A theory of cause of emotional or behavioral issues based on the once revelatory idea that rather than being driven by unconscious factors, we behave as we do due to how we interpret stimuli around us.

Cognitive Distortions: Types of distortions that most people have experienced at one time or another, which can be challenged and reframed. For instance, a person states, "I am going to fail this exam." When this thought, which often leads to anxiety, is based on data to the contrary, it can be challenged by identifying the type of distortion—in this case, "predicting the future"—and then challenged with a more realistic statement/thought.

Consumer: Terms such as patient, client, consumer, and survivor have all been used to describe the role of the person receiving mental-health services. "Consumer" is the term associated with the recovery perspective.

Hope: A reason to continue to try to find purpose and meaning in life.

Internalized Stigma: Feelings of unworthiness and self-directed rage internalized from societal assumptions; essentially seeing oneself in the role of "an illness" as learned from experiences in society.

Medical Perspective: A traditional medical perspective in the field of mental health looks at decrease in symptoms, decrease in hospitalizations, and increase in functional behaviors as end points in achieving mental health. From this perspective the role of the professional is elevated and hierarchical in relation to the consumer.

Recovery Perspective: A recovery perspective in mental health understands a definition of recovery to encompass a reawakening of a sense of hope, meaning, and life purpose. It suggests a more equal or level playing field in the relationship between a mental health provider and a consumer of mental health services.

Schema: Strongly and long-held beliefs based on early experiences that are often experienced as facts, and consistently influence our behaviors. For example, "I must adhere to directives of people in authority."

Chapter 6
Fighting Stigma in the Community:
Bridging Ties Through Social Innovation Interventions

Nicolina Bosco
University of Florence, Italy

Fausto Petrini
University of Florence, Italy

Susanna Giaccherini
Public Mental Health Service of Tuscany, Italy

Stefano Castagnoli
Public Mental Health Service of Tuscany, Italy

Patrizia Meringolo
University of Florence, Italy

ABSTRACT

This chapter will discuss action research conducted in Tuscany to fight stigma surrounding mental illness. Public mental health services (PMHS) in Italy are perceived as ascribing a mentally ill label to individuals who utilize these programs. Local associations, especially sports associations, can be used to fight this stigma. This chapter will present key aspects and results of a community social innovation intervention jointly performed by a PMHS and the University of Florence. The research will explore perceptions surrounding the role and value of the community sports association, participants' perceived improvements, effects of sports participation, and the role of the sports association as an instrument to promote mental health. Results will show that the sports association is perceived as an agent of social capital to reduce social barriers emerging from mental illness. In addition, stigma is deconstructed through improvements to individual and social wellbeing.

DOI: 10.4018/978-1-5225-3808-0.ch006

INTRODUCTION

This chapter will describe the role of the *La Rugiada* sports association as a powerful instrument to deconstruct stigma in mental health. First, the chapter will summarize the theoretical background. Next, the context of the intervention and its main features will be presented. The chapter will share study results related to a local community's strategies to prevent stigma surrounding mental illness.

Stigma consists of a social dimension (or public stigma) and an individual dimension (or self-stigma). Both dimensions are capable of affecting an individual's recovery from mental illness and isolation (Andrews, Issakidis, & Carter, 2001). Through individual participation, sports and teams can create a sense of community (Soundy et al., 2015).

By exploring a sports association's role in well-being, services can be identified to fight the effects of stigma and promote community mental health. This chapter will describe the role of *La Rugiada* in rural Tuscany, Italy. It will consider interventions realized through a sports association's role as a social innovation strategy.

THEORETICAL FRAMEWORK

Stigma: Threat to Others and to Self

Although it has been 50 years since Goffman's opera (1963), its contributions continue to be widely used (Bos, Pryor, Reeder, & Stutterheim, 2013). "Stigma" identifies negative characteristics attributed to others. In addition, it devalues stigmatized people. The rise of social problems causes limited citizenship and social segregation, including disqualification from daily community life (Montero, 2010). Participation in community life increases emotional connections in the community. However, a lack of participation, which is associated with disadvantaged social groups, can cause disempowerment (Christens, Speer, & Peterson, 2011; Gaebel et al., 2014; Bosco et al., 2016).

Stigma is a relational process because it is realized in social groups (Hebl, Tickle, & Heatherton, 2000). Through an individual's aversions and discredit toward others, it induces dehumanization and depersonalization for the out-group member (Dovidio, Major, & Crocker, 2000; Tajfel, 1981).

Negative social stereotypes surrounding a social group can be associated with both positive and negative value responses, which can cause different responses of power. As reported by Link and Phelan (2001), the interconnectedness of stigma and power is due to stigma's allowance of the balance of a prevarication relationship. In a psychosocial perspective, stigma's prevarication function is recognized between people who are and who are not stigmatized (Phelan, Link, & Dovidio, 2008). This function favors an imbalance between the powerful and the powerless groups (Major & O'Brien, 2005; Lukes, 2005).

Negative impacts of stigma generate several consequences in people who are stigmatized, including social discrimination and a system of low expectations (Crandall & Eshleman, 2003; Kurzban & Leary, 2001). Moreover, membership in a low-status group can negatively affect the individual level because it can lead to the perception that one's social identity may be threatened (Steele & Aronson, 1995).

The social identity theory (SIT) recognizes cognitive, social, and emotional aspects related to a sense of belonging to a social group as identified by society (Tajfel, 1981). This process involves both individual and social levels (Anderson & Lowen, 2010; Walton & Cohen, 2003). Belonging to a social group establishes significant emotional bonds and impacts positive self-image (Haslam, Jetten, Postmes, & Haslam, 2009). On the contrary, belonging to a low-status group causes a negative self-categorization (Sellers & Shelton, 2003). According to Major and O'Brien (2005), when the social identity is stigmatized, people can perceived themselves as at major risk of discrimination.

Coping strategies are tools to handle stigma's effects. The first strategy focuses on the attribution of negative events to discriminatory behaviors in a social system. Using this strategy, individuals can defend their self-esteem and self-identity (Vogel, Heimerdinger-Edwards, Hammer, & Hubbard, 2011). The second strategy is strictly associated with social identity, in which being a part of a labeled group can lead to evaluate self-identity independent from the in-group or to defend the social group from the society. However, the sense of belonging to a social group, even if stigmatized, allows an individual to obtain social support. The last strategy is associated with social groups (Major & O'Brien, 2005). People suffering from mental illness cope with pathology and stigmatized status. As reported by Link, Mirotznik, and Cullen (1991) people may adopt three specific coping strategies to avoid social rejection:

- Maintaining secrecy about their unhealthy conditions
- Limiting social interaction to those who know their psychological problems
- Using *"preventing telling"* to obviate negative attitude from others

When people are stigmatized, they use both functional and dysfunctional strategies, which may affect the self-evaluation (Link et al., 1991).

PUBLIC STIGMA AND SELF-STIGMA: NEGATIVE IMPACTS ON MENTAL HEALTH

Stigma grows in individual, interpersonal, and societal levels. According to Corrigan and Matthews (2003), public stigma is defined in a social system and self-stigma is a redefinition of the self, based on negative characteristics recognized by society.

Public stigma is a loss of status that produces discriminatory behavior toward people with mental illness (Corrigan & Boyle, 2003). According to Parcesepe and Cabassa (2013), public stigma is based on beliefs and negative attitudes shared by the social system. It may generate fear and social exclusion toward people with mental illness.

Self-stigma is the harmful impact that results from internalizing prejudice leading to diminished self-esteem, lower self-efficacy, and a sense of 'why try' self-deprecation" (Corrigan et al., 2012, p. 65). Moreover, self-stigma can lead stigmatized people to be aware of their social devaluation because of their unhealthy condition (Bos et al., 2013).

Both public stigma and self-stigma have cognitive (stereotypes), emotional (prejudice), and behavioral (discrimination) components. In mental illness, cognitive components are associated with a lack of expertise attributed to others or to one's self (Brohan, Elgie, Sartorius, & Thornicroft, 2010). This is also the case for emotional reactions. For example, that statement that "all people with mental illness are violent" causes the reactive statement that "everybody scares me" (Link & Phelan, 2001). Finally, the discrimination component can be defined as a barrier in the achievement of personal goals (Pingani et al., 2012). This affects opportunities to benefit from life experiences and can lead to a negative redefinition of social status (Corrigan, Larson, & Rüsch, 2009). The interiorization of attributes affects psychological resources and leads to social isolation (Feldman & Crandall, 2007).

Corrigan and Watson (2002) defined "three As" of self-stigma: (1) agreement; (2) awareness; and (3) application. As reported by Watson, Corrigan, Larson and Sells (2007), group identification, awareness of negative stereotypes, agreement, and application to the self allows self-stigma to impact individual self-esteem and self-efficacy.

Self-stigma may generate an individual's powerless response (or "the why try effect") (Watson, Corrigan, Larson, & Sells 2007). Disempowered people may be affected by a lack of self-efficacy, express a negative personal evaluation, and use an internal locus of control in case of failure (Huang & Lin, 2015). Thus, self-stigma may reduce an individual's quality of life and coping strategies (Vogel, Wade, & Haake, 2006).

From a clinical perspective, self-stigma appears to be associated with a serious increase of positive and negative symptoms, depressive symptoms, and reduced social functioning in people with schizophrenia (Yanos, Roe, Markus, & Lysaker, 2008). Self-stigma causes negative feelings, particularly shame, and embarrassment for the unhealthy condition and the discredited attitude by the social system. Self-stigma leads to negative feelings about the self, which causes an individual to perceive themselves as inferior to other community members (Huang & Lin, 2015; Rickwood, Deane, Wilson, & Ciarrochi, 2005).

The deconstruction of stigma must consider individual and social dimensions (i.e., health professionals, formal and informal associations, users as citizens, and the community). In doing so, community-based interventions and resources will be identified to promote empowerment, improved mental health, and social change.

SOCIAL CAPITAL TO PROMOTE MENTAL HEALTH

Mental health recovery through social engagement increases social capital (Tew et al., 2012). Promotion of social capital may result in greater integration in society and more access to opportunities for people with mental illness (Zoppei et al., 2014).

Social capital is a complex and debated concept with multiple definitions (Morgan et al., 2007). Its core can be summarized with the idea that networks and social relationships are valuable community resources (Field, 2003). Social capital studies refer to various aspects of social life, including social networks, mutuality, and social participation (Zoppei et al., 2014). In a more theoretical definition, social capital was defined as an "investment in social relations with expected returns" (Lin, 1999, p. 30). More specifically, *A Dictionary of epidemiology* (Porta, 2014), identified the concept's twofold nature with characteristics linked to both individual and group dimensions. Social capital is also described as a resource available to members of social groups (e.g., trust, norms) and a resource embedded in an individuals' social networks (e.g., social support, social credentials; Forsman et al., 2013).

Therefore, social capital is conceptualized as both an individual and community attribute. There has been considerable interest as to whether social capital is a feature of individuals, groups, or both. However, the notion has been at the center of a significant academic and policy debate on how socioeconomic disadvantages impact mental health (Bertotti et al., 2013).

A definition of its dimensions is needed to better understand the practical implications of social capital. Studies have discussed several types of social capital, such as structural and cognitive social capital (McKenzie, Whitley, & Weich, 2002). According to Ehsan and De Silva (2015, p. 1021):

...structural (participatory) social capital refers to relationships, networks, membership, organisations, associations, and institutions that may link groups or individuals together. Cognitive (perceived) social capital refers to values, norms, attitudes, beliefs, civic responsibility, altruism, and reciprocity within a community.

In other words, the structural component could be considered the quantity of social capital. It examines the extent and intensity of links between individuals, their behaviour, and their participation in group activities (Bertotti et al., 2013). On the other hand, the cognitive component could be regarded as the quality of social capital as it focuses on the types of social interaction between individuals (Harpham, Grant, & Thomas, 2002).

The structural and cognitive components influence health in different ways. The cognitive component, including perceived social support, trust, and a sense of belonging, has been strongly associated with a range of mental health outcome measures across several countries at individual and ecological levels (Phongsavan et al., 2006; Tomita & Burns, 2013). The structural component, which derives from social contacts and social participation, appears to have a more complex relation with health.

Systematic reviews using cross-sectional or experimental data found that social capital may act as a protective factor in mental health problems (De Silva, McKenzie, Harpham, & Huttly, 2005). The most recent systematic review from Ehsan and De Silva (2015) confirmed that both individual and ecological cognitive social capital reduce risks of common mental disorders. This means that these forms of social capital protect against mental illness.

At the same time, weaker associations emerge surrounding the positive influence of structural social capital on mental health. According to studies, low-resource settings (and selectively in these conditions) can impact an individual's participation in civic activities. This can be associated with an unexpected increase to the risk of mental disorders (Forsman, Nordmyr, & Wahbeck, 2011). Similar results emerged from Bertotti et al. (2013). In this work, the effects of social networks and perception of neighbourhood quality, which are components of structural social capital, change the sense of the relations to mental health depending on the socioeconomic characteristics of the environment (ibidem). Clayton et al. (2013) found similar unexpected results in their longitudinal randomized controlled study focusing on citizenship to prevent mental illness and criminal justice involvement.

Evidence reported in this work highlights the importance of innovative interventions based on the ecological community approach, the use of creative instruments to improve social capital and prevent mental illness, and caring for relationships among patients and the community (Bosco, Petrini, Giaccherini, &

Meringolo, 2014). Social innovation interventions can be useful because they are based on solidarity and reciprocity among citizens and the social system.

SPORTS TO FIGHT STIGMA

An increasing amount of research shows that sports intervention improves physical health in people with severe mental illness (Firth et al., 2015; Rosenbaum et al., 2014). People with serious mental disorders experience a premature mortality, approximately 15 to 20 years earlier with respect to the general population. This differential mortality gap has grown in recent decades (Saha, Chant, & McGrat, 2007). Two-thirds of these deaths are due to physical health risk factors from limited access to medical care, poor diet, reduced levels of physical exercise, and medication-induced weight gain. This risk particularly affects people with mental illness due to greater amounts of sedentary behavior (Stubbs et al., 2016).

Many of the physical health issues, which are related to modifiable risk factors, can be attenuated through lifestyle changes, including exercise (Curtis et al., 2016; McNamee, Mead, MacGillivrey, & Lawrie, 2013). Physical exercise programs are valuable to people with serious mental illness. Recent meta-analysis of randomized controlled trials demonstrated that physical exercise has a moderate to large effect size for individuals with depression disorders as compared to control groups (Krogh, Nordentolf, Sterne, & Lawlor, 2011; Retrhost, Wipfli, & Landers, 2009).

Research in adults with schizophrenia shows that exercise interventions reduce negative symptoms and cognitive deficit (Firth et al., 2016; Kimby et al., 2015). This also includes secondary symptoms like depression, low self-esteem, and social withdrawal (Faulkner & Biddle, 1999).

In the treatment of mental disorders, exercise may complement other interventions. It can be used as a stress management strategy to prevent recurrences and improve functional recovery, lifestyle practices, and overall health (Morgan, Parker, Alvarez-Jimenez, & Jorm, 2013).

Firth et al. (2015) found that the most prominent exercise barriers for people with mental illness is the lack of support. This was reported by 50% of those analyzed in the systematic review.

Within physical activities, sports are considered a type of leisure time (Howley, 2001). Thus, sports participation can be viewed as a pleasant way for people with mental illness to achieve physical activity recommendations (Bulut, Eren, & Halac, 2013; Howley, 2001; Vancampfort et al., 2012). Based on literature, sports participation has psychological and social benefits. As reported by Langle, Siemssen, and Hornberger (2000), sports participation can have positive psychological effects on an individual's mental health, including self-esteem, body awareness, social interactions, and time management.

Regarding individuals with schizophrenia, a recent study by Soundy et al. (2014) identified broader, more direct psychosocial benefits of sports participation. They highlighted self-initiated positive changes in behavior, increased confidence, pride in other settings, and a sense of purpose, meaning, and achievement. A sense of belonging, cohesion, and support are identified by Soundy et al. (2014) as benefits of sports participation.

In a meta-synthesis review on qualitative data, Soundy et al. (2015) emphasized the following themes associated with sports participation for individuals with mental illness:

1. Social Meaning of Sports in the Lives of Patients
   a. Positive social experiences to look forward to and be a part of
   b. Feelings of community and positive identity
   c. Activities to promote autonomous behavior and social engagement
2. Direct Benefits of Sports
   a. Places to go and things to do
   b. Normalized activities and opportunities to be in a positive group
   c. Distractions from typical worries, anxieties, or symptoms of mental health
3. Organization, Process, and Challenges of Sports
   a. Progression of tasks' difficulties and use of supported competitions
   b. Importance of environment and use of sports to foster a sense of belonging, identity, and interaction
4. Functional Social Support
   a. Esteem support, encouragement, and positive feedback
   b. Emotional support from staff and peers

Thus, sports can offer positive opportunities for social engagement to people with mental disorders. Participation in sports-related activities is a social learning experience. It can be an opportunity to feel "normal" in front of others. Moreover, sports can provide access to new social levels, as well as create a distance from institutionalized settings and identities (Soundy et al., 2014).

Voluntary sports organizations represent the largest voluntary sector in the western countries. According to literature, volunteering and active participation in society are considered crucial elements to social capital (Baum & Ziersch, 2003; Hartmann; 2003). Sports and exercise interventions can be used by mental health services as instruments to fight stigma and social isolation. Moreover, sports and exercise interventions can promote social interaction and a sense of community and connectivity (Coaffee, 2008; Hartmann, 2003). Thus, social interventions based on sports activities can promote community mental health and social capital by engaging diverse audiences and providing avenues for social inclusion in communities (Sherry & O'May, 2013).

PMHS IN ITALY: INNOVATIVE INTERVENTIONS WITHIN THE COMMUNITY

Research reported in this work took place in Tuscany, Italy.

The Italian system of mental health is founded on the Law n.180, Basaglia Law, from the name of its promoter. Realized in 1978, this psychiatric reform signified the closing of all insane asylums within the national borders. It also introduced diagnosis and care psychiatric services into general hospitals.

Psychiatric reform generated an enormous cultural change for communities and people living with mental illness. Prior to the Basaglia Law, the psychiatric system was addressed to the custody and social control of the deviance. After its approval, people with mental illness received the civil right to be cured and cared for in their community.

In 1998, a new organization of PMHS was settled following the first national mental health project. In accordance with the project, small services were founded in local communities and territorial areas, aimed to care for people with mental illness. To meet this goal, they used therapeutic and rehabilitative interventions, promoted empowerment, and increased healthy communities by means of preventive strategies.

The connection between PMHS and communities allows for planned interventions to prevent the worsening of mental illness, establishes networks of people suffering with mental illness, and improves social capital. This process can be achieved by starting from resources in the territory, promoting empowered communities, and generating well-being and mental health. Civic participation and civic engagement are key features to this perspective (Arcidiacono, Gelli, & Putton, 1999; Ehsan & De Silva, 2015).

The Italian system of mental health is based on participation. Bridging health professionals, families, and patients of PMHS promotes a proactive attitude toward health (Bentall, 2003). On the other hand, it is possible to obtain positive effects on the quality of PMHS due to the added value derived from the participatory process (Crawford et al., 2002; Simpson & House, 2003). Social innovation interventions generated a new model of organizations based on collaborative relationship between social actors, including nonprofit organizations, users, and citizens.

It is important to recognize interventions based on ecological approaches in the current Italian debate on mental health community care (Agnetti, 2007; Bosco et al., 2014; Re, 2005). The realization of social innovation interventions is required to achieve this recognition.

As reported by Stiglitz (2009,) social innovation can be defined as new responses to social problems, and as an instrument to improve individual and social well-being.

More specifically, the Bureau of European Policy Advisers (BEPA, 2011) defined social innovations as new ideas able to meet social needs, create new social relationships, and enhance society's capacity to act.

Considering the ecological community approach, social innovations can be a powerful strategy to promote positive effects on societies at both macro- and micro-levels. This empowers people by engaging them through participation as a model of intervention.

The sports associations for social integration was founded within this process. The group brings together PMHS and third sector organizations with mental illness users, their families, and their communities. Using sports to build social integration, they involve citizens in the management of activities to promote community wellness. Their purpose, which is based on the principles of welfare community and welfare mix, is to redefine the reciprocal relationship between individuals and communities as they bridge ties within the social system.

LA RUGIADA SPORTS ASSOCIATION FOR SOCIAL INTEGRATION

La Rugiada, a sports association, was founded in 1996 in partnership with a PMHS of Florence. It is situated in a rural area of 110,000 habitants. *La Rugiada* has 120 members, including people with mental illness, PMHS professionals, and volunteers. Football, volleyball, hiking, canoeing, and sailing are the main activities. The association promotes social integration for people suffering with mental illness. It maintains links between PMHS and the community.

La Rugiada was officially recognized in 1998 as a sports association for social integration. It earned formal autonomy in the improvement of sports activities, social projects, and management processes. An important evolutionary step of *La Rugiada* was the foundation of its sailing club in 2008. This represented true innovation. Figure 1 illustrates the principal steps of *La Rugiada*.

The sailing activities are carried out in a small lake near the town. Community activities included families, children, youth, high schools, and citizens in the

Figure 1. Steps of La Rugiada's evolution

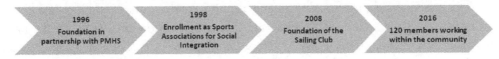

community and nearby territories. In 2016, 100 children participated in the summer activities. Three hundred young people were enrolled in sporting activities.

Members of the sailing club included individuals with mental illness, PMHS professionals, and volunteers who worked in the community. The principal innovative aspects were to:

1.   Create a sailing club in Tuscany's hilly landscape (far from the sea or basins) as an attractive community resource
2.   Establish recognize social roles for people with mental illness (e.g., patients are sailing activity instructors)
3.   Consider the sailing club as an instrument to fight stigma in mental illness, promote participation, and enrich community wellness

These new activities generated an important cultural change in the territory. Prior to the sailing club's foundation, activities promoted by PMHS and *La Rugiada* focused on people with mental illness and their social reintegration. After its foundation, as comanaged by users of PMHS, activities refocused on the community to address of social well-being. In this process, PMHS users became community resources.

The present work explores *La Rugiada*'s potential as an agent of social capital to fight stigma. It studies *La Rugiada* as an instrument to promote sports' impact on mental health in the community.

RESEARCH

The present contribution describes action research carried out by the University of Florence and a PMHS in Tuscany. The studies discussed planned effective community strategies to prevent mental illness considering the role of stigma.

The increased number of young patients led PMHS to identify new instruments and methods to care for young people with mental illness and meet their psychological needs. When faced with psychological problems or mental health episodes, young people may be reluctant to seek PMHS help due to stigma. This reluctance, which is associated with an increase of mental health problems, may generate negative consequences to future health. Moreover, it can cause drop outs, social isolation, and marginalization. This study reviews *La Rugiada*'s experience using sports participation in PMHS and the community.

The first and second studies used qualitative methods to explore sports association in the community and the effects of sport participation on people with mental illness. The third study was action research in local high schools. It investigated the role of the sports association as an instrument to prevent and promote mental health in the youth population.

The exploratory investigation used both qualitative and quantitative methods. Qualitative studies explored the perceived role of *La Rugiada* in the community. It considered the points of view of professionals and patients of PMHS. The quantitative study detected changes in the high school prior to and after the sports intervention.

Study 1: *La Rugiada* as a Change Agent in the Community

Aims

The exploratory qualitative research analyzed:

1. The perception of the role and value of the sports association in the community
2. Participants' perceived improvement from participation in the sports association

Methods

- **Participants:** Twenty-three members of *La Rugiada* (users and professionals)
- **Instruments:** Semi-structured interviews.

Qualitative content analysis was inspired by Grounded Theory approach (Glaser & Strauss, 1967) and was performed using the qualitative data analysis software Atlas.ti.

Findings

Qualitative analysis shows that user-members who participated in sports activities experienced personal change (see Figure 2).

Growth in personal and social knowledge by people with mental illness was perceived. In members' perceptions, sports participation by *La Rugiada* generated social responsibility, which positively impacted self-esteem:

Figure2. Perceived improvement

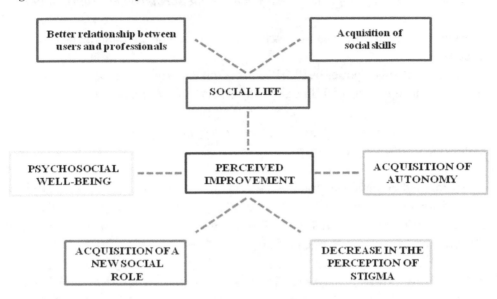

I am starting to be more independent. Now I am more confidence. (user, male)

An increase of social networking and support between members was reported, which generates "weak ties" (Granovetter, 1983) between them:

Now I have friends. Before I was alone! We can meet also outside La Rugiada. (user, male)

Before [La Rugiada] I was very shy [...] now I have another idea to stay with other people. (user, male)

Sports participation promoted by *La Rugiada* offers socialization opportunities to people with mental illness.

It brings new social opportunities like participating at national events or on summer holiday. (user, male)

According to participants, *La Rugiada* promoted specific changes in the "autonomy area of life" for people with mental illness. In particular, *La Rugiada* acquired daily organizational skills and self-care tools. Through sports participation, members could:

learn with others and apply the game's rules in the social context. (user, male)

Being a part of *La Rugiada* was perceived as a protective element in case of stressor events.

The main change reported by PMHS professionals was members' peer relationships, including those with mental illness. Being a part of *La Rugiada* meant:

they were a part of the same group ... members of the same association ... with the same rights. (professional, female)

Social and professional roles were reduced in this setting. Sports activities allowed for more spontaneous and close relationships between professionals and users. Experiencing *La Rugiada* as PMHS professionals and members reduced biases related to mental illness.

Before this experience, I used to categorize 'us' and 'them.' I used social barriers as a form of psychological defense in the professional setting. After this experience I understand that there are not differences between us. (professional, male)

Sports participation appears to reduce prejudice and barriers caused by illness. Participation also generates *"a sense of sharing and belonging":*

Through participation in sports activities, it is possible to share memories, emotions, time, and difficulties. (professional, female)

Moreover, in the participants' perception, *La Rugiada* played a valuable role in the community as a *"central instrument to promote community mental health."* As was reported by one research participant, *"it was possible to connect PMHS and the local community."*

Finally, *La Rugiada* was perceived as a powerful instrument within the social system for people with mental illness. This was due to *"the strength of the weakness ties."*

Through the participation, everyone connected with each other ... it generated the opportunity to interact with other social groups in the local community. (user, female)

La Rugiada is a possibility to interact with others in a context where the social barriers are reduced ... to create a new culture on mental health. (professional, female)

Study 2: Exploring Individual Perceptions on the Sailing Club as a Community Resource

The sailing club represents the most innovative activity promoted by *La Rugiada*. Members of the sailing club are people with mental illness, professionals of PMHS, and a great number of volunteers working together spreading their work into the community. The sports activities, sailing and canoeing, are addressed to all citizens (family, children, schools, et.)

While the first study focused on individual perceptions about the role and value of the *La Rugiada* sports association, a second study was carried out to investigate perceptions surrounding the sailing club and its peculiar function in bridging ties with the community.

- **Aims:** This study explored the effects of sports and association participation on individual well-being, as well as the value of the sailing club as a community resource.

Methods

- **Participants:** Seventeen stakeholders (directly and indirectly involved in sailing club activities)
- **Instruments:** Semi-structured interviews were analyzed using the Grounded Theory approach (Glaser & Strauss, 1967). Qualitative content analysis was performed using Atlas.ti.
- **Findings:** Data analysis showed a shared and coherent perception among stakeholders about objectives, health benefits, and community interests promoted by participation in the sailing club activities (see Figure 3).

Reduced social isolation and improved social networks appear to be an expected outcome for all stakeholders.

Before this experience, I was in a [therapeutic] community. I was just released and I did not know even where to go. My parents suggested the sailing club. (user, male)

Relationships require time. Here [in the sailing club], sports, dinners, and holidays are realized with others ... they are elements that can help to maintain contacts. People can discover positive aspects to stay with others. It is important to be part of a group. Here, I meet new people and I can spend time with people that I already know. (user, male)

Figure 3. Main effects of participation in the sailing club

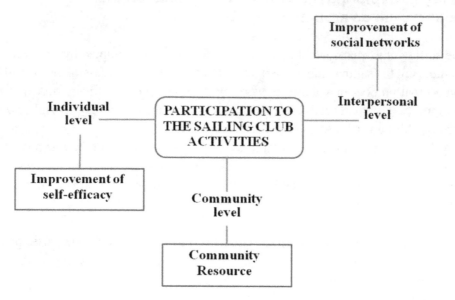

According to professionals, sports participation fosters patient autonomy, improves self-efficacy, and assists in time management.

What I see is that they [user-members] are more responsible because the club also gives them responsibilities [...] there are timetables and they learn to manage the time themselves ... they learn to do things they had never done. (professional, male)

The mutual help is a crucial dimension of the sailing club. This is recognized by all participants; they feel it reduces stigma surrounding mental illness:

When you join the club, there are no social differences. We are all equal; we are the same as a person! So, you cannot tell another 'you're problematic' or 'I have problems' and 'stay away.' On the contrary, 'I stay closer to you.' (volunteer, female)

Data suggests that the lack of competitiveness in this kind of sport could represent an added value for the recovery of people with mental illness:

This reality is special: it is not a football team or a volleyball team in which you are always with the sport team ... where you train every week, do the weekly match, and you are sharing the aim of winning more than staying together [...]. Sailing is an activity that you can do by yourself. (user, male)

The sailing club is perceived as an innovative community resource as underlined by all participants:

Sailing is an innovative activity in the community. La Rugiada promotes different sports activities, such as football and volleyball. But if you want to do sailing, you'll need to travel 90-100 km from the community. Thus, sailing is able to meet and respond to the needs of the territory. (volunteer, female)

Sailing generated a great curiosity between citizens. It generated the desire to perform sailing. There is a great interest about sailing in the community. (user, male)

The sailing activity is a very attractive sport activity, and it is perceived by participants as a *"shared dynamic movement between citizens."*

The sailing club is a place for everyone! We tried to create a place within the community. It is a sports association realized with people. So, the sailing club is an instrument and a resource for the community. (professional, female)

According to participants, another added value of the sailing club is its ability to generate relationships between members and citizens who are not involved in *La Rugiada* sports.

The sailing activity is performed by all the citizens - not only by members. This is an extraordinary wealth. (volunteer, male)

The sailing club is the spearhead of La Rugiada. It connects the community and PMHS. (professional, male)

Other institutions also perceive the sailing club as *"a resource for the community."* The social inclusion process for people with mental illness involves the community as a resource. Through interventions promoted by the sailing club, patients become resources for the territory. As reported by participants, *"this reverse of position has a strong value for the community."*

The sailing club is also perceived as a place to meet young people and an instrument to prevent mental disease:

the leisure time is important for young people. We have to take into account their needs considering that they use their extracurricular time at home or using the Internet. (user, male)

We have to include young people in the sailing club in order to realize activities able to reach their psychological needs. (professional, male)

Another important finding is the interest to spread knowledge about the sailing club. This enhances the social and solidarity dimensions, as well as characterizes the setting:

We have to stay in the community! We also have to organize meetings in the local schools. Then, students will talk with their parents, and so on. When people meet us [the sailing club], they discover a safe environment where people get involved thanks to their altruism. It's a wonderful thing that the sailing club is taken care of by all we meet. (volunteer, male)

Participants highlight their interest to work with young people. Their opinions are crucial when promoting a cultural change in the field of mental health.

We have to bring the sailing club into high schools because we need to educate youth on a culture founded on social inclusion and to change their beliefs about mental health. (professional, male)

Study 3: Preventing Mental Illness to Deconstruct Stigma

Findings from the qualitative research in the previous studies led to specific actions to prevent mental illness and promote mental health in the community. In addition, it focused on a specific setting and young people. To deconstruct stigma toward mental illness, action research was realized through *La Rugiada*'s sports activities involving Grade 12 high school students.

As reported, young people with psychological problems may avoid professional help due to prejudices toward PMHS. They may also fear receiving society's "mentally ill" label.

After considering the principal findings of the previous studies in this chapter, the third work aimed to increase knowledge about mental health. It studied how PMHS can use *La Rugiada* as an instrument of change.

- **Aims:** Action Research investigated beliefs surrounding mental illness, social and professional resources for youth with psychological problems, and the role of the sports association in promoting mental health. Moreover, the research aimed to verify if attending participatory sports activities can modify perceptions about mental illness.

Methods

- **Participants:** Three-hundred and fifty Grade 12 high school students (mean age = 17.46 years, SD = 0.66).

- **Instruments:** for each participant demographical information and data about the perception of seeking help have been collected. An ad hoc questionnaire was administered in order to explore their attitudes about mental illness and to assess perceived social support in case of psychological problems. The questionnaire had a 5-point scale ranging from 1 (strongly disagree) to 5 (strongly agree). Moreover, perceptions about the role of the sports association were collected and analyzed after the action.

- The Statistical Package for the Social Science (SPSS) was used to performed data analysis.

- **Descriptive Analysis:** One-hundred and sixty-three males (51.7%) and 152 females (48.3%).

- Almost all participants (96.8%) stated that their family had a mother and father. Participants reported that:
  - 40% of fathers held a high school diploma
  - 7.8% of fathers held a college degree
  - 45% of mothers held a high school diploma
  - 12.3% of mothers held a college degree

One-fifth of the participants (20.6%) stated that they repeated at least one school year. Of the participants, 41.5% experienced less severe educational difficulties.

Seventy-seven percent of the study participants had a friend with psychological problems. More than 53% suffered personal psychological problems. The most frequently reported issues were affective problems with partners or friends (36.4%), depression (32.6%), and anxiety (25.3%).

Among the participants, 57.6% sought help by speaking with friends for emotional support. Within the social system, participants used the social network to seek out health professionals (20.9%), peers (10.8%), and family (8.9%). Family doctors (4.1%) and teachers (2.8%) were perceived as potential helpers. The Internet was considered an instrument to seek help for 8.5% of participants. In fact, only 0.9% used social network forums for useful information.

Participants were asked to identify the time between the arising of the first symptoms and the actions to seek help. More than a quarter of participants (25.9%) consider that young people seek help after more than one year; 16.9% seek help after one year; 20.6% seek help after six months; and 5.3% seek help in one month. A low percentage (0.7%) of participants report that youth seek help in one week; 14% will not seek help (see Figure 4).

Figure 4. Time before seeking help

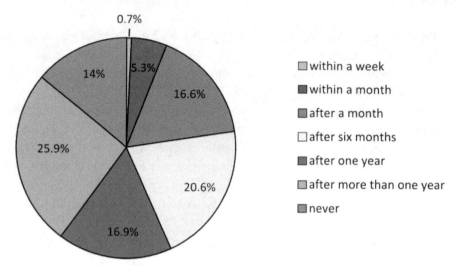

For a more accurate representation see the electronic version.

Participants believe that response time before help can be received: one week (21.8%); one month (24.8%); after one month (21.8%); and after six months (9.4%). For 12.1% and 5.7% of participants, the response time can arrive after one year or several years (see Figure 5).

Some social beliefs are associated with mental illness. Of the participants, 42.4% believed that 1 out of 10 people will suffer mental illness during their life. Lazy or weak people are perceived to be at a greater risk for mental illness (75.9%). According

Figure 5. Time before receiving help

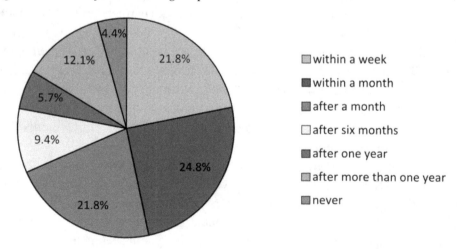

For a more accurate representation see the electronic version.

to the study, 83.2% of participants believed that people with mental illness do not seek professional help. Only 3.8% of participants believed that it was impossible to help someone with mental illness.

During the study, 8.2% of participants felt that *"it is not possible to get better from mental illness."*, which was recognized as a cause of absenteeism (34.2%) and crime (45.6%).

Difficulties to seeking help with PMHS included prejudice (M=3.54; SD=1.23), lack of knowledge about services (M=3.37; SD=1.08), and low confidence in PMHS (M=2.85; SD=1.17). Participants reported poor motivation to seek help by young people (M=2.92; SD=1.03).

Despite difficulties perceived for young people, participants considered that seeking help through PMHS would solve psychological problems (M=3.36; SD=0.80). PMHS was perceived as a social resource in the community in which family members affected by psychological distress could seek help through professional services (M=3.24; SD=1.1).

However, seeking help through PMHS was regarded as a cause of a negative social response in the peer network (M=2.96; SD=1.18). Due to this reason, young people preferred to cope with the problem by relying on their own resources (M=2.85; SD=1.32).

Psychological problems led to feelings of shame (M=3.74; SD=0.82) and self-isolation (M=3.50; SD=0.88). Participants noted youngs with psychological problems received negative responses from peers (M=3.39; SD=0.95) and may be emarginated by them (M=3.20; SD=0.89). Hence, in the participants' opinion, young people can use social resources (M=2.85; SD=0.89) to receive useful help (M=2.55; SD=0.85).

Private professionals were perceived as more competent (M=3.75; SD=1.05). Peer networks (M=3.58; SD=0.92) and family (M=3.52; SD=1.01) were the principal sources of help related to psychological distress. Participants, in fact, reported that they sought help through friends (M=3.61; SD=1.16) and family members (M=3.36; SD=1.18).

Partners were also perceived as helpful (M=3.03; SD=1.02). Significant adults (M=2.77; SD=1.04), family doctors (M=2.49; SD=1.06), and teachers were perceived as less able to provide helpful actions (M=2.41; SD=1.0). In fact, in participants' personal experiences, teachers (M=1.75; SD=0.95), family doctors (M=1.51; SD=0.87), and PMHS (M=1.51; SD=1.03) were considered less able to give support to their own psychological problems.

- **Actions in High Schools:** High school students participated in a reflection process on mental health issues. This action was realized using sports activities as an instrument to promote mental health for the community and social inclusion for people with mental illness.

A volley match (see Figure 6) and a sailing boat tour (see Figure 7) promoted the interaction and connection between students and members of the *La Rugiada* sports association.

- **Analysis of the Intervention's Outcomes:** This study aimed to explore if participation promoted changes in participants. A paired sample t-test compared the mean scores for the same group of participants in two time frames (T1 = before the intervention; T2 = after the intervention).

Table 1 shows that the intervention impacted student scores on the source of support. After the action, youth perceived parents (T1: M=2.92, SD=1.61; T2: M=3.35, SD=1.25; t=-3.41, p<.01) and teachers (T1: M=1.79, SD= 0.94; T2:M=1.94, SD=0.95; t=-1.99, p<.05) as more helpful in the case of psychological problems. Statistical differences were detected in the role of private professionals (T1: M=1.94, SD=1.36; T2: M= 2.22, SD=1.43; t=-2.20, p<.05) and PMHS (T1: M= 1.47, SD=0.90; T2: M=1.94, SD=1.28; t=-3.30, p<.01) as more effective in psychological distress after interventions.

Figure 6. Volley match with high school students

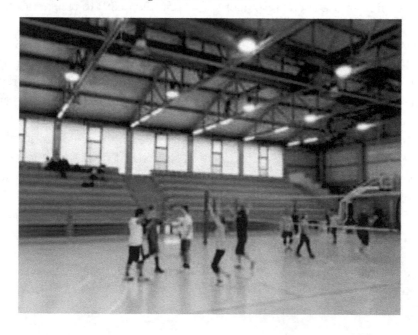

Figure 7. Sailing boat tour

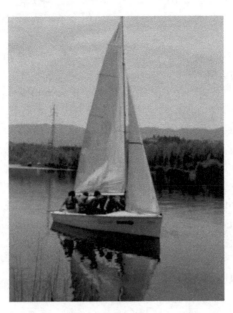

Table 1. Source of support before and after intervention

Source of Support	T1		T2		t**
	M	**SD**	**M**	**SD**	
Parents	2.92	1.61	3.35	1.25	-3.42**
Partner	2.81	1.34	2.72	1.32	0.77
Friends	3.73	1.10	3.63	1.06	1.11
Teachers	1.79	0.94	1.94	0.95	-1.99*
Family Doctor	1.50	0.86	1.39	1.12	1.14
Significant Adults	1.95	1.08	2.08	1.13	-1.1
Private Professionals	1.94	1.36	2.22	1.43	-2.2*
PMHS	1.47	0.91	1.94	1.28	-3.3**

*: $p. < 0.05$, **: $p. < 0.01$

A statistically significant change emerged in terms of difficulties perceived in a psychological problem. After the intervention, students had an increased awareness to negative attitudes and behaviors by the social system (T1: M=2.59, SD=0.96; T2:M=2.73, SD=0.94; t=-2.18, p<.05). After the intervention, students could identify adequately formal sources of support in the case of psychological problems

(T1: M=2.13, SD=0.83; T2: M=2.25, SD=0.78; *t*=-1.94, *p*=0.054). They could also receive adequate help from these sources (T1: M=2.52, SD=0.84; T2: M=2.74, SD=0.89; *t*=-3.24, *p*<.01).

Reflections related to these experiences were collected. Many participants defined the association as an important *"source of help"*. A young male noted that he *"finally knew who and how to seek help in the future in my community."* Moreover, a young female defined the sports association as *"able to take care of the community and cure people with mental illness."* Another student (female) felt that the relationship built by the sports association was based on *"non-judging attitudes ... this can really help people with an illness condition."*

Some participants found it difficult to seek help through PMHS because young people strongly recognize it as a place *"where crazy people go"*. However, the sports association is perceived as *"able to demolish prejudice that disease poses."(female)*

DISCUSSION AND CONCLUSION

La Rugiada experience is an innovative activity developed through the collaborative efforts of public organizations (a local PHMS and the University of Florence), a third sector association, users, and the community. These social actors strongly promoted a new culture of mental health founded on social inclusion for people with mental illness, and community wellness.

This contribution shows an innovative social intervention to fight stigma in mental health, as well as prevent mental illness through sports participation. Two qualitative studies explored perceptions surrounding *La Rugiada* sports association. They looked at the effects of sports participation, specifically sailing. The third study by means of an action research investigated the role of sports as an instrument to prevent mental illness and promote mental health in youth.

One of the most interesting aspects of the experience was the capacity of the intervention in linking fundamental elements in the work of mental health.

Several actions have been realized through *La Rugiada* and the sailing club: fought stigma and implemented rehabilitation pathways for people with mental illness; prevented mental illness in young people; promoted well-being in the community.

Another important outcome of this intervention was the awareness that *La Rugiada* may be a community resource, and users became active members in this process.

Fighting Stigma and Implementing Rehabilitation

Sports participation as a rehabilitative program was a powerful strategy to improve people's mental health. Consistent with the literature, findings suggest that social interventions by sports participation improved both physical health and social responsibility in people with mental illness (Firth et al., 2015). It reduced isolation and social barriers between members, as well as improved social support (Morgan et al., 2007). Both professionals and patients considered sports participation as an instrument to promote socialization for people with mental illness (Rosenbaum et al., 2014; Sherry & O'May, 2013). Active roles and perceived skills positively affected self-esteem and self-efficacy. Participation generated a sense of reciprocity between PMHS, users (considered by the community as "citizens able to"), and the community. Sports participation reduced prejudice and barriers caused by mental illness. It created of a sense of belonging.

Preventing Mental Illness in Young People

Data emerging from the third study confirmed that stigma has a central role in the decisional process of seeking help. Among young people, reluctance to seek professional help may be explained by the lack of knowledge and prejudice surrounding local mental health services. These aspects were confirmed as relevant barriers by participants (Gaebel et al., 2014; Bosco et al., 2016).

Seeking help through PMHS was considered by young people as a cause of negative social reactions in the peer network. In their opinion, people with psychological problems are stigmatized by others in the society. This process may negatively affect the Self-evaluation (Corrigan et al., 2012; Parcesepe & Cabassa, 2013).

The negative attribution derived by the society (public stigma), may categorize them as members of a powerless and stigmatized group because of their unhealthy condition. Thus, in case of psychological problems, young people do not seek professional help to avoid the social rejection, and to protect themselves by feelings of shame, self-isolation (self-stigma), and discriminatory behavior acted by the peer group.

In the case of psychological problems suffered by a friend, emotional support was the principal action realized by participants. Young people would not seek help from formal resources event when the resources were perceived as more adequate (Rickwood et al., 2005).

Actions in local high schools fostered reflections on consequences experienced by people with mental health problems. Significant changes (before and after the intervention) have been detected, particularly related to increased awareness on the consequences of stigma (public stigma and self-stigma) in social life (Vogel et al., 2006). Following the sports participation intervention, significant differences were found about the source of the support. Participants perceived formal help seekers more adequate than informal help seekers (Anderson & Lowen, 2010). Moreover, significant adults, parents, and mental health professionals were perceived as more helpful than friends in the case of psychological problems.

The reluctance of young people to seek professional help, as well as their self-reliant attitude as preferred coping strategies, required a closer connection between PMHS and young people. The example of *La Rugiada* can be effective in connecting people and institutions through sport.

Sports participation generates a sense of belonging and creates significant relationships, which may include adults. We know that stigma negatively affects PMHS: therefore, mental health services must connect with the youth population through social innovation interventions for psychological needs. *La Rugiada* can be a significant resource to promote positive attitudes toward seeking help.

Promoting Community Well-Being

La Rugiada can be an innovative intervention. It generates mutual help, creates a sense of belonging to a sports team, and boosts members' confidence. These are crucial elements to meeting a community's psychological needs.

Figure 8. Social role of La Rugiada

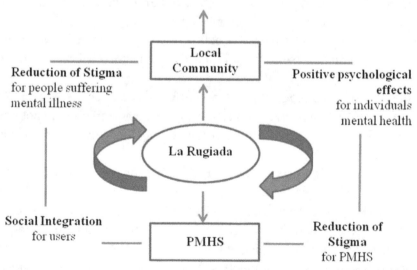

Results suggested relevant aspects to deconstruct stigma. *La Rugiada*, particularly its sailing club, may modify beliefs about mental illness. This activity allows people, including those with mental illness, to meet and connect. The community is considered a setting for everyone. People are assigned a new social role recognized by society.

Promising findings suggest that *La Rugiada* developed a powerful setting to link PMHS and the community. According to participants, the sports association functioned as an *"open workshop addressed to the whole community,* and *La Rugiada* is defined as a *"place of care"* for citizens. Thus, the intervention based on community setting and sports participation seem to be able to reduce stigma surrounding PMHS and mental illness (Soundy et al., 2015).

The social role and impact of *La Rugiada*, as suggested by results, are summarized in Figure 8.

La Rugiada may be an innovative experience to generate community participation. The capacity to promote positive change in various aspects of social life, including social networks, mutuality, and social participation (Zoppei et al., 2014), is the added value of the sailing club. It leads to consider this sports activity and *La Rugiada* as a bridging element of social capital.

As suggested by the results, *La Rugiada* connected citizens, formal and informal community networks, and the community. Thus, it can be viewed as a powerful instrument to promote healthy communities through destigmatizing strategies.

REFERENCES

Agnetti, G. (2007). Arrivano i consumatori: dove andiamo? *Psichiatria di comunità,* 6(2), 73-79.

Anderson, J. E., & Lowen, C. A. (2010). Connecting youth with health services Systematic review. *Canadian Family Physician Medecin de Famille Canadien, 56,* 778–784. PMID:20705886

Andrews, G., Issakidis, C., & Carter, G. (2001). Shortfall in mental health service utilization. *The British Journal of Psychiatry, 179*(05), 417–425. doi:10.1192/bjp.179.5.417 PMID:11689399

Arcidiacono, C., Gelli, B., & Putton, A. (1999). *Empowerment sociale. Il futuro della solidarietà: modelli di psicologia di comunità.* Milano: FrancoAngeli.

Baum, F. E., & Ziersch, A. M. (2003). A glossary of social capital. *Journal of Epidemiology and Community Health, 57*(5), 320–323. doi:10.1136/jech.57.5.320 PMID:12700212

Bentall, R. (2003). *Madness explained: Psychosis and human nature*. London: Penguin.

Bertotti, M., Watts, P., Netuveli, G., Yu, G., Schmidt, E., Tobi, P., ... Renton, A. (2013). Types of Social Capital and Mental Disorder in Deprived Urban Areas: A Multilevel Study of 40 Disadvantaged London Neighbourhoods. *PLoS One, 8*(12), e80127. doi:10.1371/journal.pone.0080127 PMID:24312459

Bos, A. E. R., Pryor, J. B., Reeder, G. D., & Stutterheim, S. E. (2013). Stigma: Advances in Theory and Research. *Basic and Applied Social Psychology, 35*(1), 1–9. doi:10.1080/01973533.2012.746147

Bosco, N., Guazzini, A., Guidi, E., Giaccherini, S., & Meringolo, P. (2016). Self-Stigma in mental health: planning effective programs for teenagers. In C. Pracana, & M. Wang (Eds.), *International Psychological Applications Conference and Trends* (pp. 36-39). Lisbon: W.I.A.R.S.

Bosco, N., Petrini, F., Giaccherini, S., & Meringolo, P. (2014). Theater as instrument to promote inclusion of mental health patients: an innovative experience in a local community. In C. Pracana (Eds.), Psychology Applications & Developments (pp. 55-66). Lisbon: InSciencePress.

Brohan, E., Elgie, R., Sartorius, N., & Thornicroft, G. (2010). Self-stigma, empowerment and perceived discrimination among people with schizophrenia in 14 European countries: The GAMIAN-Europe study. *Schizophrenia Research, 122*(1-3), 232–238. doi:10.1016/j.schres.2010.02.1065 PMID:20347271

Bulut, C., Eren, H., & Halac, D. S. (2013). Social innovation and psychometric analysis. *Procedia: Social and Behavioral Sciences, 82*, 122–130. doi:10.1016/j.sbspro.2013.06.235

Bureau of European Policy Advisors (BEPA). (2011). *Empowering people, driving change: Social innovation in the European Union*. Luxembourg: BEPA.

Christens, B. D., Speer, P. W., & Peterson, N. A. (2011). Social class as moderator of the relationship between (dis)empowering processes and psychological empowerment. *Journal of Community Psychology, 39*(2), 170–182. doi:10.1002/jcop.20425

Clayton, A., O'Connell, M. J., Bellamy, C., Benedict, P., & Rowe, M. (2013). The Citizenship Project Part II: Impact of a Citizenship Intervention on Clinical and Community Outcomes for Persons with Mental Illness and Criminal Justice Involvement. *American Journal of Community Psychology, 51*(1-2), 114–122. doi:10.100710464-012-9549-z PMID:22869206

Coaffee, J. (2008). Sport, Culture and the Modern State: Emerging Themes in Stimulating urban Regeneration in the UK. *International Journal of Cultural Policy*, *14*(4), 377–397. doi:10.1080/10286630802445856

Corrigan, P. W., & Boyle, M. G. (2003). What works for mental health system change: Evolution or revolution? *Administration and Policy in Mental Health*, *30*(5), 379–395. doi:10.1023/A:1024619913592 PMID:12940682

Corrigan, P. W., Larson, J. E., & Rüsch, N. (2009). Self-stigma and the "why try" effect: Impact on life goals and evidence-based practices. *World Psychiatry; Official Journal of the World Psychiatric Association (WPA)*, *8*(2), 75–81. doi:10.1002/j.2051-5545.2009.tb00218.x PMID:19516923

Corrigan, P. W., & Matthews, A. (2003). Stigma and disclosure: Implications for coming out of the closet. *Journal of Mental Health (Abingdon, England)*, *12*(3), 235–248. doi:10.1080/0963823031000118221

Corrigan, P. W., Michaels, P. J., Vega, E., Gause, M., Watson, A. C., & Rüsch, N. (2012). *Self-stigma* of mental illness scale-short form: Reliability and validity. *Psychiatry Research*, *199*(1), 65–69. doi:10.1016/j.psychres.2012.04.009 PMID:22578819

Corrigan, P. W., & Watson, A. C. (2002). The paradox of self-stigma and mental illness. *Clinical Psychology: Science and Practice*, *9*(1), 35–53. doi:10.1093/clipsy.9.1.35

Crandall, C. S., & Eshleman, A. (2003). A justification-suppression model of the expression and experience of prejudice. *Psychological Bulletin*, *129*(3), 414–446. doi:10.1037/0033-2909.129.3.414 PMID:12784937

Crawford, M. J., Rutter, D., Manley, C., Weaver, T., Bhui, K., Fulop, N., & Tyrer, P. (2002). Systematic review of involving patients in the planning and development of health care. *British Medical Journal*, *325*(7375), 1263. doi:10.1136/bmj.325.7375.1263 PMID:12458240

Curtis, J., Walkins, A., Rosenbaum, U. M. S., Teasdale, S., Kalucy, M., Samaras, K., & Ward, F. B. (2016). Evaluating an individualized lifestyle and life skills interventions to prevent antipsychotic-induced weight gain in first-episode psychosis. *Early Intervention in Psychiatry*, *10*(3), 267–276. doi:10.1111/eip.12230 PMID:25721464

De Silva, M. J., McKenzie, K., Harpham, T., & Huttly, S. R. A. (2005). Social Capital and mental illness: A systematic review. *Journal of Epidemiology and Community Health*, *59*(8), 619–627. doi:10.1136/jech.2004.029678 PMID:16020636

Dovidio, J. F., Major, B., & Crocker, J. (2000). Stigma: Introduction and overview. In The social psychology of stigma (pp. 1-28). New York: Guilford Press.

Ehsan, A. M., & De Silva, M. J. (2015). Social capital and common mental disorder: A systematic review. *Journal of Epidemiology and Community Health, 69*(10), 1021–1028. doi:10.1136/jech-2015-205868 PMID:26179447

Faulkner, G., & Biddle, S. (1999). Exercise as an adjunct treatment for schizophrenia: A review of the literature. *Journal of Mental Health (Abingdon, England), 23*, 355–359.

Feldman, D. B., & Crandall, C. S. (2007). Dimensions of mental illness stigma: What about mental illness causes social rejection? *Journal of Social and Clinical Psychology, 26*(2), 137–154. doi:10.1521/jscp.2007.26.2.137

Field, J. (2003). *Social capital*. London: Routledge.

Firth, J., Cottr, J., Jerome, I., Elliott, R., French, P., & Yung, A. R. (2015). A systematic review and meta-analysis of exercise interventions in schizophrenic patients. *Psychological Medicine, 45*(07), 1343–1361. doi:10.1017/S0033291714003110 PMID:25650668

Firth, J., Rosenbaum, S., Strubbs, B., Gorcynski, P., Yung, A. R., & Vancampfort, D. (2016). Motivating factors and barriers towards exercise in severe mental illness: A systematic review and meta-analysis. *Psychological Medicine, 46*(14), 2869–2881. doi:10.1017/S0033291716001732 PMID:27502153

Forsman, A. K., Nordmyr, J., & Wahlbeck, K. (2011). Psychosocial interventions for the promotion of mental health and the prevention of depression among older adults. *Health Promotion International, 26*(suppl_1), S85–S107. doi:10.1093/heapro/dar074 PMID:22079938

Forsman, A. K., Nyqvist, F., Schierenbeck, I., Gustafson, Y., & Wahlbeck, K. (2013). Structural and cognitive social capital and depression among older adults in two Nordic regions. *Aging & Mental Health, 16*(6), 771–779. doi:10.1080/13607863.2012.667784 PMID:22486561

Gaebel, W., Muijen, M., Baumann, A. E., Bhugra, D., Wasserman, D., Van Der Gaag, R. J., ... Zielesek, J. (2014). EPA guidance on building trust in mental health service. *European Psychiatry, 29*(2), 83–100. doi:10.1016/j.eurpsy.2014.01.001 PMID:24506936

Glaser, B. G., & Strauss, A. L. (1967). *The Discovery of Grounded Theory: Strategies for Qualitative Research*. Chicago: Aldine.

Goffman, E. (1963). *Stigma: Notes on the Management of Spoiled Identity*. Englewood Cliffs, NJ: Prentice-Hall.

Granovetter, M. (1983). The strength of weak ties: A network theory revisited. *Sociological Theory*, *1*, 201–233. doi:10.2307/202051

Harpham, T., Grant, E., & Thomas, E. (2002). Measuring social capital within health surverys: Key issues. *Health Policy and Planning*, *17*(1), 106–111. doi:10.1093/heapol/17.1.106 PMID:11861592

Hartmann, D. (2003). Theorizing sport as social intervention: A view from the grassroots. *Quest.*, *55*(2), 118–140. doi:10.1080/00336297.2003.10491795

Haslam, S. A., Jetten, J., Postmes, T., & Haslam, C. (2009). Social Identity, Health and Well-Being: An Emerging Agenda for Applied Psychology. *Applied Psychology*, *58*(1), 1–23. doi:10.1111/j.1464-0597.2008.00379.x

Hebl, M. R., Tickle, J., & Heatherton, T. F. (2000). Awkward moments in interactions between nonstigmatized and stigmatized individuals. In T. F. Heatherton, R. E. Kleck, M. R. Hebl, & J. G. Hull (Eds.), *The social psychology of stigma* (pp. 243–272). New York: Guilford Press.

Howley, E. T. (2001). Type of activity: Resistance, aerobic and leisure versus occupational physical activity. *Medicine and Science in Sports and Exercise*, *33*(Supplement), 364–369. doi:10.1097/00005768-200106001-00005 PMID:11427761

Huang, W. Y., & Lin, C. Y. (2015). The relationship between *Self-stigma* and quality of life among people with mental illness who participated in a community program. *Journal of Nature and Science*, *1*(7), e135.

Kimby, D., Vakhrushev, J., Bartels, M. N., Armstrong, H. F., Ballon, J. S., Khan, S., ... Ayanruoh, I. (2015). The impact of aerobic exercise on brain-derived neurothropic factor and neurocognition in individuals with schizoprenia: A single-blind randomized clinical trial. *Schizophrenia Bulletin*, *41*(4), 859–868. doi:10.1093chbulbv022 PMID:25805886

Krogh, J., Nordentolf, M., Sterne, J. A., & Lawlor, D. A. (2011). The effect of exercise in clinically depressed adults: Systematic review and meta-analysis of randomized contolled trials. *The Journal of Clinical Psychiatry*, *72*(04), 529–538. doi:10.4088/JCP.08r04913blu PMID:21034688

Kurzban, R., & Leary, M. R. (2001). Evolutionary origins of stigmatization: The functions of social exclusion. *Psychological Bulletin*, *127*(2), 187–208. doi:10.1037/0033-2909.127.2.187 PMID:11316010

Langle, G., Siemssen, G., & Hornberger, S. (2000). The role of sport in the treatment and rehabilitation of schizophrenic patients. *Rehabilitation*, *39*(5), 276–282. doi:10.1055-2000-7863 PMID:11089261

Lin, N. (1999). Building a Network Theory of Social Capital. *Connections*, *22*(1), 28–51.

Link, B. G., Mirotznik, J., & Cullen, F. (1991). The Effectiveness of Stigma Coping Orientations: Can Negative Consequences of Mental Illness Labeling be Avoided? *Journal of Health and Social Behavior*, *32*(3), 302–320. doi:10.2307/2136810 PMID:1940212

Link, B. G., & Phelan, J. C. (2001). Conceptualizing stigma. *Annual Review of Sociology*, *27*(1), 363–385. doi:10.1146/annurev.soc.27.1.363

Lukes, S. (2005). *Power: A radical view*. Hampshire, UK: Palgrave McMillan. doi:10.1007/978-0-230-80257-5

Major, B., & O'Brien, L. T. (2005). The Social Psychology of Stigma. *Annual Review of Psychology*, *56*(1), 393–421. doi:10.1146/annurev.psych.56.091103.070137 PMID:15709941

McKenzie, K., Whitley, R., & Weich, S. (2002). Social capital and mental health. *The British Journal of Psychiatry*, *181*(04), 280–283. doi:10.1192/bjp.181.4.280 PMID:12356653

McNamee, I., Mead, G., MacGillivrey, S., & Lawrie, S. M. (2013). Schizophrenia, poor physical health and physical activity: Evidence-based interventions are required to reduce major health inequalities. *The British Journal of Psychiatry*, *203*(04), 912–918. doi:10.1192/bjp.bp.112.125070 PMID:24085733

Montero, M. (2010). Fortalecimiento de la Ciudadanía y Transformación Social: Área de Encuentro entre la Psicología Política y la Psicología Comunitaria. *Psykhe (Santiago)*, *19*(2), 51–63. doi:10.4067/S0718-22282010000200006

Morgan, A. J., Parker, A. G., Alvarez-Jimenez, A., & Jorm, A. F. (2013). Exercise and mental Health: An exercise and sport science Australia commisioned review. *Journal of Exercise Physiology*, *16*(4), 64–73.

Morgan, C., Burns, T., Fitzpatrick, R., Pinfold, V., & Priebe, S. (2007). Social exclusion and mental health: Conceptual and methodological review. *The British Journal of Psychiatry*, *191*(06), 477–483. doi:10.1192/bjp.bp.106.034942 PMID:18055950

Parcesepe, A. M., & Cabassa, L. J. (2013). Public stigma of mental illness in the United States: A systematic literature review. *Administration and Policy in Mental Health, 40*(5), 384–399. doi:10.100710488-012-0430-z PMID:22833051

Phelan, J. C., Link, B. G., & Dovidio, J. F. (2008). Stigma and prejudice: One animal or two? *Social Science & Medicine, 67*(3), 358–367. doi:10.1016/j.socscimed.2008.03.022 PMID:18524444

Phongsavan, P., Chey, T., Bauman, A., Brooks, R., & Silove, D. (2006). Social capital, socio-economic status and psychological distress among Australian adults. *Social Science & Medicine, 63*(10), 2546–2561. doi:10.1016/j.socscimed.2006.06.021 PMID:16914244

Pingani, L., Forghieri, M., Ferrari, S., Ben-Zeev, D., Artoni, P., Mazzi, F., ... Corrigan, P. W. (2012). Stigma and discrimination toward mental illness: Translation and validation of the Italian version of the Attribution Questionnaire-27 (AQ-27-I). *Social Psychiatry and Psychiatric Epidemiology, 47*(6), 993–999. doi:10.100700127-011-0407-3 PMID:21688158

Porta, M. (2014). *A dictionary of epidemiology.* Oxford University Press. doi:10.1093/acref/9780199976720.001.0001

Re, E. (2005). L'associazionismo degli utenti psichiatrici tra difficoltà e possibilità. *Prospettive Sociali e Sanitarie, 35*, 1–3.

Rethrost, C. D., Wipfli, B. M., & Landers, D. M. (2009). The antidepressive effects of exsercise: A meta-analysis of Randomized trials. *Sports Medicine (Auckland, N.Z.), 39*, 491–511. PMID:19453207

Rickwood, D., Deane, F., Wilson, C., & Ciarrochi, J. (2005). Young people's help-seeking for mental health problems. *Australian e-Journal for the Advancement of Mental Health, 4*(3), 218–251. doi:10.5172/jamh.4.3.218

Rosenbaum, S., Tiederman, A., Sherrington, C., Curtis, J., & Ward, P. B. (2014). Physical activity interventions for people with mental illness: A systematic review and meta-analyses. *The Journal of Clinical Psychiatry, 75*(09), 964–974. doi:10.4088/JCP.13r08765 PMID:24813261

Saha, S., Chant, D., & McGrat, J. (2007). A systematic review on mortality in schizophrenia: Is the differential mortality gap worsenig over time? *Archives of General Psychiatry, 64*(10), 1123–1131. doi:10.1001/archpsyc.64.10.1123 PMID:17909124

Sellers, R. M., & Shelton, J. N. (2003). The role of racial identity in perceived racial discrimination. *Journal of Personality and Social Psychology, 84*(5), 1079–1092. doi:10.1037/0022-3514.84.5.1079 PMID:12757150

Sherry, E., & O'May, F. (2013). Exploring the impact of sport participation in the Homeless World Cup on individuals with substance abuse or mental health disorders. *Journal of Sports for Development, 1*, 1-9.

Simpson, E. L., & House, A. O. (2003). User and carer involvement in mental health services: From rhetoric to science. *The British Journal of Psychiatry, 183*(02), 89–91. doi:10.1192/bjp.183.2.89 PMID:12893657

Soundy, A., Freeman, P., Stubbs, B., Probst, M., Roskell, C., & Vancampfort, D. (2015). The psychosocial consequences of sports participation for individuals with severe mental illness: a metasynthesis review. *Advances in Psychiatry*, 1-8.

Soundy, A., Freeman, P., Stubbs, R., Probst, M., Coffee, P., & Vancmpfort, D. (2014). The trascending benefits of physical activity for indoividuals with schizoprenia: A systematic review and meta ethnography. *Psychiatry Research, 220*(1-2), 11–19. doi:10.1016/j.psychres.2014.07.083 PMID:25149128

Steele, C. M., & Aronson, J. (1995). Stereotype threat and the intellectual test performance of African Americans. *Journal of Personality and Social Psychology, 69*(5), 797–811. doi:10.1037/0022-3514.69.5.797 PMID:7473032

Stiglitz, J. E. (2009). Selected Works: Vol. 1. *Information and Economic Analysis*. Oxford, UK: Oxford University Press.

Stubbs, B., Firth, J., Berry, A., Schuch, F. B., Rosenbaum, S., Ward, P. B., ... Vacampfort, D. (2016). How much physical activities do people with schizophrenia engage in? A systematic review, comparative meta-analysis and meta-regression. *Schizophrenia Research, 176*(2), 431–440. doi:10.1016/j.schres.2016.05.017 PMID:27261419

Tajfel, H. (1981). *Human groups and social categories: Studies in social psychology*. Cambridge, UK: Cambridge University Press.

Tew, J., Ramon, S., Slade, M., Bird, V., Melton, J., & Le Boutillier, C. (2012). Social factors and recovery from mental health difficulties: A review of the evidence. *British Journal of Social Work, 42*(3), 443–460. doi:10.1093/bjsw/bcr076

Tomita, A., & Burns, J. K. (2013). A multilevel analysis of association between neighbourhood social capital and depression: Evidence from the first South African National Income Dynamics Study. *Journal of Affective Disorders, 144*(1-2), 101–105. doi:10.1016/j.jad.2012.05.066 PMID:22858263

Vancampfort, D., De Hert, M., Skijevern, L. H., Lundvik Gyllensten, A., Parker, A., Mulders, N., ... Probst, M. (2012). International organization of physical therapy in mental health consensus on physical activity within multidisciplinary rehabilitation programmes for minimising cardio-metabolic risk in patients with schizophrenia. *Disability and Rehabilitation, 34*(1), 1–12. doi:10.3109/09638288.2011.587090 PMID:21957908

Vogel, D. L., Heimerdinger-Edwards, S. R., Hammer, J. H., & Hubbard, A. (2011). Boys Don't Cry": Examination of the Links Between Endorsement of Masculine Norms, *Self-stigma*, and Help-Seeking Attitudes for Men From Diverse Backgrounds. *Journal of Counseling Psychology, 58*(3), 368–382. doi:10.1037/a0023688 PMID:21639615

Vogel, D. L., Wade, N. G., & Haake, S. (2006). Measuring the *Self-stigma* Associated With Seeking Psychological Help. *Journal of Counseling Psychology, 53*(3), 325–337. doi:10.1037/0022-0167.53.3.325

Walton, G. M., & Cohen, G. L. (2003). Stereotype life. *Journal of Experimental Social Psychology, 39*(5), 456–467. doi:10.1016/S0022-1031(03)00019-2

Watson, A. C., Corrigan, P. W., Larson, J. E., & Sells, M. (2007). *Self-stigma* in people with mental illness. *Schizophrenia Bulletin, 33*(6), 1312–1318. doi:10.1093chbulbl076 PMID:17255118

Yanos, P. T., Roe, D., Markus, K., & Lysaker, P. H. (2008). Pathways between internalized stigma and outcomes related to recovery in schizophrenia spectrum disorders. *Psychiatric Services (Washington, D.C.), 59*(12), 1437–1442. doi:10.1176/ps.2008.59.12.1437 PMID:19033171

Zoppei, S., Lasalvia, A., Bonetto, C., Van Bortel, T., Nyqvist, F., Webber, M., ... Wahlbeck, K. (2014). Social capital and reported discrimination among people with depression in 15 European countries. *Social Psychiatry and Psychiatric Epidemiology, 49*(10), 1589–1598. doi:10.100700127-014-0856-6 PMID:24638892

KEY TERMS AND DEFINITIONS

Basaglia Law: A legislative reform about psychiatric services that resulted in the closing down of all insane asylums in Italy.

La Rugiada: A sports association for social integration which promote well-being and mental health through sport.

PMHS: Public mental health service aimed to care and cure people with mental illness through therapeutic and rehabilitative interventions, and to promote community mental health.

Social Capital: A social and/or individual dimension in which social networks, mutuality, and social participation are valuable resources.

Social Inclusion: A process to improve participation in the society for disadvantaged people.

Social Innovation Intervention: New strategies and/or services able to meet social needs and enhance individual and social wellbeing.

Stigma: A label attributed to others based on undesirable social characteristics.

Chapter 7
Reducing Stigma in Mental Health Through Digital Storytelling

Tatiana Davidson
Medical University of South Carolina, USA

Jennifer Winkelmann
Medical University of South Carolina, USA

Angela Moreland
Medical University of South Carolina, USA

Jessica L. Hamblen
National Center for PTSD, USA

Brian E. Bunnell
Medical University of South Carolina, USA

Kenneth J. Ruggiero
Medical University of South Carolina, USA

ABSTRACT

The authors present the use of digital storytelling with two populations that have been consistently shown to be at increased risk for developing mental health disorders: veterans and firefighters. Despite efforts to increase access to evidence-based mental health programs, stigma remains a major barrier to care. AboutFace and Firefighters Helping Firefighters are two DST resources designed to help recognize the symptoms of posttraumatic stress disorder (PTSD) and related mental health symptoms, and to encourage help-seeking. These web-based video galleries introduce the viewer to 70+ peers who have experienced PTSD and have received formal treatment. These sites use the shared bonds of service to educate and help normalize common reactions that they may have due to the stressful nature of their occupations. Visitors to the site can "meet" peers and hear how mental illness has affected them through unscripted, authentic personal stories and can learn about common symptoms, struggles regarding decisions to seek care, and detailed descriptions of what treatment was like.

DOI: 10.4018/978-1-5225-3808-0.ch007

DIGITAL STORYTELLING: A PROMISING, SCALABLE APPROACH TO REDUCE MENTAL HEALTH STIGMA

Approximately 1 in 5 adults in the U.S. (43.8 million) will experience a mental health disorder in their lifetime, yet despite the availability of efficacious mental health interventions, fewer than half (45%) of individuals with a mental health problem seek treatment (Han et al., 2015; Hedden et al., 2015). Rates of treatment seeking for Posttraumatic Stress Disorder (PTSD) are similarly low. Several barriers to care have been examined, including financial, knowledge-related, logistical (e.g., transportation, scheduling), and attitudinal-barriers. Stigma consistently has been identified as a key barrier to mental health care (Corrigan, 2004). Feelings of weakness, shame, and fear of discrimination by others are reported reasons for not seeking or engaging in mental health treatment (Corrigan, 2004; Hoge et al., 2004; Kessler et al., 2001). Widely used strategies designed to reduce mental health stigma include training interventions and educational programs that address a range of audiences (e.g., health professionals, first responders, general public) and mass media campaigns (Bahora et al., 2008; Beltran et al., 2007; Corrigan, 2004, 2011). Whereas these have been found to be successful in improving attitudes toward mental health, most of these effects are short-lived (Corrigan and Gelb, 2006). In this chapter, we will provide an overview of how digital storytelling has been used to address mental health stigma and will present two digital-storytelling resources that can serve as a model for researchers seeking to develop and/or improve other web/smartphone-based DST resources to improve relevance, interest, and effectiveness in decreasing stigma.

Research consistently demonstrates that people are most responsive to advice or education when it comes from someone they consider similar to themselves (peer education). Indeed, mental illness stigma reduction has been found most effective when targeted toward specific populations, credible (using people from the targeted population to deliver the message), and when it involves contact with peers who have experienced mental health problems (Corrigan, 2011). More specifically, peers, especially those with the same psychiatric disorder or presentation of symptoms, can provide patients with accurate information (i.e., education) as well as personal contact with a similar peer that, in turn, can challenge perceptions about mental illness. A growing body of evidence supports the effectiveness of peer educators in reducing stigma and improving treatment seeking. For example, peer educators have been shown to improve knowledge, self-efficacy, and behavioral outcomes in people with HIV (Mahat et al., 2011; Medley et al., 2009), reduce drinking in college students (White et al., 2009), and reduce stigma in depressed older adults (Conner et al., 2015). However, this is a growing area of research and there is still much to be learned about the value of peer education in addressing mental health stigma. The National Alliance of Mental Illness program, *In our Own Voice (IOOV)*, is one such program that has shown success in reducing stigmatizing attitudes (Pinto-Foltz, Logsdon, and Myers, 2011). This program involves a 90-minute group interaction led by two facilitators who have successfully managed their mental illness. The group interaction consists of watching education videos, sharing of personal experiences by group facilitators, and open discussion. A major limitation of this, and other existing programs, is that they are delivered in-person, which does not address a number of noted barriers to service use, including transportation, time-commitments, scheduling difficulties, and worries about confidentiality. Moreover, costs associated with training peers and supporting their interactions with the target population limit the scalability of these approaches.

Web-based systems have effectively used this peer education approach to relay health related information to high-risk groups. Rapid growth in the use of smartphones (now used by roughly 80% of the adult US population) has strengthened the reach of these approaches and made them even more accessible and much more user-friendly. Peer education has been used effectively in online formats to address topics ranging from healthy lifestyles to severe medical illness. More recently, Naslund and colleagues (2016) proposed that online peer networks can improve access to treatment. These authors view online peer support networks as a mechanism to challenge stigma, increase consumer activation, and ultimately increase access to mental healthcare. This low-cost, highly sustainable and scalable approach to peer education may have particular value for populations with stigmatized conditions. Naslund and colleagues further suggest that people with PTSD may be motivated to access online peer interventions because they are struggling to deal with their PTSD symptoms, feel socially isolated and tend to avoid in-person interactions, and/or are afraid to reach out for traditional face-to-face help due to concerns about how others will perceive them or concerns about social or occupational repercussions to seeking help. These factors may encourage a person with PTSD to seek out online support, which is anonymous and less anxiety provoking. The decision to visit an online peer network provides opportunities to challenge stigma or other misperceptions that are preventing an individual from accessing needed mental healthcare. Additionally, peers may help people feel less isolated and alone in their illness, more empowered, and more hopeful. These interactions can motivate interest in learning more about PTSD and demystify the treatment process resulting in an increased likelihood that evidence-based care for PTSD will be accessed.

Overview of Digital Story-Telling Approaches to Address Mental Health Stigma

Peer education through digital storytelling (DST) is a particularly efficient way for everyday people to connect with others similar to themselves in a low-burdensome and sustainable way. DST features videos of individuals sharing aspects of their own personal stories (i.e., testimonials) through the use of recorded audio, video, graphics, and text that are disseminated electronically (e.g., via the Internet or DVDs) to a target population for a particular purpose (e.g., to train, instruct, educate, and motivate). This is accomplished through several storytelling modalities, including re-telling of historical events, informational or instructional videos, and/or personal narratives. DST has been used in a number of contexts and has traditionally been used in educational settings. For example, instruction-based and student-driven digital storytelling methods have led to positive learning effects in educational settings (Robin, 2008) and, when compared to basic technology-integrated instruction, DST leads to better achievement, critical thinking, and learning motivation (Yang & Wu, 2012). DST has been used with promising results in a number of mental health settings, such as development of trauma narratives in exposure therapy for PTSD (Anderson & Wallace, 2015), promoting stress reduction in female adolescents (Goodman & Newman, 2014), and encouraging positive health practices in patients with HIV (Medley et al., 2009). Despite positive findings for the role of DST as an educational and therapeutic tool, little is known about its value in decreasing mental health stigma and increasing treatment-seeking behavior. Because DST is a low-cost, scalable peer education approach, it may have tremendous value, particularly for individuals with stigmatized conditions such as PTSD, depression, alcohol and drug use, and other chronic diseases.

In the remaining sections of this chapter, we will present the use of digital storytelling with two populations that have high risk for developing mental health disorders, Veterans and firefighters. These individuals are frequently involved in life-threatening duties and occupational impacts with respect to posttraumatic stress disorder (PTSD), depression, substance abuse, and marital discord (Hoge et al., 2006; Wagner et al., 2010). Yet, despite tremendous efforts from their respective organizations to develop and increase access to evidence-based mental health programs, misconceptions about mental health and treatment continue to be pervasive, and stigma remains a major barrier to care. *AboutFace* (http://www.ptsd.va.gov/apps/AboutFace/) and *Firefighters Helping Firefighters* (http://pocketpeer.org) are two DST resources designed to help visitors recognize the symptoms of PTSD and related mental health symptoms, and to motivate visitors to seek evidence-based assessment and treatment. These web-based video galleries introduce the viewer to a community of 100+ peers who have experienced symptoms of PTSD, depression, and/or other mental health and behavioral conditions and have received both formal treatment and other support mechanisms. These sites use the shared bonds of service to educate the user and to help normalize common reactions that they may have due to the stressful nature of their occupations. Consistent with this, visitors to the sites can "meet" peers and hear how mental illness has affected them through unscripted, authentic personal stories. Moreover, they can learn about common symptoms of PTSD and other behavioral problems, treatment opinions, struggles regarding decisions to seek care, and detailed descriptions of what treatment was like. Additional features include receiving advice from expert clinicians, hearing how PTSD can affect family members, and hearing from supervisors and other leadership the importance of seeking help.

AboutFace: A Veteran-to-Veteran Digital Storytelling Resource

Military operations frequently involve life-threatening duties, such as patrols and direct fire, witnessed violence and human suffering, and hostile responses from civilians (Hoge, Auchterlonie, & Milliken, 2006). Although the majority of Veterans are resilient and/or recover quickly, PTSD occurs in around 17% of Vietnam Veterans (Dohrenwend et al., 2006) and 13% of Veterans from Iraq and Afghanistan (Kok et al., 2012). PTSD is associated with other mental health problems such as depression and alcohol abuse (Blow et al., 2013; Cohen et al., 2010; Hoge et al., 2006; Hoge et al., 2004; Kim et al., 2010), and all of these disorders are in turn associated with high levels of distress, functional impairment, and morbidity and mortality. However, mental health treatment seeking among Veterans remains strikingly low; most Veterans with mental health problems do not seek mental health services (Han et al., 2015; Hoge et al., 2014). Stigma is frequently reported as a barrier to seeking treatment (see Clement et al., 2015; Gulliver et al., 2010 for two reviews). Stigma may be even more problematic among service members who perceive that disclosing a mental illness could negatively impact their military career. In one survey of four US combat infantry units, among those who met screening criteria for a psychiatric disorder, 65% were concerned that others would see them as weak, 63% were concerned that leadership would treat them differently, and 59% were concerned that members of their unit might have less confidence in them. Importantly, those most in need of care were also the ones most concerned about stigma (Hoge et al., 2004).

Developed by the National Center for PTSD, *AboutFace* is a web-based video gallery that introduces viewers to a community of 77 veterans, diverse with regard to military experience, age, gender, and race/ethnicity. The veterans have experienced PTSD and received treatment through the Veterans Health Administration (VHA). The site also contains testimonials from 23 family members and 22 clinicians. As such, it serves as an online peer network where Veterans can meet similar others and learn from them. *AboutFace* aims to use the shared bonds of military service to educate veterans and their families and help normalize common reactions that veterans may experience due to their military service or deployment experiences. Consistent with this, visitors to the site can "meet" veterans and hear how PTSD has affected them through unscripted, authentic personal stories. Veterans are filmed in natural settings looking directly at the camera. *AboutFace* visitors to the site can challenge their stigmatizing beliefs by choosing to engage with the Veterans on the site with whom they most closely identify. They can view the clips that are most relevant to them and learn from others how they have handled similar situations. Veterans who access *AboutFace* can learn about other veterans' military histories, the common symptoms of PTSD, treatment options, and the struggles of other veterans regarding decisions to seek care. They can get detailed descriptions about what treatment was like for other Veterans. Real life examples provide corrective information to challenge misperceptions about PTSD or the treatment process for PTSD. There is even a section where Veterans give advice on what they think fellow Veterans with PTSD should know about seeking help. Thus, through honest and open testimonials, the Veterans of *AboutFace* serve as encouraging peer supports to other Veterans as they consider their own need for mental healthcare, what the process of PTSD treatment will look like, and how they can obtain and initiate needed services through the Veterans' Health Administration. This use of a peer-to-peer approach is innovative, relevant to a wide range of healthcare conditions, and has the potential to increase access to care through trusted narratives that promote hope in recovery. *AboutFace* has an open format that allows visitors to navigate the site freely based on their own user preferences (Bunnell et al., 2017). Visitors can learn about one Veteran's experience at a time by selecting that Veteran's image and then choosing from a series of statements that represent topics addressed by the Veteran (e.g., What is PTSD?, Am I ready for help?, What is treatment like?). Alternatively, the visitor can choose a specific topic and review video clips of all Veterans, who have addressed that topic. Veterans also can receive advice from expert clinicians and hear how PTSD can affect family members, via a separate component of the *AboutFace* site. Topics addressed in the brief (~1 minute) clips are included in Table 1. We recently conducted a two-stage evaluation of *AboutFace,* which included (1)

Table 1. AboutFace video clips

CLIPS OF VETERANS	CLIPS OF CLINICIANS	CLIPS OF FAMILY MEMBERS
WHO I AM *Example: A.J., US Army (1978-1998), Germany/Korea/US*	**WHO I AM** *Example: Dr. Peter Tuerk, Clinical Psychologist, Director of PCT Clinic, Ralph H. Johnson VA Medical Center, Charleston, SC*	**WHO I AM** *Example: O.J., daughter of A.J.*
HOW I KNEW I HAD PTSD *I was waking up, sweating, [and I] couldn't go back to sleep...*	**WHAT PTSD IS** *A very, very lonely experience... People have thoughts and nightmares they experience alone. They want to isolate...*	**LIVING WITH SOMEONE WITH PTSD** *I didn't experience a childhood... I would give up going to a friend's house in case Dad needed me.*
HOW PTSD AFFECTS THE PEOPLE YOU LOVE *My daughter would ask, 'Mommy, why is Daddy crying?'*	**HOW TO KNOW YOU'RE READY FOR HELP** *Have the worst time sleeping, they isolate the most, have no relationships, extremely on edge all the time...*	**THE SIGNS THAT I SAW** *He wouldn't converse with me as much, he was a little distant, his temper...*
WHY I DIDN'T ASK FOR HELP RIGHT AWAY *I didn't think she [my therapist] could relate to what I had been exposed to...*	**WHAT TREATMENT IS LIKE** *People are asked to sort of get used to the things that are bothering them the most...*	**HOW PTSD AFFECTS A FAMILY** *When I got older, he would start isolating himself... I would talk "at him" without him saying anything.*
WHEN I KNEW I NEEDED HELP *I heard about Gulf War Vets not being able to sleep, etc. I thought "Wow, that's some of the symptoms I have."*	**WHAT TREATMENT CAN DO FOR YOU** *Set goals and target treatment to those goals. If Veteran wants to get rid of nightmares, use exposure...*	**THE HARDEST PART** *PTSD made him shelter me a lot...I couldn't go to the movies on the weekend or house parties*
WHAT TREATMENT WAS LIKE FOR ME *My homework was to go into the Walmart or crowded mall for 30-45 minutes.*	**QUESTIONS WE'VE BEEN ASKED** *Does my family have to be involved?*	**HOW TREATMENT CHANGED THINGS** *We don't argue as much. He's a different person, and I like it. He's happier and taking care of himself.*
HOW TREATMENT HELPS ME *I still have PTSD, but I'm in control of it now... I'm at peace with it, and I can talk about it [the trauma].*		
MY ADVICE TO YOU *They [the therapists] are waiting for Veterans like you and I. Try it. You won't regret it.*	**MY ADVICE TO YOU** *You really want a treatment that involves some type of exposure...*	**MY ADVICE TO YOU** *Support them [the family member] and let them know you're there for them. Most importantly - listen.*

a usability testing phase and (2) a pilot randomized controlled trial phase to explore the feasibility of incorporating *AboutFace* into a specialized outpatient clinic for PTSD (Hamblen et al., 2018). Twenty veterans participated in the usability testing phase in which they answered moderator posed questions regarding *About Face* while actively exploring the website. Sixty veterans participated in the pilot study after completing a PTSD clinic evaluation and were randomized to receive an educational booklet about PTSD treatment or to *AboutFace* prior to starting treatment. Stigma and attitudes about treatment seeking were assessed at baseline and two weeks later. Our results indicated that Veterans had positive attitudes about *AboutFace* and gave suggestions for improvement. Veterans in both conditions reported improved attitudes towards mental illness from baseline to the two-week follow-up. Future directions will include a large-scale randomized controlled trial to evaluate the efficacy and preliminary effectiveness of *AboutFace*.

Firefighters Helping Firefighters: A Digital Storytelling Resource for Firefighters

Based on the context of their job duties, firefighters are often faced with multiple and repeated life-threatening duties including direct fire, witnessed violence and human suffering, and sometimes death, which have significant impact on their physical and psychological well-being (Berninger et al., 2010; de Borros, Martins, Saitiz, Batos, & Ronzani, 2013; Mitani, Fujita, Nakata, & Shirakawa, 2006; Norwood & Rascati, 2012). Thus, firefighters are at elevated risk for trauma-related consequences such as PTSD, sleep disorders, suicide, depression and alcohol abuse (de Barros et al., 2013; Laposa & Alden, 2003; Stanley, Hom, Hagan, & Joiner, 2015); all of these disorders are in turn associated with high levels of distress, functional impairment, and morbidity and mortality. However, mental health treatment seeking among firefighters remains strikingly low; most firefighters with mental health problems do not seek mental health services (Gist et al., 2011). A primary hypothesis for this is stigma, which is frequently reported as a barrier to seeking treatment (see Clement et al., 2015; Gulliver et al., 2010 for two reviews), especially among firefighters (Del Ben et al., 2006). Specifically, firefighters report significant reluctance to discuss stress and mental health problems with coworkers, peers, and family members (Antonellis & Thompson, 2012; Norwood & Rascati, 2012), as they may be seen as a sign of weakness, vulnerability, and failure (Henderson, Van Hasselt, LeDuc, & Couwels, 2016). Further, stigma may be even more problematic among firefighters and other emergency response professionals who perceive that disclosing mental illness could negatively impact their fire service career.

Firefighters Helping Firefighters (FHF), is a video-storytelling resource that provides peer education through a video library of over 250 personal stories from firefighters and support personnel intended to reduce stigma and improve readiness to seek behavioral health care when needed. It was developed by the Technology Applications Center for Healthful Lifestyles and the National Crime Victims Research and Treatment Center at the Medical University of South Carolina, in partnership with the National Fallen Firefighters Foundation. *FHF* is committed to improving the lives of fire service members who are experiencing common behavioral health problems associated with occupational stress, such as symptoms of PTSD, depression, or anxiety. On this site, members of the fire service can learn about common behavioral health problems, discover treatment options, and hear firsthand from other fire service members as well as fire service supervisors. More specifically, *FHF* visitors have access to real life examples from fellow firefighters about the effects of stress on themselves as well as their families, various ways they tried to cope with this stress, how they knew it was time to ask for help and the types of help they considered, what getting help was like for them, and what advice and recommendations they have for other firefighters who are struggling, yet are reluctant to seek help. Similar to *AboutFace, FHF* has an open format that allows visitors to navigate the site freely by selecting what discussion topic they would like to hear and from which firefighter or support personnel. Topics addressed in the brief (~1 minute) clips are included in Table 2.

CONCLUSION

Individual and societal costs of stigmatized mental health disorders, such as PTSD, anxiety depression, suicidality, and alcohol abuse are enormous, and evidence based treatments are available to address these behavioral health problems. Benefits from career preservation, enhanced productivity, and improved quality of life are immeasurable if treatment can be accepted earlier and seen through to completion. Education may assist in addressing stigma (Dickstein et al., 2010; Finkelstein, Lapshin, & Wasserman, 2008), as well as knowledge, attitudes toward seeking mental health treatment, and service utilization (Corrigan, 2004; Pinfold et al., 2003). Education that is delivered by peers who give first-hand accounts of their experiences may be particularly effective in accomplishing these goals. Uniquely, peer education delivered via DST is a low-cost, scalable, and sustainable aid to such efforts. In this chapter, we presented two digital-storytelling resources that can serve as a model for researchers seeking to develop and/or improve other web/smartphone-based DST

Table 2. Firefighters Helping Firefighters clips

CLIPS OF FIREFIGHTERS	CLIPS OF SUPERVISORS
WHAT IS THE MOST STRESSFUL PART OF YOUR JOB? *"You get comfortable in your job and then …something happens…Everything you see in the movies… flashbacks… it's all true"*	**WHAT UNIQUE STRESSORS DO FIREFIGHTERS FACE?** *"…having a lot of different calls. We call it the Big Four: any call involving children, a mass casualty, and threat of death or injury to themselves or another firefighter"*
ARE THERE ANY PARTICULAR STRESSFUL EXPERIENCES THAT STAND OUT TO YOU? *"I was trapped in a fire and I had to be pulled out. In that 5 minutes and 18 seconds, you know, you thought you were going to die"*	**HAVE FAMILIES OF FIREFIGHTER EVER REACHED OUT TO YOU IN REGARD TO SYMPTOMS?** *"I've had some family members reach out to me, especially after they know the symptoms of stress…we encourage firefighters to talk with their families…"*
HOW DO YOU KNOW WHEN YOU ARE STRESSED? *"When I lose sleep, I love to sleep, but when I know I'm waking up at night, my body lets me know through that …"*	**WHAT ARE SOME COMMON THINGS YOU HAVE SEEN FIREFIGHTERS DO WHEN THEY ARE STRESSED?** *"… A lot of times Firefighters withdraw from their families and fellow firefighters… become isolated and unfortunately go into depression sometimes…"*
HOW DOES STRESS AFFECT YOUR FRIENDS AND FAMILY? *"I would distance myself from my wife and kids… because I didn't want them to see me in that type of stress"*	**HOW DOES STRESS AFFECT THEIR FAMILY OR FRIENDS?** *"… .they feel left out, sometimes they feel anxious like they've done something wrong to affect the firefighter"*
HOW DID YOU KNOW YOU NEEDED HELP? *"After probably the third night without sleep, with all the flashbacks… I was taking it out on my wife and kids"*	**HOW DOES A FIREFIGHTER KNOW THAT THEY NEED HELP?** *"A lot of times the firefighter don't necessarily know … talking to someone is the best way to get help."*
WHAT TYPE OF HELP DID YOU CONSIDER GETTING? *"I went to a chief who was trapped in a fire one time and got burnt also … if it wasn't for him, I probably wouldn't be sitting here in front of you. He took me to [a program called] SAVE"*	**WHAT STEPS WOULD A FIREFIGHTER TAKE TO GET HELP?** *"Like a chain of command… go to that person that you trust… we have a support group we go to… have that person know not to be afraid to ask for help"*
WAS HELP WHAT YOU EXPECTED? *"It took time, but after a few sessions, it took that burden right off my shoulders"*	**WHAT CHANGES HAVE YOU SEEN AFTER PEOPLE SEEK HELP?** *"I've seen firefighters be reunited with their families in a whole sense…and see them grow back together as a family"*
WHAT WOULD YOU TELL OTHERS WHO ARE IN A SIMILAR SITUATION? *"I would tell them my story. Let them know that it's okay…we'll get help. It helped me and it will help you"*	**WHAT WOULD YOU RECOMMEND TO FIREFIGHTERS WHO ARE THINKING ABOUT SEEKING HELP?** *"To do it. Talk to somebody, reach out to peer, a family member, someone in your department that you trust, and talk."*

resources to improve relevance, interest, and effectiveness in decreasing stigma. Promisingly, this can be accomplished on both the disease (e.g., HIV, diabetes, obesity, and eating disorders) and demographic (e.g., Veterans, civilians, and first responders) level. The use of a peer-to-peer approach through digital storytelling is innovative, relevant to a wide range of healthcare conditions, and has the potential to increase access to care through trusted narratives that promote hope in recovery. Further research is needed to measure that short and long-term value of digital storytelling approaches toward addressing stigma and increasing motivation to initiate and follow-through with mental health treatment. If found valuable, DST is a scalable and sustainable approach for that can used with a wide range of traumatic stress populations (e.g., disaster victims, traumatic injury patients, first responders) to reduce attitudinal barriers and increase access to care.

REFERENCES

Anderson, K. M., & Wallace, B. (2015). Digital storytelling as a trauma narrative intervention for children exposed to domestic violence. *Film and video-based therapy*, 95-107.

Bahora, M., Hanafi, S., Chien, V. H., & Compton, M. T. (2008). Preliminary evidence of effects of crisis intervention team training on self-efficacy and social distance. *Administration and Policy in Mental Health*, *35*(3), 159–167. doi:10.100710488-007-0153-8 PMID:18040771

Beltran, R. O., Scanlan, J. N., Hancock, N., & Luckett, T. (2007). The effect of first year mental health fieldwork on attitudes of occupational therapy students towards people with mental illness. *Australian Occupational Therapy Journal*, *54*(1), 42–48.

Berninger, A., Webber, M. P., Cohen, H. W., Gustave, J., Lee, R., Niles, J. K., ... Prezant, D. J. (2010). Trends of elevated PTSD risk in firefighters exposed to the World Trade Center disaster: 2001–2005. *Public Health Reports*, *125*(4), 556–566. doi:10.1177/003335491012500411 PMID:20597456

Blow, A. J., Gorman, L., Ganoczy, D., Kees, M., Kashy, D. A., Valenstein, M., ... Chermack, S. (2013). Hazardous drinking and family functioning in National Guard veterans and spouses postdeployment. *Journal of Family Psychology*, *27*(2), 303–313. doi:10.1037/a0031881 PMID:23544925

Bunnell, B. E., Davidson, T. M., Hamblen, J. L., Cook, D. L., Grubaugh, A. L., Lozano, B. E., ... & Ruggiero, K. J. (2017). Protocol for the evaluation of a digital storytelling approach to address stigma and improve readiness to seek services among veterans. *Pilot and Feasibility Studies, 3*(1), 7.

Clement, S., Schauman, O., Graham, T., Maggioni, F., Evans-Lacko, S., Bezborodovs, N., ... Thornicroft, G. (2015). What is the impact of mental health-related stigma on help-seeking? A systematic review of quantitative and qualitative studies. *Psychological Medicine, 45*(1), 11–27. doi:10.1017/S0033291714000129 PMID:24569086

Cohen, B. E., Gima, K., Bertenthal, D., Kim, S., Marmar, C. R., & Seal, K. H. (2010). Mental health diagnoses and utilization of VA non-mental health medical services among returning Iraq and Afghanistan Veterans. *Journal of General Internal Medicine, 25*(1), 18–24. doi:10.100711606-009-1117-3 PMID:19787409

Conner, K. O., McKinnon, S. A., Ward, C. J., Reynolds, C. F. III, & Brown, C. (2015). Peer education as a strategy for reducing internalized stigma among depressed older adults. *Psychiatric Rehabilitation Journal, 38*(2), 186–193. doi:10.1037/prj0000109 PMID:25915057

Corrigan, P. (2004). How stigma interferes with mental health care. *The American Psychologist, 59*(7), 614–625. doi:10.1037/0003-066X.59.7.614 PMID:15491256

Corrigan, P., & Gelb, B. (2006). Three programs that use mass approaches to challenge the stigma of mental illness. *Psychiatric Services (Washington, D.C.), 57*(3), 393–398. doi:10.1176/appi.ps.57.3.393 PMID:16524999

Corrigan, P. W. (2011). Best practices: Strategic stigma change (SSC): Five principles for social marketing campaigns to reduce stigma. *Psychiatric Services (Washington, D.C.), 62*(8), 824–826. doi:10.1176/ps.62.8.pss6208_0824 PMID:21807820

de Barros, V. V., Martins, L., Saitz, R., Bastos, R. R., & Ronzani, T. (2013). Mental health conditions, individual and job characteristics and sleep disturbances among firefighters. *Journal of Health Psychology, 18*(3), 350–358. doi:10.1177/1359105312443402 PMID:22517948

Dickstein, B. D., Vogt, D. S., Handa, S., & Litz, B. T. (2010). Targeting self-stigma in returning military personnel and veterans: A review of intervention strategies. *Military Psychology, 22*(2), 224–236. doi:10.1080/08995600903417399

Dohrenwend, B. P., Turner, J. B., Turse, N. A., Adams, B. G., Koenen, K. C., & Marshall, R. (2006). The psychological risks of Vietnam for US veterans: A revisit with new data and methods. *Science, 313*(5789), 979–982. doi:10.1126cience.1128944 PMID:16917066

Finkelstein, J., Lapshin, O., & Wasserman, E. (2008). Randomized study of different anti-stigma media. *Patient Education and Counseling, 71*(2), 204–214. doi:10.1016/j. pec.2008.01.002 PMID:18289823

Gist, R., Taylor, V. H., & Raak, S. (2011). *Suicide surveillance, preven- tion, and intervention measures for the US Fire Service: Findings and recommendations for the Suicide and Depression Summit* [White paper]. Retrieved from http:// lifesafetyinitiatives.com/13/suicide_whitepaper .pdf

Goodman, R., & Newman, D. (2014). Testing a digital storytelling intervention to reduce stress in adolescent females. *Storytelling, Self, Society, 10*(2), 177–193. do i:10.13110torselfsoci.10.2.0177

Gulliver, A., Griffiths, K. M., & Christensen, H. (2010). Perceived barriers and facilitators to mental health help-seeking in young people: A systematic review. *BMC Psychiatry, 10*(1), 113. doi:10.1186/1471-244X-10-113 PMID:21192795

Haigh, C., & Hardy, P. (2011). Tell me a story—a conceptual exploration of storytelling in healthcare education. *Nurse Education Today, 31*(4), 408–411. doi:10.1016/j. nedt.2010.08.001 PMID:20810195

Hamblen, J., Grubaugh, A., Davidson, T. M., Borkman, A. L., Bunnell, B., Tuerk, P. W., & Ruggiero, K. J. (2018). A feasibility and pilot evaluation of an online peer-to-peer educational campaign to reduce stigma and improve help seeking in veterans with PTSD. *Telemedicine and eHealth.*

Han, B., Hedden, S. L., Lipari, R., Copello, E. A. P., & Kroutil, L. A. (2015). *Receipt of services for behavioral health problems: results from the 2014 National Survey on Drug Use and Health.* Rockville, MD: Substance Abuse and Mental Health Services Administration.

Hedden, S. L., Kenner, J., Lipari, R., Medley, G., Tice, P., Copello, E. A. P., & Kroutil, L. A. (2015). *Behavioral health trends in the United States: Results from the 2014 National Survey on Drug Use and Health.* Rockville, MD: Center for Behavioral Statistics and Quality, Substance Abuse and Mental Health Services Administration.

Hoge, C. W., Auchterlonie, J., & Milliken, C. (2006). Mental health problems, use of mental health services, attrition from military service after returning from deployment to Iraq or Afghanistan. *Journal of the American Medical Association, 295*(9), 1023–1032. doi:10.1001/jama.295.9.1023 PMID:16507803

Hoge, C. W., Castro, C. A., Messer, S. C., McGurk, D., Cotting, D. I., & Koffman, R. L. (2004). Combat duty in Iraq and Afghanistan, mental health, barriers to care. *The New England Journal of Medicine, 351*(1), 13–22. doi:10.1056/NEJMoa040603 PMID:15229303

Kessler, R. C., Berglund, P. A., Bruce, M. L., Koch, J. R., Laska, E. M., Leaf, P. J., ... Wang, P. S. (2001). The prevalence and correlates of untreated serious mental illness. *Health Services Research, 36*(6 Pt 1), 987. PMID:11775672

Kim, P. Y., Thomas, J. L., Wilk, J. E., Castro, C. A., & Hoge, C. W. (2010). Stigma, barriers to care, and use of mental health services among active duty and National Guard soldiers after combat. *Psychiatric Services (Washington, D.C.), 61*(6), 582–588. doi:10.1176/ps.2010.61.6.582 PMID:20513681

Kok, B. C., Herrell, R. K., Thomas, J. L., & Hoge, C. W. (2012). Posttraumatic stress disorder associated with combat service in Iraq or Afghanistan: Reconciling prevalence differences between studies. *The Journal of Nervous and Mental Disease, 200*(5), 444–450. doi:10.1097/NMD.0b013e3182532312 PMID:22551799

Laposa, J. M., & Alden, L. E. (2003). Posttraumatic stress disorder in the emergency room: Exploration of a cognitive model. *Behaviour Research and Therapy, 41*(1), 49–65. doi:10.1016/S0005-7967(01)00123-1 PMID:12488119

Mahat, G., Ann Scoloveno, M., & Ayres, C. (2011). HIV/AIDS knowledge and self-efficacy among Nepalese adolescents: A peer education program. *Research and Theory for Nursing Practice, 25*(4), 271–283. doi:10.1891/1541-6577.25.4.271 PMID:22329081

Medley, A., Kennedy, C., O'Reilly, K., & Sweat, M. (2009). Effectiveness of peer education interventions for HIV prevention in developing countries: A systematic review and meta-analysis. *AIDS Education and Prevention, 21*(3), 181–206. doi:10.1521/aeap.2009.21.3.181 PMID:19519235

Mitani, S., Fujita, M., Nakata, K., & Shirakawa, T. (2006). Impact of post-traumatic stress disorder and job-related stress on burnout: A study of fire service workers. *The Journal of Emergency Medicine, 31*(1), 7–11. doi:10.1016/j.jemermed.2005.08.008 PMID:16798146

Naslund, J. A., Aschbrenner, K. A., Marsch, L. A., & Bartels, S. J. (2016). The future of mental health care: Peer-to-peer support and social media. *Epidemiology and Psychiatric Sciences*, *25*(02), 113–122. doi:10.1017/S2045796015001067 PMID:26744309

Norwood, P., & Rascati, J. (2012). Recognizing and combating firefighter stress. *Fire Engineering*, *165*, 87–90.

Pinfold, V., Toulmin, H., Thornicroft, G., Huxley, P., Farmer, P., & Graham, T. (2003). Reducing psychiatric stigma and discrimination: Evaluation of educational interventions in UK secondary schools. *The British Journal of Psychiatry*, *182*(4), 342–346. doi:10.1192/bjp.182.4.342 PMID:12668411

Pinto-Foltz, M. D., Logsdon, M. C., & Myers, J. A. (2011). Feasibility, acceptability, and initial efficacy of a knowledge-contact program to reduce mental illness stigma and improve mental health literacy in adolescents. *Social Science & Medicine*, *72*(12), 2011–2019. doi:10.1016/j.socscimed.2011.04.006 PMID:21624729

Robin, B. R. (2008). Digital storytelling: A powerful technology tool for the 21st century classroom. *Theory into Practice*, *47*(3), 220–228. doi:10.1080/00405840802153916

Stanley, I. H., Hom, M. A., Hagan, C. R., & Joiner, T. E. (2015). Career prevalence and correlates of suicidal thoughts and behaviors among firefighters. *Journal of Affective Disorders*, *187*, 163–171. doi:10.1016/j.jad.2015.08.007 PMID:26339926

Wagner, S. L., McFee, J. A., & Martin, C. A. (2010). Mental health implications of fire service membership. *Traumatology*, *16*(2), 26–32. doi:10.1177/1534765610362803

White, S., Park, Y. S., Israel, T., & Cordero, E. D. (2009). Longitudinal evaluation of peer health education on a college campus: Impact on health behaviors. *Journal of American College Health*, *57*(5), 497–506. doi:10.3200/JACH.57.5.497-506 PMID:19254890

Yang, Y. T. C., & Wu, W. C. I. (2012). Digital storytelling for enhancing student academic achievement, critical thinking, and learning motivation: A year-long experimental study. *Computers & Education*, *59*(2), 339–352. doi:10.1016/j.compedu.2011.12.012

Chapter 8
Special Issue:
Sexually Transmitted Infections – Diagnoses, Stigma, and Mental Health

Sara Bender
Central Washington University, USA

Karlie Hill
Central Washington University, USA

ABSTRACT

Misconceptions regarding the cause(s) of sexually transmitted infections (STIs) has led to a number of prejudices against those with such diagnoses. A fear of being the object of prejudicial attitudes and behaviors leaves many individuals concerned about the social stigma of a STI diagnosis. This, in turn, may leave people unwilling to get tested or hesitant to disclose their diagnosis to others, which may fuel the spread of such infections. In addition to the numerous medical concerns associated with STIs, the psychological consequences of STIs are notable as well. Understanding the stigma related to STIs is an important step towards improving the mental health of people with such diagnoses. This chapter provides the reader with an overview of STI diagnoses, and an explanation of their physical and mental health consequences. The chapter continues by examining the three types of stigma as well as their components. Finally, the chapter offers a number of suggestions regarding how to combat STI stigma, which may be extrapolated to combat other forms of stigma affecting mental health.

DOI: 10.4018/978-1-5225-3808-0.ch008

INTRODUCTION

According to the Center for Disease Control (CDC) (2016), there were 1,526,658 cases of chlamydia, 395,216 cases of gonorrhea, 23,872 cases of primary and secondary syphilis, and 487 cases of congenital syphilis reported in United States in 2015. These figures, which only include a small fraction of potential sexually transmitted infections (STIs), represent a substantial increase in reported diagnoses from the previous reporting period (2014), suggesting that the transmission of sexually transmitted infections (STIs) is on the rise. What is interesting about these figures is that they paint only a part of the picture. The CDC relies on the reports of local health authorities and other public reports to gather its data. As such, these figures are estimates, at best, and likely greatly underrepresent the STI epidemic plaguing the country. The fact is that many cases of chlamydia, gonorrhea, and syphilis go undiagnosed and/or unreported. Further, data on other STIs, such as herpes simplex virus, trichomoniasis, and human papillomavirus, are not routinely reported at the national level. As such, information regarding the pervasiveness of the current STI epidemic is based on estimates. In 2016, the CDC estimated that approximately 20 million new cases of sexually transmitted infections occur every year within the United States (CDC, 2016).

While the exact prevalence of STIs are unknown, their impact is evident. Research indicates that STI diagnoses influence people's short-term and long-term physical health and often impacts their mental health statuses as well. Additionally, STIs also contribute to a number of burdens that broadly impact society as a whole, including compromised productivity as well as economic outcomes (CDC, 2016). In 2016, the CDC estimated that the country spends over $16 billion in health care costs related to STIs (CDC). Despite these known effects, trends in the data suggest that many people remain resistant to pursuing adequate testing and/or treatment for possible STIs due to their concerns regarding the stigma of having such diagnoses (Foster & Byers, 2008). This resistance may not only compromise the health of the individual with the STI, but also has the potential to negatively impact his or her current and future sexual partners.

There remain a number of misnomers regarding STIs, including information regarding the manner in which they are contracted as well as their treatability. This misinformation may lead individuals with potential or confirmed STI diagnoses undue stress, which may compromise their overall mental health functioning. It likely also aids in the further perpetuation of inaccurate myths and subsequent stigma regarding sexuality and reproductive health.

The goals of this chapter are to:

1. Introduce the reader to the effects of a STI diagnosis and the consequences of non-disclosure,
2. Explain the types of stigma typically associated with STI diagnoses as well as their components,
3. Explore how STI stigma compares to other forms of stigma affecting wellness, and
4. Review strategies to reduce stigma

By the end of this chapter, readers will better understand the impact of stigma as it relates to sexually transmitted infection diagnoses and associated mental health functioning. Understanding the nature of STI stigma will provide insight into the nature of stigma, as a whole, thus allowing the reader to further deconstruct the stigma of mental health specifically. The ability to more fully understand the nature of stigma will allow advocates an increased capacity to combat it effectively.

BACKGROUND

Physical and Psychological Effects of an STI Diagnosis

There are over 20 different types of viruses known to be transmitted via sexual contact (NICHD, 2017). Of these, the most common include: chlamydia, gonorrhea, syphilis, herpes, HIV/AIDs, human papillomavirus (HPV), bacterial vaginosis, and viral hepatitis. While each variable in the display of its specific symptoms, STIs may have a profound impact on a person's physical health. For example, chlamydia, an infection that may spread via oral, anal, or vaginal sex, may lead to a variety of symptoms. Some with the infection will experience no symptoms while others will experience high fevers, abdominal pain, and unusual genital discharge. Chlamydia may also cause a woman to develop pelvic inflammatory disease (PID), which, if it develops, can lead permanent damage to her reproductive organs and lead to infertility. Further, there is an increased risk to the health of the fetus of women pregnant whom have this infection (NICHD).

Gonorrhea symptoms most typically include genital discharge and/or painful urination. Like chlamydia, this infection is spread via genital, anal, and oral contact and may also result in PID and its associated consequences. Research indicates that gonorrhea can spread to multiple parts of the body and eventually become a life-threatening illness. This diagnosis may also place an individual at an increased risk of contracting other STIs, such as HIV (NICHD, 2017).

Syphilis is also spread via oral, anal, or vaginal sex. Its most recognizable symptom includes painless genital sores. If left untreated, this infection may involve other organs of the body, including skin, blood vessels, the liver, and bones. Over a period of years, the infection may further spread to involve the nerves, eyes, and brain, often leading to death. Mothers carrying the infection may spread it to their fetuses, which could result in miscarriage, stillbirths, or a number of other birth deformities. Additionally, research indicates that those with syphilis are two to five times more likely to contract the HIV virus (NICHD, 2017).

There are two types of herpes, which is caused by the herpes simplex virus (HSV). This virus is typically spread via genital, anal, or oral contact. Herpes leads to the development of painful blisters, which typically appear around the genitals or anus. Fever blisters or cold sores may also develop on the lips as well. While some people with this infection may remain asymptomatic, the virus is incredibly easy to spread. Like many other STIs, herpes poses great risk to the unborn fetuses of women whom are infected (NICHD, 2017).

The human immunodeficiency virus (HIV) may lead to the development of acquired immunodeficiency syndrome) (AIDS). HIV attacks a person's immune system by killing the blood cells that fight infection, leaving those infected with the virus particularly susceptible to further illness. A few decades ago, the presence of the HIV virus would typically mean almost uncertain death, however recent research has led to a number of functional cures for the virus. Further, increased sexual education has helped curb the spread of this virus (NICHD, 2017).

The most common STI at this time is human papillomavirus (HPV). Thus far, research indicates that there are over 40 variations of this virus, which commonly lead to infections throughout the body, the development of genital warts, and the growth of certain cancers. As with HIV, scientists have developed some medical interventions aimed at minimizing the prevention of HPV, including effective screening procedures to identify the presence of the virus as well as an immunization against it (NICHD, 2017).

Women are susceptible to bacterial vaginosis, a vaginal infection that is thought to be sexually transmitted. While the symptoms associated with this particular infection tend to be minimal, its presence is of concern as it puts women at increased risk of contracting other STIs, PID, and suffering from compromised reproductive health (NICHD, 2017).

Viral hepatitis results from one of several viruses that are typically transmitted through sexual contact, exposure to infected needles, exposure during birth, or exposure to infected blood. This infection results in a serious liver disease. There are several forms of the infection. Hepatitis A typically results in a serious, but short-term liver infection. Another form of the virus, Hepatitis B, is a serious liver disease that can result in urgent illness as well as well chronic infection, which can lead to death. Like Hepatitis B, Hepatitis C can result in an immediate illness or a more chronic infection of the liver, which can contribute to one's death. Vaccination is said to help prevent the spread of Hepatitis A and B, but there is no cure or prevention for Hepatitis C (NICHD, 2017).

MAIN FOCUS OF THE CHAPTER

Issues, Controversies, Problems

Collectively, the research pertaining to these STIs indicates that they can lead to acute infection (NICHD, 2017), chronic pain (CDC, 2016), severe reproductive health obstacles, including infertility and pregnancy complications (CDC), or even death (NICHD, 2017). As such the prevalence of and efforts to prevent these infections should not be taken lightly. Luckily, as medical science has expanded so too has our understanding regarding the very nature of these infections. Medical interventions, including a number of immunizations and antibiotics, are now available to help prevent and/or combat the symptoms of these illnesses.

The impacts of STIs are not limited to physical health, however. STI diagnoses may also have a notable impact on one's mental health presentation as well. Past research confirms that those diagnosed with one or more STI diagnoses are likely to experience embarrassment, anxiety, shame, and fear both sexual and social rejection (Darroch, Myers, & Cassell, 2003; Duncan, Hart, Scoular, & Birgrigg, 2001; Osborn, King, & Weir, 2002). STI diagnoses are also correlated with depressive symptoms (Chen, Wu, Yi, Huang, & Wong, 2008; Khan et al., 2009) as well as symptoms of anxiety (Arkell, Osborn, Ivens, & King, 2006) and increased suicidal gestures (Badiee, Moore, Atkinson, Vaida, Gerard, & Duarte, 2012).

Disclosure and Non-Disclosure

There are a number of reasons a person may choose not to disclose his or her STI diagnosis to others. More often than not, the primary reason is to avoid stigma (Lichenstein, Neal, & Brodsky, 2008). Past research confirms that internalized stigma and the potential for treatment stigma often lead people to avoid seeking help for their STI-related symptoms. More specifically, people endorse concern regarding the confidentiality of their diagnosis status as a main treatment-seeking barrier (Clement, Shauman, Graham & Maggioni, 2015). Concerns regarding others' external stigma, which is often rooted in religious and cultural expectations, leads many people to avoid disclosure primarily due to the fear of social judgement, and, in some cases, fear for personal safety (Kingori, Ice, Hassan, Elmi, & Perko, 2016). Non-disclosure has several potential effects. First, it may exacerbate the cognitive and emotional toll of the diagnosis itself, causing increased stress, shame, and discomfort to the individual. Further, the failure to disclose one's symptoms to parents, medical providers, and others affecting one's healthcare may prevent access to effective treatment, which could actually help minimize symptoms and/ or prevent the infection from further developing.

The impact of an STI is not limited to the person diagnosed. In addition to the many social consequences of such infections, including high medical costs, compromised productivity in the workplace, and similar circumstances, one's sexual health also affects his or her current or future sexual partners. Individuals who learn of their partners' STI diagnosis may need to reconsider sexual practices, including what activities to engage in and to what extent as to reduce their own chances of infection. Additionally, increased protection, such as the use of condoms, may be warranted. Of course, learning of a partner's STI status after exposure may also have psychological consequences as well. Bender and Hill (2017) conducted a phenomenological study, which reveals that partners often wonder about their partners' level of sexual responsibility, commitment to their relationship, and monogamy practices secondary to learning of their partners' STI diagnoses. This, in turn, often creates situations in which the partner of the person infected experiences heightened levels of psychological distress, including anxiety, anger, and depression. Given the potential for conflict with one's partner and/or the prospect of being denied sexual intimacy, it may be tempting for some people to not disclose their STI diagnoses with their partners. Failure to disclose such diagnoses leaves the partner at an increased vulnerability to future infections and associated medical complications.

Defining Stigma

The definition of stigma is inconsistent within the literature. Most explanations of the concept refer back, in some form, to the word's Greek origin of 'a sign or a branding mark' (Sharfestin, 2012). In his seminal book on the topic, sociologist Erving Goffman (1963) defined stigma as an 'attribute that is deeply discrediting" ultimately reducing an individual "from a whole and usual person to a tainted, discounted one" (p.3). Within his explanation, Goffman (1963) highlighted three categories of stigma: tribal identities, body abominations, and blemishes of individual characters. Tribal identity (also referred to as 'group identity') refer to a person's group membership as determined by religion, nationality, sex, race, and similar characteristics. Body abominations refer to physical deformities. Finally, blemishes of individual characters refer to circumstances such as the presence of a mental health diagnosis, unemployment, addiction, etc. Each of the categories, according to Goffman, renders those with them as distinct from those whom do not have them, thus paving the way for prejudicial attitudes and subsequent discriminatory practices to occur. Goffman explained, "By definition, we believe the person with a stigma is not quite human" (p. 5). Within this framework, stigma devalues the individual and excludes him or her from societal acceptance (Goffman).

Jones and colleagues (1984) suggested that there are six stigmatizing dimensions that fuel the separation between a 'usual person' and a 'discounted one' (Goffman, 1963, p. 3). These dimensions include: Whether the stigma is visible vs. concealable, the perceived origin of the condition, the aesthetics of the condition, whether or not the condition is viewed as perilous or not, whether or not the condition is likely to be disruptive to ongoing social interaction, and the projected course of the condition over time.

Explaining Stigma

Social scientists have not only struggled to define stigma, but also to explain it. There are a number of psychological and sociological theories that help describe this phenomenon. Corrigan (2004) suggest that three paradigms exist, which help explain stigma. First, the social cultural perspective suggests that stigmas form to substantiate prevailing social injustices. The paradigm of motivational biases suggest that stigmas develop secondary to meeting basic psychological needs. Finally, social cognitive theories suggest that stigmas result as the consequence of human information processing. Of these three paradigms, the social cognitive theories are most widely accepted. They are said to be the most theoretically rich and best supported empirically out of the three.

Social cognitive theories recognize that people engage in a number of heuristics, which allow them to quickly categorize individuals into groups (Dovidio et al, 2011; Kahneman, 2011). While a normative process, this categorization likely organically leads to prejudice and discrimination. Gordon Allport (1954) suggested that this tendency to categorize others an essential element of social life. Assigning those we encounter into categories allows us to process large volumes of information about those we encounter by filtering that data into specific classifications. Categorization also allows us to cluster that information efficiently by relying on previous assessments regarding individuals and situations that we recognize as similar. This, in turn, may also allow us increased access to emotions more easily, as we tend to develop distinct like or dislike for those things we have categorized. Finally, categorizing people also allows us to identify them with speed and efficiency. Prejudice, it is suggested, is an organic consequence of this categorization. Prejudicial beliefs, often lead to discriminatory behaviors associated with stigma.

Stigma Impact

Link and Phelan (2001) suggested that most common definitions of stigma are too simplistic due to the perspectives traditionally held by stigma researchers, which are rooted and limited by their participants' experiences, as well as the individualistic focus of the research dedicated to understanding the phenomenon. They argue that a larger cultural focus must also be considered when operationalizing stigma. Link and Pehan expand the term stigma to refer to "when the elements of labeling, stereotyping, separation, status loss, and discrimination co-occur in a power situation..." (p. 367). They assert that stigma likely serves as a "key determinant of many of the life chances...from psychological well-being to employment, housing and life itself" (382).

There are four commonly accepted manifestations of stigma, including: 1.) public stigma, which refers to people's social and psychological reactions to someone with a perceived stigma, 2.) self-stigma, which refers to how an individual reacts to the possession of a stigma, 3) stigma-by-association, or courtesy stigma, refers to the social and psychological reactions to people associated with a stigmatized person or how people react to their own associations with a stigmatized person, and 4.) institutional stigma, which essentially is the legitimatization and perpetuation of a stigmatized status by society's ideological systems and institutional practices. Each of these manifestations is likely to impact a person's wellness and functioning. Public stigma and stigma-by-association, lead to biases, negative stereotyping, and negative judgment (Kendra et al., 2014). Similarly, institutional stigmatization may lead to increased difficulties securing employment, social status, or housing (Sickel, Seacat, & Nabors, 2014). These factors may serve as barriers to treatment, contribute to increased isolation, and facilitate a variety of negative psychological effects. Further, self-stigma may impact an individual's self-esteem and opportunities (Watson, Corrigan, Larson, & Sells, 2007). All forms of felt and enacted stigma are likely to negatively affect a person's quality of life (Gerrida-Hernansaiz, Helyen, Bharat, Ramakrishna, & Ekstrand, 2016).

STI and Mental Health Stigma

STI-related stigma refers to an individual's awareness that a STI diagnosis is accompanied by a negative social judgement (Foster & Byers, 2008). Historically, the acquisition of an STI has been misattributed to deviant behavior and immorality rather than a consequence of normal sexual activity. Misperceptions regarding the cause(s) of STIs has led to a number of prejudicial attitudes and beliefs against those with such diagnoses. A fear of being the object of prejudicial attitudes and corresponding behaviors leaves many individuals concerned about the social implications and general stigma of such diagnoses. This fear of social stigma secondary to a STI diagnosis leads a high proportion of people unwilling to get tested for STIs and/or to disclose their confirmed diagnoses. This, of course, not only compromises their own health, but also increases the likely transmission of STIs to others, further fueling the STI epidemic.

There are three components of STI stigma, including: shame, sexual anxiety and social desirability. STI-related shame is a "negative affect that an individual experiences as a result of internalizing stigma" (Foster & Byers, 2008, 194). This relates to feelings of immorality and often leads people to think of themselves and themselves as "dirty". Secondary to this label of being 'dirty' due to their diagnosis, those suffering experiencing shame related to the STIs assume that they will be viewed negatively by others (Foster & Byers). Foster and Byers (2008) found that those who reported higher levels of shame were less likely to get tested for STIs and less likely to disclose their diagnosis; again, risking their future health and that of those with whom they are sexually intimate.

While the shame associated with having a STI may affect anyone at any time, research suggests that it is especially prevalent among women. East and colleagues (2011) report that women typically attribute other women's STI diagnoses as a consequence of promiscuity or sexual deviance. This perspective changes, however, when women receive a STI diagnosis themselves. Instead, the literature suggests that women in such scenarios shift their perspectives to internalize new feelings of self-blame and denial, which lead to shame. This shame is often experienced at a deep personal level upon the time of diagnosis and may cause physical and psychological burdens on the individual, which, in turn, places pressure and strain on intimate relationships (East et al., 2011). Research also suggests that there is a positive correlation between sexual conservatism and dissatisfaction with school-based sexual education with high levels of shame due to STI diagnoses (Foster & Byers, 2008).

The second component of STI stigma, sexual anxiety, occurs when a person fears sexual rejection secondary to his or her STI diagnosis. Sexual anxiety is category of sexual dysfunctions, defined as persistent impairment of sexual interest or response cycle. This dysfunction can be physiological or psychological (Adekeye, Sheikh, & Adekeye, 2012). It can create biological and interpersonal conflicts, and can be affected by stress, emotional disorders, ignorance of sexual function, and basic physiology (Adekeye, Sheikh, & Adekeye). Foster and Byers (2008) determined that people with more traditional values are more likely to associate STIs with stigma and shame and are more likely to experience sexual anxiety (Foster & Byers). This sexual anxiety, in turn, may facilitate lower levels of sexual pleasure and satisfaction (Brassard, Dupuy, Bergeron, & Shaver, 2013).

Social Desirability Theory indicates that humans retain an innate desire to please and be accepted by others. Social norms, perceived negative consequences, and fear of rejection all affect social desirability. The desire to remain socially desirable, in combination with fear of rejection, leads many people to resist seeking STI testing as well as disclosing STI diagnoses (Cunningham, 2009). A fear of rejection seems to serve as the common denominator between shame, sexual anxiety, and social desirability in relation to sexuality. This fear of rejection leads many people to avoid seeking STI testing, procuring STI treatment, and disclosing STI diagnoses to their partners. Lichtenstein and colleagues (2005) found that many people reported being embarrassed regarding their STI diagnoses, which contributed to the delay or complete avoidance of treatment for the same. Barth and colleagues (2002) asserted that people sometimes also avoid pursuing initial STI testing due to their own preconceived biases regarding what a STI diagnosis might mean. In their study of undergraduate students, they found that in an effort to avoid negative emotions, deny the possibility of even having a STI, or even a simple preference to not have such a hypothesis confirmed, some individuals would not participate in STI screenings.

While the stigma associated with STI diagnoses is formidable, research demonstrates that the stigma associated with mental health diagnoses is stronger than that associated with physical health diagnoses (Corrigan, 2004). Further, the stigma associated with various mental health diagnoses seems to be further stratified by the perceived severity of dysfunction commonly allocated to a diagnoses (Stuber, Rocha, Christian, & Link, 2014). For example, those with psychotic diagnoses, such as schizophrenia, are typically evaluated more harshly than those with a more common mental health diagnosis such as depression or anxiety (Corrigan, 2004).

In line with the behaviors of those with suspected STI diagnoses, those experiencing mental health symptoms also often avoid or delay seeking clinical assistance. A systematic review of studies completed from 2008-2011 revealed that stigma was the fourth highest ranked barrier to help-seeking. Within the collection of studies reviewed, the potential to have one's mental health diagnosis revealed was the most notable stigma barrier (Clement, Shauman, Gram, & Maggioni, 2014). Via their study of undergraduate student experiences, Eisenberg, Downs, Golberstein and Zivin (2009) confirmed that perceived stigma or bias affected help-seeking behaviors. Corrigan, Druss, and Perlick (2014) also recognize mental health stigma as a primary barrier to care, but note that the dynamics involved in avoiding such treatment are not that simple. They suggest that one must also consider personal barriers (beliefs about treatment effectiveness, lack of a support network, lack of mental health literacy, etc.) and provider and system-level barriers (lack of insurance, financial constraints, staff incompetence, etc.) affecting the quest for care, too.

THE ROLE OF STIGMA IN PERPETUATING PREJUDICIAL BEHAVIORS AND DISCRIMINATION

Perpetuating Stigma

Stigma, regardless of its focus, is frequently fueled by media's attention on the negative attributes of a situation or diagnosis and via the public's subsequent understanding of the visible minority. For example, one only need to look at the coverage of mass shootings over the past decade to note the media's propensity to focus on whether or not the shooters associated with each horrific incident had some sort of mental health diagnosis. Rarely, did these outlets examine current the offender's stressors, ongoing drug abuse, extreme ideological beliefs, personal victimization, or other factors as potential root causes of their actions. Instead, more often than not, mainstream media often learned of these individuals' diagnoses and dismissed their extreme actions as the result of such diagnoses. Such conclusions fail to portray a comprehensive picture of the various intersecting factors likely propelling these offenders to such acts of horror. The news media's propensity to reduce and oversimplify the dynamics at play in these situations often portrays an inaccurate, or at very least, incomplete depiction of such events, which then leaves the consumers of this media with negative impressions regarding those with mental health issues. Further, due to their own fear of being the victims of such atrocities, those whom consume these media portrayals may feel an increased need to distance themselves from those whom they know or perceive to have a mental health diagnosis as a way to increase their perceived physical safety and in an unconscious effort to protect their own psychological safety (McGinty, Webster, & Barry, 2013). These beliefs trickle down into other areas of society as well. For example, researchers found that most employers report that they are less likely to hire someone with a known mental health diagnosis, as they assume such individuals are more likely to be absent, disengaged, dangerous, or otherwise unpredictable (Overton & Medina, 2008).

The perpetuation of mental health stigma is not the sole responsibility of a misinformed media, however. Research indicates that those within the medical profession also perpetuate stigma related to various physical and mental health diagnoses. In one study, up to 31% of patients surveyed believed that they were discriminated against by medical professionals secondary to their mental health diagnoses (Henderson, Boblett, Parke, Clement, Caffrey, & Gale-Grant, 2014). Crapanzano and Vath (2015) suggest that such discrimination could affect clinical decision making. For example, one's physical symptoms may be dismissed as a manifestation of one's mental health diagnosis, thus compromising a thorough diagnostic process or medical treatment regimen. Closely related to this, the researchers also found that medical providers who stigmatize mental health diagnoses often failed to provide appropriate referrals, were less likely to pursue inpatient hospitalization for their patients with known mental health symptoms, and also maintained the assumption that their patients with mental health diagnoses were less likely to be compliant with treatment recommendations. Corrigan (2005) asserted that the known presence of a mental health disorder may lead providers to provide substandard medical care, even if that is not the providers' intention. His conclusion echoes that of previous researchers whom concluded that those with mental health disorders rarely receive adequate treatment for their medical ailments in general practitioner environments (Wang, Demler, & Kessler, 2002).

Similarly, research indicates that some mental health professionals also maintain prejudicial ideologies pertaining to those they perceive to be 'mentally ill', which further perpetuates mental health stigma (Smith & Cahswell, 2010). Past surveys have found that individuals with mental health disorders often feel as if their mental health providers focus only on their diagnosis while dismissing them as people (Pinfold, Byrne, & Toulman, 2005). Other studies found that mental health professionals sometimes reinforce misnomers regarding the nature of mental health diagnoses by perpetuating the beliefs that the presence of a mental health diagnosis may be correlated with dangerousness or unpredictability (Kingdon, Sharmer, & Hart, 2004) or by insinuating the recovery from one's mental health symptoms is not plausible (Magliano, Fiorillo, De Rosa, Malangone, & Maj, 2004). Smith and Cahswell (2010) suggest that a lack of training and preparedness among mental health professionals sometimes contributes to their negative attitudes regarding some diagnoses. Similarly, Crowe and Averett (2015) indicate that increased educational involvement improved mental health professionals' perspectives regarding likely recovery, effectiveness of treatment, etc. This coincides with research of the general public, which indicates that the more contact one has with those diagnosed with mental health issues, the less dangerous he or she would perceive those with mental health issues to be (Penn et al., 1994).

The patterns and impact of stigma associated with mental health diagnoses is similar to stigma accompanying potential STI diagnoses. For example, via their survey of men who have sex with men, Ross, Larson, Nyoni, and Agardh (2016) found that most patients felt that their health care providers were 'impolite' regarding their symptoms, which served as a barrier to seeking further or comprehensive treatment. Researchers also found that women seeking healthcare from a public health clinic for STI-related issues felt judged by medical staff. This disapproval, it seemed, was compounded in cases in which the patients did not view their symptoms as something to be ashamed of, but rather as a normative consequence of being sexually active (Lichtenstein, 2003). Similarly, a qualitative study conducted by Scheim and Travers (2016) revealed that medical providers' lack of competency regarding gender and sexual identity issues, coupled with lack of trust for those providers, negatively affected individuals' willingness to seek STI testing and subsequent treatment. Even in the instances in which patients desired additional medical intervention for their symptoms despite their perceptions of providers' attitudes regarding their symptoms, these treatments were not always offered or provided.

CHALLENGES AND SUGGESTED SOLUTIONS

The CDC (2017) offers a comprehensive outline that serves as a national response to the current STI epidemic. It suggests that numerous parties must be engaged to effectively treat current STIs and prevent the future spread of such diseases. First, the CDC suggests that all medical providers make screening for STIs a part of their regular medical care protocol. More precisely the CDC calls for physicians to 'integrate STD prevention and treatment into prenatal care and other routine visits' (CDC, 2016, p.3). Next, the public must discuss the topics of gender, sexuality, and reproductive health. There must be an open dialogue regarding the need for those whom are sexually active to receive routine STI tests and to practice mutual monogamy and engage in contraceptive use. Further, parents and medical professional are called upon to proactively discuss the topic of sexual health with younger people to provide them with the information they need to protect themselves and potential sexual partners. Sexual health literacy, in particular, is an important step in the quest to reduce stigma. The CDC calls upon state and local health departments to allocate resources and other support to those impacted by this epidemic. Another important step in reducing stigma is to maintain interpersonal contact with those perceived to be different. Exposure to people of varying backgrounds and statuses allow each individual increased insight into the commonalities held across people making their perceived differences less threatening and more valuable. A final component to reducing stigma includes social activism. Professionals and members of the general public alike are called upon to advocate for increased attention, funding, and care towards sexual and reproductive healthcare issues (Corigan, Morris, Michale, Rafaacz, & Rush, 2012).

CONCLUSION

The aim of this chapter was to introduce the role of stigma in the identification and prevention of STI diagnoses. As the content of the chapter indicates, STIs have the potential to greatly affect one's physical health, mental health, interpersonal relationships, and overall quality of life. As such, it is imperative that individuals are aware of their STI status as not to compromise their own health or that of others. A principal reason many people avoid addressing their STI status is due to the stigma that shrouds such diagnoses. There are a number of interrelated factors that contribute to stigma, including: group identity, perceived blemishes of character, and visible deformations of the body. Collectively, these elements service to differentiate those with a designation or stigma, from those whom do not. STI stigma, specifically, seems to persist due to an intermingling of factors, including shame, sexual anxiety, and social desirability, which are deeply embedded in one's culture. Stigma contributes to the oppression of those diagnosed with STI diagnoses, often resulting in prejudicial beliefs and discriminatory acts against those with them. As with other social justice issues, the most effective advocacy efforts towards STI stigma seem to include a recognition of such circumstances, an active dialogue regarding the same, and a commitment to increased education and funding towards sexual and reproductive issues.

REFERENCES

Allport, G. W. (1954). *The nature of prejudice*. New York, NY: Perseus.

Arkell, J., Osborn, D., Ivens, D., & King, M. (2006). Factors associated with anxiety in patients attending a sexually transmitted infection clinic: Qualitative survey. *International Journal of STD & AIDS*, *17*(5), 299–303. doi:10.1258/095646206776790097 PMID:16643678

Badiee, J., Moore, D. J., Atkinson, J. H., Vaida, F., Gerard, M., Duarte, N. A., ... Grant, I. (2012). Lifetime suicidal ideation and attempt are common among HIV+ individuals. *Journal of Affective Disorders*, *136*(3), 993–999. doi:10.1016/j. jad.2011.06.044 PMID:21784531

Barth, K., Cook, R., Downs, S., Switzer, G., & Fischhoff, B. (2002). Social stigma and negative consequences: Factors that influence college students' decisions to seek testing for sexually transmitted infections. *Journal of American College Health*, *50*(4), 153–159. doi:10.1080/07448480209596021 PMID:11910948

Bender, S., & Hill, K. (2017). *The Experience of STI Exposure Discovery in the Context of Monogamous Relationships.* Manuscript in Preparation.

Center for Disease Control (CDC). (2016). *Reported STDs in the United States: 2015 National Data for Chlamydia, Gonorrhea, and Syphilis.* Retrieved from: https://www.cdc.gov/nchhstp/newsroom/2016.std-suvelliance-report

Chen, Y., Wu, J., Yi, Q., Huang, G., & Wong, T. (2008). Depression associated with sexually transmitted infection in Canada. *Sexually Transmitted Infections*, *84*(7), 535–540. doi:10.1136ti.2007.029306 PMID:18550695

Clement, S., Shauman, O., Graham, T., & Maggioni, F. (2015). What is the impact of mental health-related stigma on help-seeking? A systematic review of quantitative and qualitative studies. *Psychological Medicine*, *45*(1), 11–27. doi:10.1017/S0033291714000129 PMID:24569086

Corrigan, P. (2004). How stigma interferes with mental health care. *The American Psychologist*, *59*(7), 614–625. doi:10.1037/0003-066X.59.7.614 PMID:15491256

Corrigan, P. W., Morris, S. B., Michaels, P. J., Rafacz, J. D., & Rüsch, N. (2012). Challenging the public stigma of mental illness: A meta-analysis of outcome studies. *Psychiatric Services (Washington, D.C.)*, *63*(10), 963–973. doi:10.1176/appi.ps.201100529 PMID:23032675

Corrigan, P. W., River, L. P., Lundin, R. K., Uphoff Wasowski, K., Campion, J., Mathisen, J., & ... . (2000). Stigmatizing attributions about mental illness. *Journal of Community Psychology*, *28*(1), 91–102. doi:

Crapanzano, K., & Vath, R. J. (2015). Observations: Confronting physician attitudes towards the mentally ill: A challenge to medical educators. *Journal of Graduate Medical Education*, *7*(4), 686. doi:10.4300/JGME-D-15-00256.1 PMID:26692993

Crowe, A., & Averett, P. (2015). Attitudes of Mental Health Professionals toward Mental Illness: A Deeper Understanding. *Journal of Mental Health Counseling*, *37*(1), 47–62. doi:10.17744/mehc.37.1.l23251h783703q2v

Darroch, J., Myers, L., & Cassell, J. (2003). Sex differences in the experiences of testing positive for genital chlamydia infection: A qualitative study with implications for public health and for a national screening programme. *Sexually Transmitted Infections*, *79*(5), 372–376. doi:10.1136ti.79.5.372 PMID:14573831

Dovidio, J. R., Pagotto, L., & Hebl, M. R. (2011). Implicit attitudes and discrimination against people with disabilities. In R. L. Wiener & S. L. Wilborn (Eds.), *Disability and age discrimination: Perspectives in law and psychology* (pp. 157–184). New York, NY: Springer; doi:10.1007/978-1-4419-6293-5_9

Duncan, B., Hart, G., Scoular, A., & Bigrigg, A. (2001). Qualitative analysis of psychosocial impact of diagnosis of chlamydia trachomatis: Implication for screening. *British Medical Journal*, *27*(7280), 195–199. doi:10.1136/bmj.322.7280.195 PMID:11159612

Foster, L., & Byers, E. (2008). Predictors of stigma and shame related to sexually transmitted infections: Attitudes, education, and knowledge. *The Canadian Journal of Human Sexuality*, *17*(4), 193–202.

Garrido-Hernansaiz, H., Heylen, E., Bharat, S., Ramakrishna, J., & Ekstrand, M.L. (2016). Stigmas, symptom severity and perceived social support predict quality of life for PLHIC in urban Indian Context. *Health Quality Life Outcomes, 3*(14), 152. doi: 10.1186/s12955-016-0556-x

Goffma, E. (1963). *Stigma: Notes from the Management of a Spoiled Identity*. London: Penguin Books.

Henderson, C., Noblett, J., Parke, H., Clement, S., Caffrey, A., Gale-Grant, O., ... Thornicroft, G. (2014). Mental health-related stigma in health care and mental health-care settings. *The Lancet. Psychiatry*, *1*(6), 467–482. doi:10.1016/S2215-0366(14)00023-6 PMID:26361202

Jones, E., Farina, A., Hastorf, A., Markus, H., Miller, D. T., & Scott, R. (1984). *Social Stigma: The Psychology of Marked Relationships*. New York, NY: Freeman.

Kahneman, D. (2011). *Thinking, fast and slow*. New York, NY: Farar, Straus, and Giroux.

Khan, M. R., Kaufman, J. S., Pence, B. W., Gaynes, B. N., Adimora, A. A., Weir, S. S., & Miller, W. C. (2009). Depression, sexually transmitted infection, and sexual risk behavior among young adults in the United States. *Archives of Pediatrics & Adolescent Medicine, 163*(7), 644–652. doi:10.1001/archpediatrics.2009.95 PMID:19581548

Kingdon, D., Sharma, T., & Hart, D. (2004). What attitudes do psychiatrist hold towards people with mental illness? *Psychiatric Bulletin, 28*(11), 401–406. doi:10.1192/pb.28.11.401

Kingori, C., Ice, G. H., Hassan, Q., Elmi, A., & Perko, E. (2016). 'If I went to mom with that information, I'm dead': Sexual health knowledge barriers among immigrant and refugee Somali young adults in Ohio. *Ethnicity & Health, 22*(4), 1–14. doi:10.1080/13557858.2016.1263285 PMID:27350450

Lichentenstein, B. (2003). Stigma as a barrier treatment of sexually transmitted infection in the American Deep South: Issues of races, gender, and poverty. *Social Science & Medicine, 57*(12), 2435–2445. doi:10.1016/j.socscimed.2003.08.002 PMID:14572849

Lichtenstein, B., Neal, T. M., & Brodsky, S. L. (2008). The stigma of sexually transmitted infections: Knowledge, attitudes, and an educationally-based intervention. *Health Educ. Monogr. ser, 25*, 28-33.

Link, B. G., & Phelan, J. C. (2001). Conceptualizing stigma. *Annual Review of Sociology, 27*(1), 363–385. doi:10.1146/annurev.soc.27.1.363

Magliano, L., Fiorillo, A., De Rosa, C., Malangone, C., & Maj, M. (2004). Beliefs about schizophrenia in Italy" A comparative nationwide survey of the general public, mental health professionals, and patients' relatives. *Canadian Journal of Psychiatry, 49*(5), 323–331. doi:10.1177/070674370404900508 PMID:15198469

McGinty, E. E., Webster, D. W., & Barry, C. L. (2013). Effects of news media messages about mass shootings on attitudes toward persons with serious mental illness and public support for gun control policies. *The American Journal of Psychiatry, 170*(5), 494–501. doi:10.1176/appi.ajp.2013.13010014 PMID:23511486

National Institute of Childhood and Human Development (NICHD). (2017). *What are some types of sexually transmitted diseases or sexually transmitted infections (STDs/STIs)?* Retrieved from: https://www.nichd.nih.gov/topics/stds/conditioninfo/pages

Osborn, D. P. J., King, M. B., & Weir, M. (2002). Psychiatric health in a sexually transmitted infections clinic: Effect on reattendence. *Journal of Psychosomatic Research, 52*(4), 267–272. doi:10.1016/S0022-3999(01)00299-9 PMID:11943245

Overton, S. L., & Medina, S. L. (2008). The stigma of mental illness. *Journal of Counseling and Development, 86*(2), 143–151. doi:10.1002/j.1556-6678.2008.tb00491.x

Penn, D. L., Guynan, K., Daily, T., Spaulding, W. D., Garbin, C. P., & Sullivan, M. (1994). Dispelling the stigma of schizophrenia: What sort of information is best? *Schizophrenia Bulletin, 20*(3), 567–578. doi:10.1093chbul/20.3.567 PMID:7973472

Pinfold, V., Byrne, P., & Toulman, H. (2005). Challenging stigma and discrimination in communities: A focus group study identifying UK mental health services users? Main campaign priorities. *The International Journal of Social Psychiatry, 51*(2), 128–138. doi:10.1177/0020764005056760 PMID:16048242

Ross, M.W., Larsson, M., Nyoni, J.E., Agardh, A. (2016). Prevalence of STI symptoms and high levels of stigma in STI healthcare among men who have sex with men in Dar es Salaam, Tanzania: a respondent-driven sampling study. *International Journal of STD and AIDS, 28*(9), 925-928. doi: 10.1177/0956462416683625

Scheim, A., & Travers, R. (2016). Barriers and facilitators to HIV and sexually transmitted infections testing for gay, bisexual, and other transgender men who have sex with men. *AIDS Care, 27*, 1–6. doi:10.1080/09540121.2016.1271937 PMID:28027664

Sharfstein, S. S. (2012). Status of stigma. *Psychiatric Services (Washington, D.C.), 63*(10), 953. doi:10.1176/appi.ps.631011 PMID:23032671

Sickel, A. E., Seacat, J. D., & Nabors, N. A. (2014). Mental health stigma update: A review of consequences. *Advances in Mental Health, 12*(3), 202–215. doi:10.1080/18374905.2014.11081898

Smith, A. L., & Cahswell, C. S. (2010). Stigma and mental illness: Investigating attitudes of mental health and non-mental health professionals and trainees. *The Journal of Humanistic Counseling, Education and Development, 49*(2), 189–202. doi:10.1002/j.2161-1939.2010.tb00097.x

Wang, P.S., Demler, O, & Kessler, R.C. (2002). Adequacy of treatment for serious mental illness in the United States. *American Journal of Public Health, 92*, 92-98. doi: 10.2105-AJPH.92.1.92

Watson, A. C., Corrigan, P., Larson, J. E., & Sells, M. (2007). Self-stigma in people with mental illness. *Schizophrenia Bulletin, 33*(6), 1312–1318. doi:10.1093chbulbl076 PMID:17255118

ADDITIONAL READING

Arboleda-Flórez, J., & Stuart, H. (2012). From sin to science: Fighting the stigmatization of mental illnesses. *Canadian Journal of Psychiatry, 57*(8), 457–463. doi:10.1177/070674371205700803 PMID:22854027

Aromaa, E., Tolvanen, A., Tuulari, J., & Wahlbeck, K. (2011). Predictors of stigmatizing attitudes towards people with mental disorders in a general population in Finland. *Nordic Journal of Psychiatry, 65*(2), 125–132. doi:10.3109/08039488. 2010.510206 PMID:20735187

Brown, C., Conner, K. O., Copeland, V. C., Grote, N., Beach, S., Battista, D., & Reynolds, C. III. (2010). Depression stigma, race, and treatment seeking behavior and attitudes. *Journal of Community Psychology, 38*(3), 350–368. doi:10.1002/jcop.20368 PMID:21274407

Chacko, M., von Sternberg, K., Velasquez, M. M., Wiemann, C. M., Smith, P., & DiClemente, R. (2008). Young women's perspective of the pros and cons to seeking screening for chlamydia and gonorrhea: An exploratory study. *Journal of Pediatric and Adolescent Gynecology, 21*(4), 187–193. doi:10.1016/j.jpag.2007.08.009 PMID:18656072

Chandra, A., & Minkovitz, C. S. (2006). Stigma starts early: Gender differences in teen willingness to use mental health services. *The Journal of Adolescent Health, 38*(6), 754.e751–754.e758. doi:10.1016/j.jadohealth.2005.08.011 PMID:16730608

Coles, M. E., & Coleman, S. L. (2010). Barriers to treatment seeking for anxiety disorders: Initial data on the role of mental health literacy. *Depression and Anxiety, 27*(1), 63–71. doi:10.1002/da.20620 PMID:19960488

Cook, C. (2013). Diagnostic classification, viral sexually transmitted infections and discourses of femininity: Limits of normalization to erase stigma. *Nursing Inquiry, 20*(2), 145–155. doi:10.1111/j.1440-1800.2012.00593.x PMID:22333002

Cooper-Patrick, L., Powe, N., Jenckes, M., Gonzales, J., Levine, D., & Ford, D. (1997). Identification of patient attitudes and preferences regarding treatment of depression. *Journal of General Internal Medicine, 12*(7), 431–438. doi:10.1046/j.1525-1497.1997.00075.x PMID:9229282

Corrigan, P. (2004). How stigma interferes with mental health care. *The American Psychologist, 59*(7), 614–625. doi:10.1037/0003-066X.59.7.614 PMID:15491256

Corrigan, P., River, L., Lundin, R., Penn, D., Uphoff-Wasowski, K., Campion, J., ... Kubiak, M. A. (2001). Three strategies for changing attributions about severe mental illness. *Schizophrenia Bulletin, 27*(2), 187–195. doi:10.1093/oxfordjournals. schbul.a006865 PMID:11354586

Corrigan, P. W. (2007). How clinical diagnosis might exacerbate the stigma of mental illness. *Social Work, 52*(1), 31–39. doi:10.1093w/52.1.31 PMID:17388081

Corrigan, P. W., & O'Shaughnessy, J. R. (2007). Changing mental illness stigma as it exists in the real world. *Australian Psychologist, 42*(2), 90–97. doi:10.1080/00050060701280573

Corrigan, P. W., Watson, A. C., Otey, E., Westbrook, A. L., Gardner, A. L., Lamb, T. A., & Fenton, W. S. (2007). How do children stigmatize people with mental illness? *Journal of Applied Social Psychology, 37*(7), 1405–1417. doi:10.1111/j.1559-1816.2007.00218.x PMID:18181355

Cunningham, S., Kerrigan, D., Jennings, J., & Ellen, J. (2009). Relationships between perceived STD-related stigma, STD-related shame and STD screening among a household sample of adolescents. *Perspectives on Sexual and Reproductive Health, 41*(4), 225–230. doi:10.1363/4122509 PMID:20444177

DasGupta, S., & Charon, R. (2004). Personal illness narratives: Using reflective writing to teach empathy. *Academic Medicine, 79*(4), 351–356. doi:10.1097/00001888-200404000-00013 PMID:15044169

de Araújo, L. F., Alvarez, I. T., & Sánchez, M. P. B. (2014). Psychological and socio-demographic variables associated with sexual risk behavior for sexually transmitted infections/HIV. *International Journal of Clinical and Health Psychology, 14*(2), 120–127. doi:10.1016/S1697-2600(14)70045-6

East, L., Jackson, D., Peters, K., & O'Brien, L. (2010). Disrupted sense of self: Young women and sexually transmitted infections. *Journal of Clinical Nursing, 19*(13-14), 1995–2003. doi:10.1111/j.1365-2702.2009.03183.x PMID:20920025

Eisenberg, D., Downs, M. F., Golberstein, E., & Zivin, K. (2009). Stigma and help seeking for mental health among college students. *Medical Care Research and Review: MCRR, 66*(5), 522–541. doi:10.1177/1077558709335173 PMID:19454625

Fair, C., & Vanyur, J. (2011). Sexual coercion, verbal aggression, and condom use consistency among college students. *Journal of American College Health*, *59*(4), 273–280. doi:10.1080/07448481.2010.508085 PMID:21308587

Fife, B., & Wright, E. (2000). The dimensionality of stigma: A comparison of its impact on the self of persons with HIV/AIDS and cancer. *Journal of Health and Social Behavior*, *41*(1), 50–67. doi:10.2307/2676360 PMID:10750322

Flanagan, E. H., Miller, R., & Davidson, L. (2009). "Unfortunately, we treat the chart:" Sources of stigma in mental health settings. *The Psychiatric Quarterly*, *80*(1), 55–64. doi:10.100711126-009-9093-7 PMID:19191027

Gaynes, B. N., Pence, B. W., Eron, J. J. Jr, & Miller, W. C. (2008). Prevalence and comorbidity of psychiatric diagnoses based on reference standard in an HIV+ patient population. *Psychosomatic Medicine*, *70*(4), 505–511. doi:10.1097/PSY.0b013e31816aa0cc PMID:18378865

Greene, K., & Banerjee, S. (2006). Disease-related stigma: Comparing predictors of AIDS and cancer stigma. *Journal of Homosexuality*, *50*(4), 185–209. doi:10.1300/J082v50n04_08 PMID:16723345

Hackler, A. (2012). Contact and stigma toward mental illness: Measuring the effectiveness of two video interventions. *Dissertation Abstracts International*, *72*, 7716.

Henderson, C., Evans-Lacko, S., & Thornicroft, G. (2013). Mental illness stigma, help seeking, and public health programs. *American Journal of Public Health*, *103*(5), 777–780. doi:10.2105/AJPH.2012.301056 PMID:23488489

Hudson, W., Murphy, G., & Nurius, R. S. (1983). A short-form scale to measure liberal vs. conservative orientations towards human sexual expression. *Journal of Sex Research*, *19*(3), 258–272. doi:10.1080/00224498309551186

Klin, A., & Lemish, D. (2008). Mental disorders stigma in the media: Review of studies on production, content, and influences. *Journal of Health Communication*, *13*(5), 434–449. doi:10.1080/10810730802198813 PMID:18661386

LaBrie, J., Pederson, E., Thompson, A., & Earleywine, M. (2008). A brief decisional balance intervention increases motivation and behavior regarding condom use in high-risk heterosexual college men. *Archives of Sexual Behavior*, *37*(2), 330–339. doi:10.100710508-007-9195-y PMID:17653840

Lauber, C., Nordt, C., Braunschweig, C., & Rössler, W. (2006). Do mental health professionals stigmatize their patients? *Acta Psychiatrica Scandinavica, 113*(s429), 51–59. doi:10.1111/j.1600-0447.2005.00718.x PMID:16445483

Leal, C. C. (2005). Stigmatization of Hispanic children, pre-adolescents, and adolescents with mental illness: Exploration using a national database. *Issues in Mental Health Nursing, 26*(10), 1025–1041. doi:10.1080/01612840500280695 PMID:16283997

Lichtenstein, B., Hook, E. I., & Sharma, A. K. (2005). Public tolerance, private pain: Stigma and sexually transmitted infections in the American Deep South. *Culture, Health & Sexuality, 7*(1), 43–57. doi:10.1080/13691050412331271416 PMID:16864187

Link, B. G. (1987). Understanding labeling effects in the area of mental disorders: An assessment of the effects of expectations of rejection. *American Sociological Review, 52*(1), 96–112. doi:10.2307/2095395

Link, B. G., Cullen, F. T., Struening, E. L., Shrout, P. E., & Dohrenwend, B. P. (1989). A modified labeling theory approach to mental disorders: An empirical assessment. *American Sociological Review, 54*(3), 400–423. doi:10.2307/2095613

Link, B. G., & Phelan, J. C. (2001). Conceptualizing Stigma. *Annual Review of Sociology, 27*(1), 363–385. doi:10.1146/annurev.soc.27.1.363

Link, B. G., Phelan, J. C., Bresnahan, M., Stueve, A., & Pescosolido, B. A. (1999). Public conceptions of mental illness: Labels, causes, dangerousness, and social distance. *American Journal of Public Health, 89*(9), 1328–1333. doi:10.2105/AJPH.89.9.1328 PMID:10474548

Link, B. G., Struening, E. L., Neese-Todd, S., Asmussen, S., & Phelan, J. C. (2001). Stigma as a barrier to recovery: The consequences of stigma for the self-esteem of people with mental illnesses. *Psychiatric Services (Washington, D.C.), 52*(12), 1621–1626. doi:10.1176/appi.ps.52.12.1621 PMID:11726753

Link, B. G., Yang, L. H., Phelan, J. C., & Collins, P. Y. (2004). Measuring Mental Illness Stigma. *Schizophrenia Bulletin, 30*(3), 511–541. doi:10.1093/oxfordjournals.schbul.a007098 PMID:15631243

Nadeem, E., Lange, J. M., Edge, D., Fongwa, M., Belin, T., & Miranda, J. (2007). Does stigma keep poor young immigrant and US-born black and Latina women from seeking mental health care? *Psychiatric Services (Washington, D.C.), 58*(12), 1547–1554. doi:10.1176/ps.2007.58.12.1547 PMID:18048555

Pescosolido, B. A., Jensen, P. S., Martin, J. K., Perry, B. L., Olafsdottir, S., & Fettes, D. (2008). Public knowledge and assessment of child mental health problems: Findings from the National Stigma Study-Children. *Journal of the American Academy of Child and Adolescent Psychiatry, 47*(3), 339–349. doi:10.1097/CHI.0b013e318160e3a0 PMID:18216729

Prior, S. (2012). Overcoming stigma: How young people position themselves as counselling service users. *Sociology of Health & Illness, 34*(5), 697–713. doi:10.1111/j.1467-9566.2011.01430.x PMID:22026466

Spagnolo, A. B., Murphy, A. A., & Librera, L. A. (2008). Reducing stigma by meeting and learning from people with mental illness. *Psychiatric Rehabilitation Journal, 31*(3), 186–193. doi:10.2975/31.3.2008.186.193 PMID:18194945

Spence, J. T., Helmreich, R., & Stapp, J. (1973). A short version of the attitudes toward women scale (AWS). *Bulletin of the Psychonomic Society, 2*(4), 219–222. doi:10.3758/BF03329252

Spitzer, R. L., Kroenke, K., & Williams, J. B. (1999). Validation and utility of a self-report version of PRIME-MD: The PHQ primary care study. *Journal of the American Medical Association, 282*, 1737–1744. doi:10.1001/jama.282.18.1737 PMID:10568646

Stuart, H. (2006). Media portrayal of mental illness and its treatments. *CNS Drugs, 20*(2), 99–106. doi:10.2165/00023210-200620020-00002 PMID:16478286

Stuber, J. P., Rocha, A., Christian, A., & Link, B. G. (2014). Conceptions of mental illness: Attitudes of mental health professionals and the general public. *Psychiatric Services (Washington, D.C.), 65*(4), 490–497. doi:10.1176/appi.ps.201300136 PMID:24430508

Sun, X., Liu, X., Shi, Y., Wang, Y., Wang, P., & Chang, C. (2013). Determinants of risky sexual behavior and condom use among college students in China. *AIDS Care, 25*(6), 775–783. doi:10.1080/09540121.2012.748875 PMID:23252705

Toyoki, S., & Brown, A. D. (2013). Stigma, identity and power: Managing stigmatized identities through discourse. *Human Relations, 67*(6), 715–737. doi:10.1177/0018726713503024

Vauth, R., Kleim, B., Wirtz, M., & Corrigan, P. W. (2007). Self-efficacy and empowerment as outcomes of self-stigmatizing and coping in schizophrenia. *Psychiatry Research, 150*(1), 71–80. doi:10.1016/j.psychres.2006.07.005 PMID:17270279

Vogel, D. L., Wade, N. G., & Haake, S. (2006). Measuring the self-stigma associated with seeking psychological help. *Journal of Counseling Psychology, 53*(3), 325–337. doi:10.1037/0022-0167.53.3.325

Vogel, D. L., Wade, N. G., & Hackler, A. H. (2007). Perceived public stigma and the willingness to seek counseling: The mediating roles of self-stigma and attitudes toward counseling. *Journal of Counseling Psychology, 54*(1), 40–50. doi:10.1037/0022-0167.54.1.40

Wahl, O. F. (1999). Mental health consumers' experience of stigma. *Schizophrenia Bulletin, 25*(3), 467–478. doi:10.1093/oxfordjournals.schbul.a033394 PMID:10478782

Wahl, O. F. (1999). Mental health consumers' experience of stigma. *Schizophrenia Bulletin, 25*(3), 467–478. doi:10.1093/oxfordjournals.schbul.a033394 PMID:10478782

Waller, J., Marlow, L. A., & Wardle, J. (2006). Mothers' attitudes towards preventing cervical cancer through human papillomavirus vaccination: A qualitative study. *Cancer Epidemiology, Biomarkers & Prevention, 15*(7), 1257–1261. doi:10.1158/1055-9965. EPI-06-0041 PMID:16835320

Wells, K., Sturm, R., & Burnam, M. A. (2003). *Healthcare for Communities Household Survey public use files: Revised codebook.* Ann Arbor, MI: ICPSR.

Wong, J. P. H., Chan, K. B., Boi-Doku, R., & McWatt, S. (2012). Risk discourse and sexual stigma: Barriers to STI testing, treatment and care among young heterosexual women in disadvantaged neighbourhoods in Toronto. *The Canadian Journal of Human Sexuality, 21*(2), 75–89.

KEY TERMS AND DEFINITIONS

Bias: Prejudice against or in favor of a person, thing, or situation.

Institutionalized Stigma: Stigma that is embedded within organizational culture.

Mental Health Diagnosis: A collection of behaviors meeting the criteria set forth by the DSM-5, typically resulting in distress, dysfunction, or deviance.

Prejudice: A preconceived opinion regarding a person, thing, or situation based primarily on group membership.

Self-Stigma: Beliefs about one's self and one's status based on perceived stigma pertaining to a feature, group membership, or situation maintained by that individual.

Sexual Anxiety: Anxiety regarding the possibility of being sexually rejected.

Sexually Transmitted Infection (STI): An infection transmitted via sexual activity, either via anal contact, oral contact, or vaginal contact.

Shame: A social emotion tied to one's experiences or status.

Social Desirability: The innate desire to please and be accepted by others.

Stigma: Disproval based on perceived group membership.

Stigma by Association: Being the object of actual or perceived stigma secondary to a relationship with a person that maintains a particular group membership.

Chapter 9

Stamped Life:
Stigmatization Stories of Women Who Care for Patients With Schizophrenia

Fulya Akgül Gök
Ankara University, Turkey

Elif Gökçearslan Çifci
Ankara University, Turkey

ABSTRACT

This research was conducted with a view to ascertaining the perceptions, feelings, and thoughts of the women who care for patients with schizophrenia regarding the challenges they face and stigma. This research was conducted by using qualitative research method. To this end, in-depth interviews were made with 10 women who care for schizophrenia patients. As a result of the research, it was found out that the women who care for patients often care of the patient on their own, and thus, they have some psychosocial challenges. The disease negatively affects family relationships, but some families, on the contrary, have positive changes in their relationships. The parents accuse themselves as they are the cause of the disease and they are accused by the social circles. The women who care for patients are exposed to stigma during almost the all processes of the disease and some women internalize being stigmatized and they mostly tend to hide the disease in order to cope with the stigma.

DOI: 10.4018/978-1-5225-3808-0.ch009

INTRODUCTION

Mental diseases affect not only the patient but also the family of the patient and the systems they are affiliated to. Particularly the patient's family and the individuals who care for the patient are physically, economically, psychologically and socially affected by the process. Negative attitude and behaviours of the society towards mental illnesses make this process harder. Lack of adequate information and awareness of the society about the mental diseases cause the individuals who are mentally ill and their family to be marginalised. Fear of being marginalised and stigmatised prevents the patient who is going through a tough disease and his/her family from taking social benefit and, as a result, cause the family members to isolate themselves from the society. This may either strengthen the family relationships or cause deterioration in in-family relations. Bartol et al. (1994) stated that having a family member being diagnosed with schizophrenia in the family might change family life.

Stigma may increase the families' burden which is caused by the disease process. Gülseren et. al (2010) stated that the families' burden might increase because of the stigmatisation. Schizophrenia disease affects family system and may cause great stress in the family (Öztürk, 2001). Disease process may cause the family members to feel depressed, stressed, embarrassed, guilty, scared, desperate and angry (Saunders & Byrne 2002; Gülseren, 2002). The name of the disease is a label (Angermeyer and Matschinger, 2003). While this definition is a labelling for many diseases, it reaches stigmatisation level for some diseases (Yıldız et. al., 2011). Schizophrenia is one of them.

As for the stigmatisation which is among the problems faced by the families during disease, firstly some mindscapes about these patients develop. Then, these mindscapes turn into prejudices which is followed by negative thoughts and feelings. A power balance is in place in stigmatisation which goes towards the weak from the strong one (Corrigan ve Watson, 2002). The families may feel that the sick person and they are, along with him or her, are being trivialised (Struening et. al., 2001), and the family members face stigma together with the mentally ill person (Larson and Corrigan, 2008). Therefore, stigma affects not only the mentally sick individuals but also their families. Dardas and Simmons (2015) stated that some authors considered the stigma as an information problem while some considered the same thing as a form of negative attitudes, and some considered it as a result of discriminative behaviours.

Stigma affects the individuals' life quality and social interaction (Yanos et al., 2001; Lundberg at al., 2008). Whereas communicating and interacting with mental health services have a positive impact on some aspects of life quality such as family relationships, financial situation, security and health; stigma has a negative impact on these aspects (Rosenfield, 1997; Lundberg et al., 2008).

Being one of the important factors which affect family life, stigma causes psychological problems in family members, particularly those caring for the patient. Corrigan et al. (2006) stated that stigma affects not only the person with mental illness but also the family members of the patient. Yang and Pearson (2002) stated in a study they conducted that the families of the individuals with mental illnesses experience stigmatisation and their prestige in the society would be negatively affected. Chinese families who participated in the research stated that they do not participate in the social activities in order to minimise stigmatization.

Since the first-degree caregiver of the patient is at the heart of the patient's daily life, giving care may turn into a long-run intensive and dependant obligation which cause trouble in the caregiver's life as the responsibilities increase (Atagün et al. 2011). It is stated in the study of Madianos et al. (2004) that social isolation stemming from the decrease and change in social activities, financial problems and fear of being stigmatised is among the reasons of the psychological problems experienced by the caregivers of schizophrenia patients. In Turkey where gender point of view prevails, the role of caregiving is considered as the extension of the women's domestic role. The women spend almost whole day with their relative to whom they give care. Depending on the symptoms of the disease, they cannot leave the patient at home alone, they are worried even if they leave them alone, and they cannot spend quality time. Subjective and objective burden of the female caregivers increase as the society stigmatise the mentally ill person and his or her family. This may result in the women staying at home, ending their social relations, reducing their social activities, making them unable to talk with their social circles about the disease and about the things they are experiencing. All these factors cause these individuals being alienated to themselves and to society, family relations being deteriorated and internalising this even if there is no stigma towards them.

METHOD

Qualitative research method was used in this research which aims at ascertaining how the women who care for (female caregivers) the mentally ill living in Turkey experience and internalise stigma considering cultural structure of Turkey. Framework of the research was formed with a phenomenological approach. This study intended to understand the stigmatisation process of the women who care for the mentally ill because of the disease both in the society and in their internal processes in line with their own lives and perceptions.

This research was conducted with the married women who live in Ankara and have a mentally ill child. These persons were reached with snowball sampling method. The interviews continued until they reached saturation point.

The women participating in the research were included in the research process without seeking any age requirement. Main purpose of interviewing with women at different ages is the belief that the women at different ages may experience stigma in different forms. The women included in the research are between 43-60 years old and they are all legally married. However, 3 of them are separated from their husbands although they are legally married, and they live with their children. Considering their education level, four of these women hold high school degree, two of them hold bachelor's degree and four of them hold primary school degree. Considering their professional life, one of these women works in a government agency and one of them works as a housekeeper. The children of all of the women participating in the research were diagnosed with schizophrenia. Due to ethical reasons, the names of the women participating in the research were not disclosed, instead, their names were expressed with alphabetical letters.

In-depth interviews and observation notes were used during data collection. Interview forms include questions aiming at ascertaining the women's and children's socio-demographic, socio-economic knowledge, family relationships, women's internal and external perception of stigma and reflections of stigma on daily life. Moreover, observation notes taken during the interviews were used.

While determining the place of interview, importance was attached to ensuring the individuals participating in the research feel comfortable. In this scope, two interviews were made in the interviewee's house and eight interviews were made in quiet cafés.

In this respect, semi-conducted in-depth interviews were made with 10 female caregivers of mentally ill individuals. Interviews last between 30 and 65 minutes. Research data were collected between April and May in 2016. After the interviews made with the participants are deciphered, they were read by the researchers and also by two experts in depth.

FINDINGS

This research includes stigmatisation/being stigmatised experienced by the women who care for patients with schizophrenia both in society and in their internal processes. In this context, the results were addressed under three categories. The first category is "mental illness from the point of view of the female caregivers"; the second category is "mental illness from the point of view of the family" and the third category is "mental illness from the point of view of the parent". Sub-themes of the first category "mental illness from the point of view of the female caregivers" are "feeling of sadness, embarrassment and desperateness", "internalised stigmatisation". Sub-themes of the third category "mental illness from the point of view of the parent" are "self-accusation as a parent", "being accused by the others" and "coping with the stigma".

Category 1: Mental Illness From the Point of View of Caregivers

The people who care for the mentally ill are often women. While the women meet various needs of the mentally ill, they may forget their own lives, ignore their personal grooming, and their social relations may break off. Some of these female caregivers spend almost all their time with the sick person, whereas some men spend most of their time outside. This exacerbates negative feelings of the women. In this study, the women who are assisted and supported by their husbands stated that they managed to control the process more easily. Considering all these processes, female caregivers either fight against the process or move on with negative feelings and thoughts.

One of the participants stated that she had no support during the disease, and the thing that hurt the most was that her husband did not support her.

She is not only my daughter but also his. It hurts so much. It is me who care for everything about my daughter. Of course, I will take care of her, she is my daughter, she is my precious, but what if he gave a hand, what if he let me rest, what if he comforted me when I cry. Is that too much to ask? I swear you I am sick of living. (E, 45)

The spouse's support may physically, socially and psychologically ease the female caregiver's life. A female caregiver describes her happiness about her husband's support as below.

I understood that nobody can help in this situation. I also have mother-in-law, I am already overbusy, I do all the work. But my husband is an understanding person. May God bless him. My only luck in this world is my husband. The most important thing in one's life is your spouse. I am satisfied with his support. (I, 56)

The families mostly have to fight against the disease alone (Gülseren, 2002). In the studies conducted, it is stated that the women are mostly responsible for the care of the patient. (Gülseren et. al. 2010; Awad and Voruganti, 2008). Researches on the sex of the caregiver revealed that compared to men, the female caregivers have much burden; whereas the men do not claim caregiving responsibility as much (Atagün et. al., 2011).

Sub-Category A: Sadness, Embarrassment and Desperateness

The women who care for the mentally ill cannot accept the disease during the first symptoms, and they feel sad, embarrassed and desperate when they accept it.

It is very hard. I would not wish that on my worst enemy. That moment, I wanted to die. It was as if my child was gone and someone else came. I cannot explain that situation. You cannot understand it without experiencing. I was desperate, sad. I could not know what to do. Where should I go? From whom should I ask for help? (A, 57)

As some relatives of the patients are not informed about the symptoms of mental diseases, they ignore the symptoms for some time and think that they are results of the development process of the puberty. However, some time later, the family members realise that there was something wrong and decide to go to a psychiatrist. They expressed their sadness, desperateness and shock after the diagnosis as below.

...He was not talking and wanted to sleep all the time. And I thought that he was just feeling blue. All in all, he is an adolescent. You know, they behave different at puberty. But he began to do things he had never done before. Then I understood that there was something wrong. When he began to hit me, I took him to the doctor and the rest is history: a life full of disappointment and desperateness. (B, 45)

In the qualitative study conducted by Liegghio (2013), it was stated that the people who care for the mentally ill might have problems in realising whether their children's behaviour stemmed from a mental illness or they are just normal adolescent behaviour.

One of the female caregivers stated that she could not do anything against the disease, could not find a way out and she expressed her desperateness as below.

I let it flow. You cannot do anything. You sit just like this as if you are sick. You brood. How can I find a way out? You will give a lead? Will I able to find a way out? What will I do? How will I manage it? (E, 45)

Being stigmatised by the society and the negative attitude and behaviours of the society towards the mentally ill and their families may cause the family members to hide the illness and feel embarrassed. In this context, we can say that stigma and embarrassment is related to each other.

At first, I could not tell anyone. I cried every time I thought about what I would do. I thought that everybody would pity me and would not see me. Can you imagine a mother being ashamed of her child's illness? But I was. Then, I always blamed myself as I thought this way. It is so hard, really hard. (D, 60)

Embarrassment and stigma are the concepts associated with each other especially in terms of "self-stigma" (Patrick, Corrigan and Frederick, 2004). Some researches indicate that having a mentally ill family member makes the family feel embarrassed and thus, they hide it (Veltman et al., 2002; Shibre et al., 2001).

Most of these individuals take the caregiving role on their own. The female caregivers feel hopeless, embarrassed and frustrated due to lack of adequate information about the illness, lack of adequate support from their husbands and others, negative attitude and judgments of the society, uncertain future and other problems that come with the process.

Sub-Category B: "Internalised Stigmatisation"

Negative attitude and behaviours of the society towards mental diseases cause the caregivers feel embarrassed and tendency to hide the illness. During this process, some of the caregivers isolate themselves from social environment and start to live a life just inside four walls.

I did not want to share my family life with anyone; I had not shared before. My husband acts quite the opposite way and talks to everybody, his siblings. I wanted to tell one of my close friends at the office and I did. She said she was sorry and wished me recovery, but then she started to stay away from me day by day. I have worried so much and got so exhausted that I do not talk to even my mother or father, anybody. I do not want anybody to feel pity for me or my family. As a consequence, now I see almost nobody. (D, 60)

How many people have a psychological disease? Very few. In other words, you can only know these people if you have a close relationship. After my son got sick, the people said that 'do not tell anybody, but my older brother has the same illness'. In other words, this illness is kept secret. Then, other said that their father and brother had the same illness. I used to act the same way. I did not want to share this because of the thing in society. Because my son has to graduate from high school. This must be kept secret. I feel as if everybody will feel pity for us. (E, 45)

The families of the people with a mental illness sometimes feel embarrassed and guilty. Some family members even blame themselves for the illness. All these feelings may result in the family members stigmatise themselves (Larson and Corrigan, 2008).

Category 2: Mental Illness From the Point of View of Family

Having a mentally ill person in the family affects the family system as a whole and the sub- systems. The symptoms of the disease and the disease process may cause a crisis for the family members and particularly for the individuals who give care. During this process, the relationships between the children and the parents may deteriorate, and in some cases, family members may support each other and their already tainted relationships may improve. Any mental disease of the children may affect the family as a whole, and it may also deteriorate the relationship between the spouses. Family members' having inadequate information about the disease may cause wrong beliefs and thoughts between the spouses.

As those who take caring responsibility are mostly the women, this may cause them not to be able to spare some time to themselves and others. Inability or unwillingness to share the challenges of the disease with the others, the men not supporting or helping their wives during this process and the spouses accusing one another may damage the relationship between the spouses.

After our son's illness we could not find any solution. We already had some problems. At last we came to blows. (E, 45)

Having a mentally ill person in the family cause changes in balances of the family and some differences in the relationships between the spouses, parent-children and siblings. Particularly; intensive anxiety, sadness, desperateness and other negative feelings may cause conflict between the spouses.

We were not good before, as well. But we used to go out, visit friends and relatives, he used to ask why I was sad when I was feeling blue. Now we are worse than before. We don't even see our faces at times. He does not want to stay at home. He sometimes takes the child out for maximum one hour, then he goes. (A, 57)

In addition to these problems, the families with mentally ill individuals are exposed to stigmatisation as a system, which results in a different cycle in the family and alienation of the family as a whole or individual alienation of the family members to each other. To the opposite of this situation, some families manage to partially move on with their existing routine, or they can support each other more.

Indeed, I did not want to talk about this with anybody. But I cannot help telling my mother. Then everybody heard about it. Nobody said anything to my face, but they spoke behind me. My daughter did not tell anything to her friends, and my husband to his reliable friends. We are all afraid; there is nothing worse than being excluded.

At home, nobody talks to each other. We cannot adequately take care of our other daughter. I am worried about it. My husband turned in on himself, keep his hands off everything. (B, 45)

When you go through this, you understand that you have nothing but your family. I am grateful that my husband supports me. If he did not support me, I could not manage. Therefore, what others say does not affect me. The only important thing is that your family is okay. (I, 56)

Family stigma includes some judgement patterns such as feeling guilty and embarrassed. Although the opinion which defends inadequacy of the family lags behind, the society may still find the family guilty for mental illnesses. Therefore, the family members being accused by the society may feel embarrassed. This feeling may negatively affect the relationships of the family members with their social circles. Furthermore, this may cause the family to hide the disease (Larson and Corrigan, 2008). The study conducted by Struening et al. (2001) with the family members of 461 individuals with mental diseases indicated that being stigmatised and rejected by the society, these families have a harder life.

In the study conducted by Liegghio (2013), some of the family members stated that they argue with their husbands more than usual. Furthermore, the caregivers stated that they became distant from other family members and could not take care of their needs while they were trying to meet the needs of the mentally ill individual. This cause the husband or other child/children to be ignored and thus, feeling guilty.

As seen in this study, a mental disease in the family may cause the balances in the family to change. As the female caregiver focus on the sick person, emotional needs of the husband and other family members, if any, cannot be met.

Category 3: Mental Illness From the Point of View of Parents

Mental diseases affect the family in different ways both with the parenting and caregiving role. In terms of being a parent, the families think that they have done something wrong with regard to mental illness, they question being a parent, and as a result of this questioning, they think that they were not able to be "good parents". This may cause the parents to accuse themselves and one another regarding the occurrence of mental illness.

Some parents face some accusations from their social circles about the occurrence of mental illnesses. In countries such as Turkey where gender point of view prevails, the women may be accused by alleging that she cannot raise her child well and spoil him/her. Besides, both female and male parents may be accused by alleging that they cannot be a good couple, argue too much and have problems.

Sub-Category A: Self-Accusation as a Parent

Some parents of the mentally ill see themselves as the cause of their child's disease. The initial questionings such as "Why me?" turn into a detailed review of the past. It was found out that more than half of the women participating in the research ask these questions and they stated that they had made some mistakes regarding their past, childcare and in-family relations.

I grumbled many times on my own. I asked 'My God, what did I do wrong?' Then, I thought that if I had spared more time to my child when he was young, this would not be the case. At first, these thoughts worried me to death. Regrets... (F, 55)

Some parents may accuse themselves as they think that the arguments and problems with their spouses have caused mental illness of their child.

We used to argue with my husband for a reason from the day we got married. There was no reason to fight, but we happened to fight tooth and nail. Now when I give a thought and believe that the blame is on me for our child's illness. If a child grows in the middle of fights, this will be the result (cries).(G, 43).

As it is obvious, the first thing the caregivers do in such a crisis is to question themselves. Particularly the female caregivers think where they did wrong and associate the illness with unreal incidents and situations. This cause feeling guilty and increase the burden of these individuals.

Sub-Category B: Being Accused by the Others

In many societies, the people are not informed about the mental illnesses as much as they are about other diseases. The families tend to hide the illness due to the society's lack of information about the illness, self-stigmatisation and the intention to be protected from some negativities. The people to whom the illness is told or who are somehow informed of the illness may tend to accuse the parents of the sick person. These accusations are that they are not good parents, they conflict all the time, they spoil their children, or they are indifferent to their child. As a result of study he conducted, Liegghio (2013) stated that the caregivers tend to either hide the disease to avoid from being stigmatised or to share information to raise awareness about the disease.

Some parents can keep nonreactive to the accusations of the others; whereas, some internalise these accusations and thus, they accuse themselves.

When this child was first diagnosed with the disease, my mother-in-law said that I was the reason. I asked what I did and she said that I spoiled the child. And much more… At first, I pretended not to have heard, but then I thought I was the reason. Once I felt suspicious, then I thought about it all the time. (H, 52).

People having an individual with a mental illness in the family sometimes put up walls against social circles while in some cases social circles put up walls against these families. Family members being exposed to some accusations regarding the illness can be seen as stigmatisation. Because of the social walls put up between the two people, they may withdraw themselves from social life. Some researches revealed that the society accuse family members and especially the parents for any mental disease of their family (Corrigan et al., 2000; Shibre et al., 2001). The parents are accused for not being good parents. In addition, some argue that the child has mental disorders due to inadequacy of the mother.

Subcategory C: Coping With the Stigma

Low awareness and knowledge level of the society about the mental illnesses in Turkey cause people to avoid the mentally ill persons, to be scared of them, to avoid being friends with them, and the ill people to be called "insane" or "demonical". In this process, the families may be exposed to stigmatisation by the society, or they may avoid social life, isolate themselves from outside world, hide the illness and even not take the mentally ill person outside as a result of the fear of stigmatisation. Some families hide the illness even from their extended family. Main reason of this includes the fear of being excluded from the society, having inadequate information about the disease and feeling embarrassed because of the illness/patient. On the contrary, there are some family members who read in order to have information about the illness and how to approach the patient, get information from the professionals and go to the foundations who help people with mental illnesses and their relatives. Moreover, some families act to raise awareness and knowledge of the society and media about mental illnesses. Both methods are the family members' processes of coping with the illness and managing the stigma. The factors affecting the individuals' applying different methods during this process include socio-economic level, personal characteristics, social support, family relationships and personal characteristics of the patient.

Some of the female caregivers participating in the research stated that they had hard time coping with the process on their own, and even though they tend to share this situation with the others, they hesitated to take social support due to the fear of stigmatisation of themselves or their children.

I cannot share this with anyone. They would call my child psychiatric patient. As I think this way, I ended my connection with everybody. I used to have women's gathering days, but now I meet neither my neighbours nor my parents. There is no place for me other than my home. (B, 45)

In the further processes of the illness, the caregivers may tend to share the illness with someone else, when compared to the beginning. A woman participating in the research stated that at first, stigmatisation on the mental illnesses prevented her, at first, from talking to someone else, but then her need to share increased in the further stages.

I did not share it with anybody. Because, as I observed, the society see the people taking medicines insane. Therefore, I did not tell anybody at first. But now I cannot stand. I want to tell no matter who as long he/she does not look down on me. (C, 41)

Stigmatisation/being stigmatised may be in the form of nonverbal attitude and behaviours, apart from verbal behaviours. Although the families expect support particularly from their close circle and relatives, sometimes those who first respond to them may be from close circle. One of the participants explained this as below:

...The father was secretly telling the illness to everybody. Then everybody changed. I even saw my relatives avoiding from and being afraid of my daughter. I understood this from what they said and how they looked at her. For example, some of them did not want my daughter to go to their home. For example, there was a women's gathering day in my aunt's daughter's home, and we went there. I told my daughter that I was going to E. When I went there, I saw her sitting in the garden. My aunt's daughter had not allowed her come in. I felt very bad when I saw her there. I thought if she was thinking that my daughter was normal, then she would have allowed her to come in. (D, 60)

One of the women participating in the research stated that she obtained information about the illness after the diagnosis from the books, television shows, magazines and professional experts.

I was devastated when I first learned about what this illness was. Words fail to describe that. Then I told to myself that this happened. I should learn what it was exactly. I should tell my neighbours, relatives. Let them know; in fact, I wanted them to realise there was nothing to be afraid of. (İ, 56).

As it is clear from the statements of the women participating in the research who give care to the patients, the caregivers of the mentally ill develop some coping methods and manage stigma and try to cope with it. Terschinsky (2000) stated that instead of going to hospital for treatment, the families tried to overcome the illness on their own due to their fear of stigmatisation and embarrassment.

CONCLUSION

The lives of the female caregivers of those diagnosed with schizophrenia which change along with the illness process were intended to be analysed in the context of being a woman, family and parent. In this respect, the challenges and stigmatisation being exposed by the caregivers experienced as a woman, parent and family member were examined particularly from the point of view of the female caregivers in line with their perception.

In this study, mental illness process and the challenges experienced in this process as well as stigma were intended to be explained in line with the feelings, thoughts and perceptions of the female caregivers. During caregiving process, it is observed that the women face huge challenges and stigma makes this process harder.

Particularly in countries such as Turkey where the women are more active in assuming the caregiving role, the studies on the families with regard to mental illnesses and relevant response programs should be increased. These programs should be applied by a multi-disciplinary team, and it should be ensured that both men and women participate in these studies. Another important point is that such studies which raise the knowledge of the society about mental illnesses should be focused. To this end, informative programs about mental illnesses should be made through media, courses on mental illnesses should be given by the professionals in primary school, effort should be made in order to ensure the patients' and their families' social integration, acting with the aim of ensuring treatment of the mentally ill people under better conditions, ensuring government's support, and rehabilitating both the patients and their families.

REFERENCES

Angermeyer, M. C., & Matschinger, H. (2003). The stigma of mental illness: Effects of labelling on public attitudes towards people with mental disorder. *Acta Psychiatrica Scandinavica*, *108*(4), 304–309. doi:10.1034/j.1600-0447.2003.00150.x PMID:12956832

Atagün, M. İ., Balaban, Ö. D., Atagün, Z., Elagöz, M., & Özpolat, A. Y. (2011). Burden on the caregivers in chronic diseases. *Psikiyatride Güncel Yaklasimlar, 3*(3), 513–552. doi:10.5455/cap.20110323

Awad, A. G., & Voruganti, L. N. (2008). The burden of schizophrenia on caregivers. *PharmacoEconomics, 26*(2), 149–162. doi:10.2165/00019053-200826020-00005 PMID:18198934

Barney, L. J., Griffiths, K. M., Jorm, A. F., & Christensen, H. (2006). Stigma about depression and its impact on help-seeking intentions. *The Australian and New Zealand Journal of Psychiatry, 40*(1), 51–54. doi:10.1080/j.1440-1614.2006.01741.x PMID:16403038

Bartol, G. M., Moon, E., & Linton, M. (1994). Nursing assistance for families of patients. *Journal of Psychosocial Nursing, 32*(12), 27–29. PMID:7714849

Corrigan, P. W., & Miller, F. E. (2004). Shame, blame, and contamination: A review of the impact of mental illness stigma on family members. *Journal of Mental Health (Abingdon, England), 13*(6), 537–548. doi:10.1080/09638230400017004

Corrigan, P. W., River, L. P., Lundin, R. K., Wasowski, K. U., Campion, J., Mathisen, J., ... Kubiak, M. A. (2000). Stigmatizing attributions about mental illness. *Journal of Community Psychology, 28*(1), 91–102. doi:

Corrigan, P. W., & Watson, A. C. (2002). Understanding the impact of stigma on people with mental illness. *World Psychiatry; Official Journal of the World Psychiatric Association (WPA), 1*(1), 16–20. PMID:16946807

Corrigan, P. W., Watson, A. C., & Miller, F. E. (2006). The impact of mental illness and drug dependence stigma on family members. *Journal of Family Psychology, 20*(2), 239–246. doi:10.1037/0893-3200.20.2.239 PMID:16756399

Dardas, L. A., & Simmons, L. A. (2015). The stigma of mental illness in Arab families: A concept analysis. *Journal of Psychiatric and Mental Health Nursing, 22*(9), 668–679. doi:10.1111/jpm.12237 PMID:26118332

Gülseren, L. (2002). Schizophrenia and family: Challenges, feelings, needs. *Türk Psikiyatri Dergisi, 13*(2), 143–151. PMID:12794667

Gülseren, L., Çam, B., Karakoç, B., Yiğit, T., Danacı, A. E., Çubukçuoğlu, Z., ... Mete, L. (2010). The factors affecting the burden n the family in schizophrenia. *Turkish Journal of Psychiatry, 21*, 203–212. PMID:20818508

Kamal, R. (2013). *A Narrative Study of the Lived Experiences of Family Caregivers Through Different Stages of Mental Illness* (Unpublished Doctoral Dissertation). Department of Counselor Education, New Mexico.

Larson, J. E., & Corrigan, P. (2008). The stigma of families with mental illness. *Academic Psychiatry, 32*(2), 87–91. doi:10.1176/appi.ap.32.2.87 PMID:18349326

Liegghio, M. (2013). *The Stigma of Mental of Illness: Learning from the Situated Knowledge of Psychiatrized Youth, Caregivers, and Young Siblings* (Unpublished doctoral thesis). Wilfrid Laurier University, Canada.

Lundberg, B., Hansson, L., Wentz, E., & Björkman, T. (2008). Stigma, discrimination, empowerment and social networks: A preliminary investigation of their influence on subjective quality of life in a Swedish sample. *The International Journal of Social Psychiatry, 54*(1), 47–55. doi:10.1177/0020764007082345 PMID:18309758

Madianos, M., Economou, M., Dafni, O., Koukia, E., Palli, A., & Rogakou, E. (2004). Family disruption, economic hardship and psychological distress in schizophrenia: Can they be measured? *European Psychiatry, 19*(7), 408–414. doi:10.1016/j.eurpsy.2004.06.028 PMID:15504647

Öztürk, O. (2001). *Mental Health and Disorders. Eight edition.* Ankara: Feryal Printing House.

Phelan, J. C. (2002). Genetic bases of mental illness–a cure for stigma? *Trends in Neurosciences, 25*(8), 430–431. doi:10.1016/S0166-2236(02)02209-9 PMID:12127761

Rosenfield, S. (1997). Labeling mental illness: The effects of received services and perceived stigma on life satisfaction. *American Sociological Review, 62*(4), 660–672. doi:10.2307/2657432

Saunders, J. C., & Byrne, M. M. (2002). A thematic analysis of families living with schizophrenia. *Archives of Psychiatric Nursing, 16*(5), 217–223. doi:10.1053/apnu.2002.36234 PMID:12434327

Shibre, T., Negash, A., Kullgren, G., Kebede, D., Alem, A., Fekadu, A., ... Jacobsson, L. (2001). Perception of stigma among family members of individuals with schizophrenia and major affective disorders in rural Ethiopia. *Social Psychiatry and Psychiatric Epidemiology, 36*(6), 299–303. doi:10.1007001270170048 PMID:11583460

Struening, E. L., Perlick, D. A., Link, B. G., Hellman, F., Herman, D., & Sirey, J. A. (2001). Stigma as a barrier to recovery: The extent to which caregivers believe most people devalue consumers and their families. *Psychiatric Services (Washington, D.C.)*, *52*(12), 1633–1638. doi:10.1176/appi.ps.52.12.1633 PMID:11726755

Teschinsky, U. (2000). Living with schizophrenia: The family illness experience. *Issues in Mental Health Nursing*, *21*(4), 387–396. doi:10.1080/016128400248004 PMID:11249357

Veltman, A., Cameron, J. I., & Stewart, D. E. (2002). The experience of providing care to relatives with chronic mental illness. *The Journal of Nervous and Mental Disease*, *190*(2), 108–114. doi:10.1097/00005053-200202000-00008 PMID:11889365

Yang, L. H., & Pearson, V. J. (2002). Understanding families in their own context: Schizophrenia and structural family therapy in Beijing. *Journal of Family Therapy*, *24*(3), 233–257. doi:10.1111/1467-6427.00214

Yıldız, M., Özten, E., Işık, S., Özyıldırım, İ., Karayün, D., Cerit, C., & Üçok, A. (2012). Self-stigmatisation of schizophrenia patients, relatives of the patients and patients with major depressive disorders. *Anatolian Journal of Psychiatry*, *13*(1), 1–7.

Related References

To continue our tradition of advancing academic research, we have compiled a list of recommended IGI Global readings. These references will provide additional information and guidance to further enrich your knowledge and assist you with your own research and future publications.

Abdelaziz, H. A. (2013). From content engagement to cognitive engagement: Toward an immersive web-based learning model to develop self-questioning and self-study skills. *International Journal of Technology Diffusion*, *4*(1), 16–32. doi:10.4018/jtd.2013010102

Acha, V., Hargiss, K. M., & Howard, C. (2013). The relationship between emotional intelligence of a leader and employee motivation to job performance. *International Journal of Strategic Information Technology and Applications*, *4*(4), 80–103. doi:10.4018/ijsita.2013100105

Agrawal, P. R. (2014). Digital information management: preserving tomorrow's memory. In S. Dhamdhere (Ed.), *Cloud computing and virtualization technologies in libraries* (pp. 22–35). Hershey, PA: IGI Global. doi:10.4018/978-1-4666-4631-5.ch002

Akram, H. A., & Mahmood, A. (2014). Predicting personality traits, gender and psychopath behavior of Twitter users. *International Journal of Technology Diffusion*, *5*(2), 1–14. doi:10.4018/ijtd.2014040101

Akyol, Z. (2013). Metacognitive development within the community of inquiry. In Z. Akyol & D. Garrison (Eds.), *Educational communities of inquiry: Theoretical framework, research and practice* (pp. 30–44). Hershey, PA: IGI Global. doi:10.4018/978-1-4666-2110-7.ch003

Albers, M. J. (2012). How people read. In *Human-information interaction and technical communication: Concepts and frameworks* (pp. 367–397). Hershey, PA: IGI Global. doi:10.4018/978-1-4666-0152-9.ch011

Albers, M. J. (2012). What people bring with them. In *Human-information interaction and technical communication: Concepts and frameworks* (pp. 61–113). Hershey, PA: IGI Global. doi:10.4018/978-1-4666-0152-9.ch003

Ally, M. (2012). Designing mobile learning for the user. In B. Khan (Ed.), *User interface design for virtual environments: Challenges and advances* (pp. 226–235). Hershey, PA: IGI Global. doi:10.4018/978-1-61350-516-8.ch014

Almeida, L., Menezes, P., & Dias, J. (2013). Augmented reality framework for the socialization between elderly people. In M. Cruz-Cunha, I. Miranda, & P. Gonçalves (Eds.), *Handbook of research on ICTs for human-centered healthcare and social care services* (pp. 430–448). Hershey, PA: IGI Global. doi:10.4018/978-1-4666-3986-7.ch023

Alonso, E., & Mondragón, E. (2011). Computational models of learning and beyond: Symmetries of associative learning. In E. Alonso & E. Mondragón (Eds.), *Computational neuroscience for advancing artificial intelligence: Models, methods and applications* (pp. 316–332). Hershey, PA: IGI Global. doi:10.4018/978-1-60960-021-1.ch013

Ancarani, A., & Di Mauro, C. (2013). The human side of supply chains: A behavioural perspective of supply chain risk management. In *Supply chain management: Concepts, methodologies, tools, and applications* (pp. 1453–1476). Hershey, PA: IGI Global. doi:10.4018/978-1-4666-2625-6.ch086

Andres, H. P. (2013). Collaborative technology and dimensions of team cognition: Test of a second-order factor model. *International Journal of Information Technology Project Management*, *4*(3), 22–37. doi:10.4018/jitpm.2013070102

Arora, A. S., Raisinghani, M. S., Leseane, R., & Thompson, L. (2013). Personality scales and learning styles: Pedagogy for creating an adaptive web-based learning system. In M. Raisinghani (Ed.), *Curriculum, learning, and teaching advancements in online education* (pp. 161–182). Hershey, PA: IGI Global. doi:10.4018/978-1-4666-2949-3.ch012

Ashcraft, D., & Treadwell, T. (2010). The social psychology of online collaborative learning: The good, the bad, and the awkward. In web-based education: concepts, methodologies, tools and applications (pp. 1146-1161). Hershey, PA: IGI Global. doi:10.4018/978-1-61520-963-7.ch078

Aston, J. (2013). Database narrative, spatial montage, and the cultural transmission of memory: An anthropological perspective. In D. Harrison (Ed.), *Digital media and technologies for virtual artistic spaces* (pp. 150–158). Hershey, PA: IGI Global. doi:10.4018/978-1-4666-2961-5.ch011

Asunka, S. (2013). Collaborative online learning in non-formal education settings in the developing world: A best practice framework. In V. Wang (Ed.), *Technological applications in adult and vocational education advancement* (pp. 186–201). Hershey, PA: IGI Global. doi:10.4018/978-1-4666-2062-9.ch015

Attia, M. (2014). The role of early learning experience in shaping teacher cognition and technology use. In P. Breen (Ed.), *Cases on teacher identity, diversity, and cognition in higher education* (pp. 1–21). Hershey, PA: IGI Global. doi:10.4018/978-1-4666-5990-2.ch001

Ávila, I., Menezes, E., & Braga, A. M. (2014). Strategy to support the memorization of iconic passwords. In K. Blashki & P. Isaias (Eds.), *Emerging research and trends in interactivity and the human-computer interface* (pp. 239–259). Hershey, PA: IGI Global. doi:10.4018/978-1-4666-4623-0.ch012

Bachvarova, Y., & Bocconi, S. (2014). Games and social networks. In T. Connolly, T. Hainey, E. Boyle, G. Baxter, & P. Moreno-Ger (Eds.), *Psychology, pedagogy, and assessment in serious games* (pp. 204–219). Hershey, PA: IGI Global. doi:10.4018/978-1-4666-4773-2.ch010

Bagley, C. A., & Creswell, W. H. (2013). The role of social media as a tool for learning. In E. McKay (Ed.), *ePedagogy in online learning: New developments in web mediated human computer interaction* (pp. 18–38). Hershey, PA: IGI Global. doi:10.4018/978-1-4666-3649-1.ch002

Balogh, Š. (2014). Forensic analysis, cryptosystem implementation, and cryptology: Methods and techniques for extracting encryption keys from volatile memory. In S. Sadkhan Al Maliky & N. Abbas (Eds.), *Multidisciplinary perspectives in cryptology and information security* (pp. 381–396). Hershey, PA: IGI Global. doi:10.4018/978-1-4666-5808-0.ch016

Banas, J. R., & Brown, C. A. (2012). Web 2.0 visualization tools to stimulate generative learning. In D. Polly, C. Mims, & K. Persichitte (Eds.), *Developing technology-rich teacher education programs: Key issues* (pp. 77–90). Hershey, PA: IGI Global. doi:10.4018/978-1-4666-0014-0.ch006

Bancroft, J., & Wang, Y. (2013). A computational simulation of the cognitive process of children knowledge acquisition and memory development. In Y. Wang (Ed.), *Cognitive informatics for revealing human cognition: Knowledge manipulations in natural intelligence* (pp. 111–127). Hershey, PA: IGI Global. doi:10.4018/978-1-4666-2476-4.ch008

Bartsch, R. A. (2011). Social psychology and instructional technology. In *Instructional design: Concepts, methodologies, tools and applications* (pp. 1237–1244). Hershey, PA: IGI Global. doi:10.4018/978-1-60960-503-2.ch508

Bertolotti, T. (2013). Facebook has it: The irresistible violence of social cognition in the age of social networking. In R. Luppicini (Ed.), *Moral, ethical, and social dilemmas in the age of technology: Theories and practice* (pp. 234–247). Hershey, PA: IGI Global. doi:10.4018/978-1-4666-2931-8.ch016

Berwick, R. C. (2013). Songs to syntax: Cognition, combinatorial computation, and the origin of language. In Y. Wang (Ed.), *Cognitive informatics for revealing human cognition: Knowledge manipulations in natural intelligence* (pp. 70–80). Hershey, PA: IGI Global. doi:10.4018/978-1-4666-2476-4.ch005

Best, C., O'Neill, B., & Gillespie, A. (2014). Assistive technology for cognition: An updated review. In G. Naik & Y. Guo (Eds.), *Emerging theory and practice in neuroprosthetics* (pp. 215–236). Hershey, PA: IGI Global. doi:10.4018/978-1-4666-6094-6.ch011

Bhattacharya, A. (2014). Organisational justice perception: A work attitude modifier. In N. Ray & K. Chakraborty (Eds.), *Handbook of research on strategic business infrastructure development and contemporary issues in finance* (pp. 296–322). Hershey, PA: IGI Global. doi:10.4018/978-1-4666-5154-8.ch021

Biggiero, L. (2012). Practice vs. possession: Epistemological implications on the nature of organizational knowledge and cognition. In M. Mora, O. Gelman, A. Steenkamp, & M. Raisinghani (Eds.), *Research methodologies, innovations and philosophies in software systems engineering and information systems* (pp. 82–105). Hershey, PA: IGI Global. doi:10.4018/978-1-4666-0179-6.ch005

Bishop, J. (2014). The psychology of trolling and lurking: The role of defriending and gamification for increasing participation in online communities using seductive narratives. In J. Bishop (Ed.), *Gamification for human factors integration: Social, education, and psychological issues* (pp. 162–179). Hershey, PA: IGI Global. doi:10.4018/978-1-4666-5071-8.ch010

Blasko, D. G., Lum, H. C., White, M. M., & Drabik, H. B. (2014). Individual differences in the enjoyment and effectiveness of serious games. In T. Connolly, T. Hainey, E. Boyle, G. Baxter, & P. Moreno-Ger (Eds.), *Psychology, pedagogy, and assessment in serious games* (pp. 153–174). Hershey, PA: IGI Global. doi:10.4018/978-1-4666-4773-2.ch008

Borah, P. (2014). Interaction of incivility and news frames in the political blogosphere: Consequences and psychological mechanisms. In A. Solo (Ed.), *Handbook of research on political activism in the information age* (pp. 407–424). Hershey, PA: IGI Global. doi:10.4018/978-1-4666-6066-3.ch024

Borri, D., & Camarda, D. (2011). Spatial ontologies in multi-agent environmental planning. In J. Yearwood & A. Stranieri (Eds.), *Technologies for supporting reasoning communities and collaborative decision making: Cooperative approaches* (pp. 272–295). Hershey, PA: IGI Global. doi:10.4018/978-1-60960-091-4.ch015

Boukhobza, J. (2013). Flashing in the cloud: Shedding some light on NAND flash memory storage systems. In D. Kyriazis, A. Voulodimos, S. Gogouvitis, & T. Varvarigou (Eds.), *Data intensive storage services for cloud environments* (pp. 241–266). Hershey, PA: IGI Global. doi:10.4018/978-1-4666-3934-8.ch015

Boyle, E. (2014). Psychological aspects of serious games. In T. Connolly, T. Hainey, E. Boyle, G. Baxter, & P. Moreno-Ger (Eds.), *Psychology, pedagogy, and assessment in serious games* (pp. 1–18). Hershey, PA: IGI Global. doi:10.4018/978-1-4666-4773-2.ch001

Boyle, E., Terras, M. M., Ramsay, J., & Boyle, J. M. (2014). Executive functions in digital games. In T. Connolly, T. Hainey, E. Boyle, G. Baxter, & P. Moreno-Ger (Eds.), *Psychology, pedagogy, and assessment in serious games* (pp. 19–46). Hershey, PA: IGI Global. doi:10.4018/978-1-4666-4773-2.ch002

Breen, P. (2014). Philosophies, traditional pedagogy, and new technologies: A report on a case study of EAP teachers' integration of technology into traditional practice. In P. Breen (Ed.), *Cases on teacher identity, diversity, and cognition in higher education* (pp. 317–341). Hershey, PA: IGI Global. doi:10.4018/978-1-4666-5990-2.ch013

Buchanan, A. (2014). Protective factors in family relationships. In M. Merviö (Ed.), *Contemporary social issues in east Asian societies: Examining the spectrum of public and private spheres* (pp. 76–85). Hershey, PA: IGI Global. doi:10.4018/978-1-4666-5031-2.ch004

Burke, M. E., & Speed, C. (2014). Knowledge recovery: Applications of technology and memory. In M. Michael & K. Michael (Eds.), *Uberveillance and the social implications of microchip implants: Emerging technologies* (pp. 133–142). Hershey, PA: IGI Global. doi:10.4018/978-1-4666-4582-0.ch005

Burusic, J., & Karabegovic, M. (2014). The role of students' personality traits in the effective use of social networking sites in the educational context. In G. Mallia (Ed.), *The social classroom: Integrating social network use in education* (pp. 224–243). Hershey, PA: IGI Global. doi:10.4018/978-1-4666-4904-0.ch012

Caixinha, A., Magalhães, V., & Alexandre, I. M. (2013). Do you remember, or have you forgotten? In R. Martinho, R. Rijo, M. Cruz-Cunha, & J. Varajão (Eds.), *Information systems and technologies for enhancing health and social care* (pp. 136–146). Hershey, PA: IGI Global. doi:10.4018/978-1-4666-3667-5.ch009

Carbonaro, N., Cipresso, P., Tognetti, A., Anania, G., De Rossi, D., Pallavicini, F., ... Riva, G. (2014). Psychometric assessment of cardio-respiratory activity using a mobile platform. *International Journal of Handheld Computing Research*, 5(1), 13–29. doi:10.4018/ijhcr.2014010102

Castellani, M. (2011). Cognitive tools for group decision making: The repertory grid approach revisited. In J. Yearwood & A. Stranieri (Eds.), *Technologies for supporting reasoning communities and collaborative decision making: Cooperative approaches* (pp. 172–192). Hershey, PA: IGI Global. doi:10.4018/978-1-60960-091-4.ch010

Cawthon, S. W., Harris, A., & Jones, R. (2010). Cognitive apprenticeship in an online research lab for graduate students in psychology. *International Journal of Web-Based Learning and Teaching Technologies*, 5(1), 1–15. doi:10.4018/jwltt.2010010101

Cederborg, T., & Oudeyer, P. (2014). Learning words by imitating. In *Computational linguistics: Concepts, methodologies, tools, and applications* (pp. 1674–1704). Hershey, PA: IGI Global. doi:10.4018/978-1-4666-6042-7.ch084

Cervantes, J., Rodríguez, L., López, S., Ramos, F., & Robles, F. (2013). Cognitive process of moral decision-making for autonomous agents. *International Journal of Software Science and Computational Intelligence*, 5(4), 61–76. doi:10.4018/ijssci.2013100105

Chadwick, D. D., Fullwood, C., & Wesson, C. J. (2014). Intellectual disability, identity, and the internet. In *Assistive technologies: Concepts, methodologies, tools, and applications* (pp. 198–223). Hershey, PA: IGI Global. doi:10.4018/978-1-4666-4422-9.ch011

Chan, E. C., Baciu, G., & Mak, S. C. (2010). Cognitive location-aware information retrieval by agent-based semantic matching. *International Journal of Software Science and Computational Intelligence, 2*(3), 21–31. doi:10.4018/jssci.2010070102

Chen, C. (2014). Differences between visual style and verbal style learners in learning English. *International Journal of Distance Education Technologies, 12*(1), 91–104. doi:10.4018/ijdet.2014010106

Chen, K., & Barthès, J. A. (2012). Giving personal assistant agents a case-based memory. In Y. Wang (Ed.), *Developments in natural intelligence research and knowledge engineering: Advancing applications* (pp. 287–304). Hershey, PA: IGI Global. doi:10.4018/978-1-4666-1743-8.ch021

Chen, S., Tai, C., Wang, T., & Wang, S. G. (2011). Social simulation with both human agents and software agents: An investigation into the impact of cognitive capacity on their learning behavior. In S. Chen, Y. Kambayashi, & H. Sato (Eds.), *Multi-agent applications with evolutionary computation and biologically inspired technologies: Intelligent techniques for ubiquity and optimization* (pp. 95–117). Hershey, PA: IGI Global. doi:10.4018/978-1-60566-898-7.ch006

Chiriacescu, V., Soh, L., & Shell, D. F. (2013). Understanding human learning using a multi-agent simulation of the unified learning model. *International Journal of Cognitive Informatics and Natural Intelligence, 7*(4), 1–25. doi:10.4018/ijcini.2013100101

Christen, M., Alfano, M., Bangerter, E., & Lapsley, D. (2013). Ethical issues of 'morality mining': Moral identity as a focus of data mining. In H. Rahman & I. Ramos (Eds.), *Ethical data mining applications for socio-economic development* (pp. 1–21). Hershey, PA: IGI Global. doi:10.4018/978-1-4666-4078-8.ch001

Cipresso, P., Serino, S., Gaggioli, A., & Riva, G. (2014). Modeling the diffusion of psychological stress. In J. Rodrigues (Ed.), *Advancing medical practice through technology: Applications for healthcare delivery, management, and quality* (pp. 178–204). Hershey, PA: IGI Global. doi:10.4018/978-1-4666-4619-3.ch010

Code, J. (2013). Agency and identity in social media. In S. Warburton & S. Hatzipanagos (Eds.), *Digital identity and social media* (pp. 37–57). Hershey, PA: IGI Global. doi:10.4018/978-1-4666-1915-9.ch004

Combs, R. M., & Mazur, J. (2014). 3D modeling in a high school computer visualization class: Enacting a productive, distributed social learning environment. In *K-12 education: Concepts, methodologies, tools, and applications* (pp. 1020–1040). Hershey, PA: IGI Global. doi:10.4018/978-1-4666-4502-8.ch061

Cook, R. G., & Sutton, R. (2014). Administrators' assessments of online courses and student retention in higher education: Lessons learned. In S. Mukerji & P. Tripathi (Eds.), *Handbook of research on transnational higher education* (pp. 138–150). Hershey, PA: IGI Global. doi:10.4018/978-1-4666-4458-8.ch008

Correa, T., Bachmann, I., Hinsley, A. W., & Gil de Zúñiga, H. (2013). Personality and social media use. In E. Li, S. Loh, C. Evans, & F. Lorenzi (Eds.), *Organizations and social networking: Utilizing social media to engage consumers* (pp. 41–61). Hershey, PA: IGI Global. doi:10.4018/978-1-4666-4026-9.ch003

Cowell, R. A., Bussey, T. J., & Saksida, L. M. (2011). Using computational modelling to understand cognition in the ventral visual-perirhinal pathway. In E. Alonso & E. Mondragón (Eds.), *Computational neuroscience for advancing artificial intelligence: Models, methods and applications* (pp. 15–45). Hershey, PA: IGI Global. doi:10.4018/978-1-60960-021-1.ch002

Crespo, R. G., Martíne, O. S., Lovelle, J. M., García-Bustelo, B. C., Díaz, V. G., & Ordoñez de Pablos, P. (2014). Improving cognitive load on students with disabilities through software aids. In *Assistive technologies: Concepts, methodologies, tools, and applications* (pp. 1255–1268). Hershey, PA: IGI Global. doi:10.4018/978-1-4666-4422-9.ch066

Cró, M. D., Andreucci, L., Pinho, A. M., & Pereira, A. (2013). Resilience and psychomotricity in preschool education: A study with children that are socially, culturally, and economically disadvantaged. In M. Cruz-Cunha, I. Miranda, & P. Gonçalves (Eds.), *Handbook of research on ICTs for human-centered healthcare and social care services* (pp. 366–378). Hershey, PA: IGI Global. doi:10.4018/978-1-4666-3986-7.ch019

Cummings, J. J., & Ross, T. L. (2013). Optimizing the psychological benefits of choice: information transparency and heuristic use in game environments. In R. Ferdig (Ed.), *Design, utilization, and analysis of simulations and game-based educational worlds* (pp. 142–157). Hershey, PA: IGI Global. doi:10.4018/978-1-4666-4018-4.ch009

Curumsing, M. K., Pedell, S., & Vasa, R. (2014). Designing an evaluation tool to measure emotional goals. *International Journal of People-Oriented Programming*, *3*(1), 22–43. doi:10.4018/ijpop.2014010102

Cuzzocrea, F., Murdaca, A. M., & Oliva, P. (2013). Using precision teaching method to improve foreign language and cognitive skills in university students. In A. Cartelli (Ed.), *Fostering 21st century digital literacy and technical competency* (pp. 201–211). Hershey, PA: IGI Global. doi:10.4018/978-1-4666-2943-1.ch014

DaCosta, B., & Seok, S. (2010). Human cognition in the design of assistive technology for those with learning disabilities. In S. Seok, E. Meyen, & B. DaCosta (Eds.), *Handbook of research on human cognition and assistive technology: Design, accessibility and transdisciplinary perspectives* (pp. 1–20). Hershey, PA: IGI Global. doi:10.4018/978-1-61520-817-3.ch001

DaCosta, B., & Seok, S. (2010). Multimedia design of assistive technology for those with learning disabilities. In S. Seok, E. Meyen, & B. DaCosta (Eds.), *Handbook of research on human cognition and assistive technology: Design, accessibility and transdisciplinary perspectives* (pp. 43–60). Hershey, PA: IGI Global. doi:10.4018/978-1-61520-817-3.ch003

Danielsson, U., & Öberg, K. D. (2011). Psychosocial life environment and life roles in interaction with daily use of information communication technology boundaries between work and leisure. In D. Haftor & A. Mirijamdotter (Eds.), *Information and communication technologies, society and human beings: Theory and framework (Festschrift in honor of Gunilla Bradley)* (pp. 266–282). Hershey, PA: IGI Global. doi:10.4018/978-1-60960-057-0.ch020

Daradoumis, T., & Lafuente, M. M. (2014). Studying the suitability of discourse analysis methods for emotion detection and interpretation in computer-mediated educational discourse. In H. Lim & F. Sudweeks (Eds.), *Innovative methods and technologies for electronic discourse analysis* (pp. 119–143). Hershey, PA: IGI Global. doi:10.4018/978-1-4666-4426-7.ch006

De Simone, C., Marquis, T., & Groen, J. (2013). Optimizing conditions for learning and teaching in K-20 education. In V. Wang (Ed.), *Handbook of research on teaching and learning in K-20 education* (pp. 535–552). Hershey, PA: IGI Global. doi:10.4018/978-1-4666-4249-2.ch031

Deka, G. C. (2014). Significance of in-memory computing for real-time big data analytics. In P. Raj & G. Deka (Eds.), *Handbook of research on cloud infrastructures for big data analytics* (pp. 352–369). Hershey, PA: IGI Global. doi:10.4018/978-1-4666-5864-6.ch014

Demirbilek, M. (2010). Cognitive load and disorientation issues in hypermedia as assistive technology. In S. Seok, E. Meyen, & B. DaCosta (Eds.), *Handbook of research on human cognition and assistive technology: Design, accessibility and transdisciplinary perspectives* (pp. 109–120). Hershey, PA: IGI Global. doi:10.4018/978-1-61520-817-3.ch007

Derrick, M. G. (2013). The inventory of learner persistence. In M. Bocarnea, R. Reynolds, & J. Baker (Eds.), *Online instruments, data collection, and electronic measurements: Organizational advancements* (pp. 271–290). Hershey, PA: IGI Global. doi:10.4018/978-1-4666-2172-5.ch016

Doolittle, P. E., McNeill, A. L., Terry, K. P., & Scheer, S. B. (2011). Multimedia, cognitive load, and pedagogy. In *Instructional design: Concepts, methodologies, tools and applications* (pp. 1564–1585). Hershey, PA: IGI Global. doi:10.4018/978-1-60960-503-2.ch706

Dourlens, S., & Ramdane-Cherif, A. (2013). Cognitive memory for semantic agents architecture in robotic interaction. In Y. Wang (Ed.), *Cognitive informatics for revealing human cognition: Knowledge manipulations in natural intelligence* (pp. 82–97). Hershey, PA: IGI Global. doi:10.4018/978-1-4666-2476-4.ch006

Dubbels, B. (2011). Cognitive ethnography: A methodology for measure and analysis of learning for game studies. *International Journal of Gaming and Computer-Mediated Simulations*, *3*(1), 68–78. doi:10.4018/jgcms.2011010105

Dunbar, N. E., Wilson, S. N., Adame, B. J., Elizondo, J., Jensen, M. L., Miller, C. H., ... Burgoon, J. K. (2013). MACBETH: Development of a training game for the mitigation of cognitive bias. *International Journal of Game-Based Learning*, *3*(4), 7–26. doi:10.4018/ijgbl.2013100102

Dunham, A. H., & Burt, C. D. (2012). Mentoring and the transfer of organizational memory within the context of an aging workforce: Cultural implications for competitive advantage. In *Organizational learning and knowledge: Concepts, methodologies, tools and applications* (pp. 3076–3099). Hershey, PA: IGI Global. doi:10.4018/978-1-60960-783-8.ch817

Durrington, V. A., & Du, J. (2013). Learning tasks, peer interaction, and cognition process an online collaborative design model. *International Journal of Information and Communication Technology Education*, *9*(1), 38–50. doi:10.4018/jicte.2013010104

Duțu, A. (2014). Understanding consumers' behaviour change in uncertainty conditions: A psychological perspective. In F. Musso & E. Druica (Eds.), *Handbook of research on retailer-consumer relationship development* (pp. 45–69). Hershey, PA: IGI Global. doi:10.4018/978-1-4666-6074-8.ch004

Dwyer, P. (2013). Measuring collective cognition in online collaboration venues. In N. Kock (Ed.), *Interdisciplinary applications of electronic collaboration approaches and technologies* (pp. 46–61). Hershey, PA: IGI Global. doi:10.4018/978-1-4666-2020-9.ch004

Egan, R. G., & Zhou, M. (2011). Re-conceptualizing calibration using trace methodology. In G. Dettori & D. Persico (Eds.), *Fostering self-regulated learning through ICT* (pp. 71–88). Hershey, PA: IGI Global. doi:10.4018/978-1-61692-901-5.ch005

El-Farargy, N. (2013). Refresher training in clinical psychology supervision: A blended learning approach. In A. Benson, J. Moore, & S. Williams van Rooij (Eds.), *Cases on educational technology planning, design, and implementation: A project management perspective* (pp. 295–317). Hershey, PA: IGI Global. doi:10.4018/978-1-4666-4237-9.ch016

El Louadi, M., & Tounsi, I. (2010). Do organizational memory and information technology interact to affect organizational information needs and provision? In M. Jennex (Ed.), *Ubiquitous developments in knowledge management: Integrations and trends* (pp. 1–20). Hershey, PA: IGI Global. doi:10.4018/978-1-60566-954-0.ch001

Estrada-Hernández, N., & Stachowiak, J. R. (2010). Evaluating systemic assistive technology needs. In S. Seok, E. Meyen, & B. DaCosta (Eds.), *Handbook of research on human cognition and assistive technology: Design, accessibility and transdisciplinary perspectives* (pp. 239–250). Hershey, PA: IGI Global. doi:10.4018/978-1-61520-817-3.ch016

Fitzpatrick, M., & Theoharis, R. (2010). Assistive technology for deaf and hard of hearing students. In S. Seok, E. Meyen, & B. DaCosta (Eds.), *Handbook of research on human cognition and assistive technology: Design, accessibility and transdisciplinary perspectives* (pp. 179–191). Hershey, PA: IGI Global. doi:10.4018/978-1-61520-817-3.ch012

Francis, A. G. Jr, Mehta, M., & Ram, A. (2012). Emotional memory and adaptive personalities. In *Machine learning: Concepts, methodologies, tools and applications* (pp. 1292–1313). Hershey, PA: IGI Global. doi:10.4018/978-1-60960-818-7.ch507

Gagliardi, F. (2014). A cognitive machine-learning system to discover syndromes in erythemato-squamous diseases. In J. Rodrigues (Ed.), *Advancing medical practice through technology: Applications for healthcare delivery, management, and quality* (pp. 66–101). Hershey, PA: IGI Global. doi:10.4018/978-1-4666-4619-3.ch005

Gaines, B. R., & Shaw, M. L. (2013). Sociocognitive inquiry. In *Data mining: Concepts, methodologies, tools, and applications* (pp. 1688–1708). Hershey, PA: IGI Global. doi:10.4018/978-1-4666-2455-9.ch088

Gardner, M. K., & Hill, R. D. (2013). Training older adults to improve their episodic memory: Three different approaches to enhancing numeric memory. In R. Zheng, R. Hill, & M. Gardner (Eds.), *Engaging older adults with modern technology: Internet use and information access needs* (pp. 191–211). Hershey, PA: IGI Global. doi:10.4018/978-1-4666-1966-1.ch010

Ghili, S., Nazarian, S., Tavana, M., Keyvanshokouhi, S., & Isaai, M. T. (2013). A complex systems paradox of organizational learning and knowledge management. *International Journal of Knowledge-Based Organizations*, *3*(3), 53–72. doi:10.4018/ijkbo.2013070104

Gibson, D. (2012). Designing a computational model of learning. In *Machine learning: Concepts, methodologies, tools and applications* (pp. 147–174). Hershey, PA: IGI Global. doi:10.4018/978-1-60960-818-7.ch203

Gibson, M., Renaud, K., Conrad, M., & Maple, C. (2013). Music is the key: Using our enduring memory for songs to help users log on. In *IT policy and ethics: Concepts, methodologies, tools, and applications* (pp. 1018–1037). Hershey, PA: IGI Global. doi:10.4018/978-1-4666-2919-6.ch046

Godine, N., & Barnett, J. E. (2013). The use of telepsychology in clinical practice: Benefits, effectiveness, and issues to consider. *International Journal of Cyber Behavior, Psychology and Learning*, *3*(4), 70–83. doi:10.4018/ijcbpl.2013100105

Gökçay, D. (2011). Emotional axes: Psychology, psychophysiology and neuroanatomical correlates. In D. Gökçay & G. Yildirim (Eds.), *Affective computing and interaction: Psychological, cognitive and neuroscientific perspectives* (pp. 56–73). Hershey, PA: IGI Global. doi:10.4018/978-1-61692-892-6.ch003

Goswami, R., Jena, R. K., & Mahapatro, B. B. (2013). Psycho-social impact of shift work: A study of ferro-alloy industries in Orissa. In P. Ordóñez de Pablos (Ed.), *Business, technology, and knowledge management in Asia: Trends and innovations* (pp. 166–174). Hershey, PA: IGI Global. doi:10.4018/978-1-4666-2652-2.ch013

Graff, M. (2011). Can cognitive style predict how individuals use web-based learning environments? In *Instructional design: Concepts, methodologies, tools and applications* (pp. 1553–1563). Hershey, PA: IGI Global. doi:10.4018/978-1-60960-503-2.ch705

Griffiths, M., Kuss, D. J., & Ortiz de Gortari, A. B. (2013). Videogames as therapy: A review of the medical and psychological literature. In M. Cruz-Cunha, I. Miranda, & P. Gonçalves (Eds.), *Handbook of research on ICTs and management systems for improving efficiency in healthcare and social care* (pp. 43–68). Hershey, PA: IGI Global. doi:10.4018/978-1-4666-3990-4.ch003

Guger, C., Sorger, B., Noirhomme, Q., Naci, L., Monti, M. M., & Real, R. ... Cincotti, F. (2014). Brain-computer interfaces for assessment and communication in disorders of consciousness. In G. Naik & Y. Guo (Eds.), Emerging theory and practice in neuroprosthetics (pp. 181-214). Hershey, PA: IGI Global. doi:10.4018/978-1-4666-6094-6.ch010

Güngör, H. (2014). Adolescent suicides as a chaotic phenomenon. In Ş. Erçetin & S. Banerjee (Eds.), *Chaos and complexity theory in world politics* (pp. 306–324). Hershey, PA: IGI Global. doi:10.4018/978-1-4666-6070-0.ch022

Hai-Jew, S. (2013). Interpreting "you" and "me": Personal voices, PII, biometrics, and imperfect/perfect electronic memory in a democracy. In C. Akrivopoulou & N. Garipidis (Eds.), *Digital democracy and the impact of technology on governance and politics: New globalized practices* (pp. 20–37). Hershey, PA: IGI Global. doi:10.4018/978-1-4666-3637-8.ch003

Hainey, T., Connolly, T. M., Chaudy, Y., Boyle, E., Beeby, R., & Soflano, M. (2014). Assessment integration in serious games. In T. Connolly, T. Hainey, E. Boyle, G. Baxter, & P. Moreno-Ger (Eds.), *Psychology, pedagogy, and assessment in serious games* (pp. 317–341). Hershey, PA: IGI Global. doi:10.4018/978-1-4666-4773-2.ch015

Hainey, T., Soflano, M., & Connolly, T. M. (2014). A randomised controlled trial to evaluate learning effectiveness using an adaptive serious game to teach SQL at higher education level. In T. Connolly, T. Hainey, E. Boyle, G. Baxter, & P. Moreno-Ger (Eds.), *Psychology, pedagogy, and assessment in serious games* (pp. 270–291). Hershey, PA: IGI Global. doi:10.4018/978-1-4666-4773-2.ch013

Haque, J., Erturk, M., Arslan, H., & Moreno, W. (2011). Cognitive aeronautical communication system. *International Journal of Interdisciplinary Telecommunications and Networking*, 3(1), 20–35. doi:10.4018/jitn.2011010102

Hauge, J. B., Boyle, E., Mayer, I., Nadolski, R., Riedel, J. C., Moreno-Ger, P., ... Ritchie, J. (2014). Study design and data gathering guide for serious games' evaluation. In T. Connolly, T. Hainey, E. Boyle, G. Baxter, & P. Moreno-Ger (Eds.), *Psychology, pedagogy, and assessment in serious games* (pp. 394–419). Hershey, PA: IGI Global. doi:10.4018/978-1-4666-4773-2.ch018

Haykin, S. (2013). Cognitive dynamic systems. In Y. Wang (Ed.), *Cognitive informatics for revealing human cognition: Knowledge manipulations in natural intelligence* (pp. 250–260). Hershey, PA: IGI Global. doi:10.4018/978-1-4666-2476-4.ch016

Henderson, A. M., & Sabbagh, M. A. (2014). Learning words from experience: An integrated framework. In *Computational linguistics: Concepts, methodologies, tools, and applications* (pp. 1705–1727). Hershey, PA: IGI Global. doi:10.4018/978-1-4666-6042-7.ch085

Hendrick, H. W. (2011). Cognitive and organizational complexity and behavior: Implications for organizational design and leadership. In D. Haftor & A. Mirijamdotter (Eds.), *Information and communication technologies, society and human beings: Theory and framework (Festschrift in honor of Gunilla Bradley)* (pp. 147–159). Hershey, PA: IGI Global. doi:10.4018/978-1-60960-057-0.ch013

Henrie, K. M., & Miller, D. W. (2013). An examination of mediation: Insights into the role of psychological mediators in the use of persuasion knowledge. In R. Eid (Ed.), *Managing customer trust, satisfaction, and loyalty through information communication technologies* (pp. 106–117). Hershey, PA: IGI Global. doi:10.4018/978-1-4666-3631-6.ch007

Ho, W. C., Dautenhahn, K., Lim, M., Enz, S., Zoll, C., & Watson, S. (2012). Towards learning 'self' and emotional knowledge in social and cultural human-agent interactions. In *Virtual learning environments: Concepts, methodologies, tools and applications* (pp. 1426–1445). Hershey, PA: IGI Global. doi:10.4018/978-1-4666-0011-9.ch705

Holt, L., & Ziegler, M. F. (2013). Promoting team learning in the classroom. In V. Wang (Ed.), *Technological applications in adult and vocational education advancement* (pp. 94–105). Hershey, PA: IGI Global. doi:10.4018/978-1-4666-2062-9.ch008

Honey, R. C., & Grand, C. S. (2011). Application of connectionist models to animal learning: Interactions between perceptual organization and associative processes. In E. Alonso & E. Mondragón (Eds.), *Computational neuroscience for advancing artificial intelligence: Models, methods and applications* (pp. 1–14). Hershey, PA: IGI Global. doi:10.4018/978-1-60960-021-1.ch001

Hoppenbrouwers, S., Schotten, B., & Lucas, P. (2012). Towards games for knowledge acquisition and modeling. In R. Ferdig & S. de Freitas (Eds.), *Interdisciplinary advancements in gaming, simulations and virtual environments: Emerging trends* (pp. 281–299). Hershey, PA: IGI Global. doi:10.4018/978-1-4666-0029-4.ch018

Huang, C., Liang, C., & Lin, E. (2014). A study on emotion releasing effect with music and color. In F. Cipolla-Ficarra (Ed.), *Advanced research and trends in new technologies, software, human-computer interaction, and communicability* (pp. 23–31). Hershey, PA: IGI Global. doi:10.4018/978-1-4666-4490-8.ch003

Huang, W. D., & Tettegah, S. Y. (2014). Cognitive load and empathy in serious games: A conceptual framework. In J. Bishop (Ed.), *Gamification for human factors integration: Social, education, and psychological issues* (pp. 17–30). Hershey, PA: IGI Global. doi:10.4018/978-1-4666-5071-8.ch002

Huijnen, C. (2011). The use of assistive technology to support the wellbeing and independence of people with memory impairments. In J. Soar, R. Swindell, & P. Tsang (Eds.), *Intelligent technologies for bridging the grey digital divide* (pp. 65–79). Hershey, PA: IGI Global. doi:10.4018/978-1-61520-825-8.ch005

Huseyinov, I. N. (2014). Fuzzy linguistic modelling in multi modal human computer interaction: Adaptation to cognitive styles using multi level fuzzy granulation method. In *Assistive technologies: Concepts, methodologies, tools, and applications* (pp. 1481–1496). Hershey, PA: IGI Global. doi:10.4018/978-1-4666-4422-9.ch077

Hussey, H. D., Fleck, B. K., & Richmond, A. S. (2014). Promoting active learning through a flipped course design. In J. Keengwe, G. Onchwari, & J. Oigara (Eds.), *Promoting active learning through the flipped classroom model* (pp. 23–46). Hershey, PA: IGI Global. doi:10.4018/978-1-4666-4987-3.ch002

Ilin, R., & Perlovsky, L. (2010). Cognitively inspired neural network for recognition of situations. *International Journal of Natural Computing Research*, *1*(1), 36–55. doi:10.4018/jncr.2010010102

Ilin, R., & Perlovsky, L. (2011). Cognitive based distributed sensing, processing, and communication. In B. Igelnik (Ed.), *Computational modeling and simulation of intellect: Current state and future perspectives* (pp. 131–161). Hershey, PA: IGI Global. doi:10.4018/978-1-60960-551-3.ch006

Jenkins, J. L., Durcikova, A., & Burns, M. B. (2013). Simplicity is bliss: Controlling extraneous cognitive load in online security training to promote secure behavior. *Journal of Organizational and End User Computing*, *25*(3), 52–66. doi:10.4018/joeuc.2013070104

Jennings, D. J., Alonso, E., Mondragón, E., & Bonardi, C. (2011). Temporal uncertainty during overshadowing: A temporal difference account. In E. Alonso & E. Mondragón (Eds.), *Computational neuroscience for advancing artificial intelligence: Models, methods and applications* (pp. 46–55). Hershey, PA: IGI Global. doi:10.4018/978-1-60960-021-1.ch003

Jin, S., DaCosta, B., & Seok, S. (2014). Social skills development for children with autism spectrum disorders through the use of interactive storytelling games. In B. DaCosta & S. Seok (Eds.), *Assistive technology research, practice, and theory* (pp. 144–159). Hershey, PA: IGI Global. doi:10.4018/978-1-4666-5015-2.ch010

Johnson, R. D., De Ridder, D., & Gillett, G. (2014). Neurosurgery to enhance brain function: Ethical dilemmas for the neuroscientist and society. In S. Thompson (Ed.), *Global issues and ethical considerations in human enhancement technologies* (pp. 96–118). Hershey, PA: IGI Global. doi:10.4018/978-1-4666-6010-6.ch006

Johnson, V., & Price, C. (2010). A longitudinal case study on the use of assistive technology to support cognitive processes across formal and informal educational settings. In S. Seok, E. Meyen, & B. DaCosta (Eds.), *Handbook of research on human cognition and assistive technology: Design, accessibility and transdisciplinary perspectives* (pp. 192–198). Hershey, PA: IGI Global. doi:10.4018/978-1-61520-817-3.ch013

Kalyuga, S. (2012). Cognitive load aspects of text processing. In C. Boonthum-Denecke, P. McCarthy, & T. Lamkin (Eds.), *Cross-disciplinary advances in applied natural language processing: Issues and approaches* (pp. 114–132). Hershey, PA: IGI Global. doi:10.4018/978-1-61350-447-5.ch009

Kammler, D., Witte, E. M., Chattopadhyay, A., Bauwens, B., Ascheid, G., Leupers, R., & Meyr, H. (2012). Automatic generation of memory interfaces for ASIPs. In S. Virtanen (Ed.), *Innovations in embedded and real-time systems engineering for communication* (pp. 79–100). Hershey, PA: IGI Global. doi:10.4018/978-1-4666-0912-9.ch005

Khan, T. M. (2011). Theory of mind in autistic children: multimedia based support. In P. Ordóñez de Pablos, J. Zhao, & R. Tennyson (Eds.), *Technology enhanced learning for people with disabilities: Approaches and applications* (pp. 167–179). Hershey, PA: IGI Global. doi:10.4018/978-1-61520-923-1.ch012

Khetrapal, N. (2010). Cognition meets assistive technology: Insights from load theory of selective attention. In S. Seok, E. Meyen, & B. DaCosta (Eds.), *Handbook of research on human cognition and assistive technology: Design, accessibility and transdisciplinary perspectives* (pp. 96–108). Hershey, PA: IGI Global. doi:10.4018/978-1-61520-817-3.ch006

Khetrapal, N. (2010). Cognitive science helps formulate games for moral education. In K. Schrier & D. Gibson (Eds.), *Ethics and game design: Teaching values through play* (pp. 181–196). Hershey, PA: IGI Global. doi:10.4018/978-1-61520-845-6.ch012

Kickmeier-Rust, M. D., Mattheiss, E., Steiner, C., & Albert, D. (2011). A psycho-pedagogical framework for multi-adaptive educational games. *International Journal of Game-Based Learning, 1*(1), 45–58. doi:10.4018/ijgbl.2011010104

Kiel, L. D., & McCaskill, J. (2013). Cognition and complexity: An agent-based model of cognitive capital under stress. In S. Banerjee (Ed.), *Chaos and complexity theory for management: Nonlinear dynamics* (pp. 254–268). Hershey, PA: IGI Global. doi:10.4018/978-1-4666-2509-9.ch012

Kiili, K., & Perttula, A. (2013). A design framework for educational exergames. In S. de Freitas, M. Ott, M. Popescu, & I. Stanescu (Eds.), *New pedagogical approaches in game enhanced learning: Curriculum integration* (pp. 136–158). Hershey, PA: IGI Global. doi:10.4018/978-1-4666-3950-8.ch008

Kiliç, F. (2011). Structuring of knowledge and cognitive load. In G. Kurubacak & T. Yuzer (Eds.), *Handbook of research on transformative online education and liberation: Models for social equality* (pp. 370–382). Hershey, PA: IGI Global. doi:10.4018/978-1-60960-046-4.ch020

Kim, E. B. (2011). Student personality and learning outcomes in e-learning: An introduction to empirical research. In S. Eom & J. Arbaugh (Eds.), *Student satisfaction and learning outcomes in e-learning: An introduction to empirical research* (pp. 294–315). Hershey, PA: IGI Global. doi:10.4018/978-1-60960-615-2.ch013

Kinsell, C. (2010). Investigating assistive technologies using computers to simulate basic curriculum for individuals with cognitive impairments. In S. Seok, E. Meyen, & B. DaCosta (Eds.), *Handbook of research on human cognition and assistive technology: Design, accessibility and transdisciplinary perspectives* (pp. 61–75). Hershey, PA: IGI Global. doi:10.4018/978-1-61520-817-3.ch004

Kirwan, G., & Power, A. (2012). Can forensic psychology contribute to solving the problem of cybercrime? In G. Kirwan & A. Power (Eds.), *The psychology of cyber crime: Concepts and principles* (pp. 18–36). Hershey, PA: IGI Global. doi:10.4018/978-1-61350-350-8.ch002

Klippel, A., Richter, K., & Hansen, S. (2013). Cognitively ergonomic route directions. In *Geographic information systems: Concepts, methodologies, tools, and applications* (pp. 250–257). Hershey, PA: IGI Global. doi:10.4018/978-1-4666-2038-4.ch017

Knafla, B., & Champandard, A. J. (2012). Behavior trees: Introduction and memory-compact implementation. In A. Kumar, J. Etheredge, & A. Boudreaux (Eds.), *Algorithmic and architectural gaming design: Implementation and development* (pp. 40–66). Hershey, PA: IGI Global. doi:10.4018/978-1-4666-1634-9.ch003

Kokkinos, C. M., Antoniadou, N., Dalara, E., Koufogazou, A., & Papatziki, A. (2013). Cyber-bullying, personality and coping among pre-adolescents. *International Journal of Cyber Behavior, Psychology and Learning, 3*(4), 55–69. doi:10.4018/ijcbpl.2013100104

Konrath, S. (2013). The empathy paradox: Increasing disconnection in the age of increasing connection. In R. Luppicini (Ed.), *Handbook of research on technoself: Identity in a technological society* (pp. 204–228). Hershey, PA: IGI Global. doi:10.4018/978-1-4666-2211-1.ch012

Kopp, B., & Mandl, H. (2012). Supporting virtual collaborative learning using collaboration scripts and content schemes. In *Virtual learning environments: Concepts, methodologies, tools and applications* (pp. 470–487). Hershey, PA: IGI Global. doi:10.4018/978-1-4666-0011-9.ch303

Kumar, S., Singhal, D., & Murthy, G. R. (2013). Doubly cognitive architecture based cognitive wireless sensor networks. In N. Chilamkurti (Ed.), *Security, design, and architecture for broadband and wireless network technologies* (pp. 121–126). Hershey, PA: IGI Global. doi:10.4018/978-1-4666-3902-7.ch009

Kutaula, S., & Talwar, V. (2014). Integrating psychological contract and service-related outcomes in emerging economies: A proposed conceptual framework. In A. Goyal (Ed.), *Innovations in services marketing and management: Strategies for emerging economies* (pp. 291–306). Hershey, PA: IGI Global. doi:10.4018/978-1-4666-4671-1.ch016

Kyriakaki, G., & Matsatsinis, N. (2014). Pedagogical evaluation of e-learning websites with cognitive objectives. In D. Yannacopoulos, P. Manolitzas, N. Matsatsinis, & E. Grigoroudis (Eds.), *Evaluating websites and web services: Interdisciplinary perspectives on user satisfaction* (pp. 224–240). Hershey, PA: IGI Global. doi:10.4018/978-1-4666-5129-6.ch013

Kyritsis, M., Gulliver, S. R., & Morar, S. (2014). Cognitive and environmental factors influencing the process of spatial knowledge acquisition within virtual reality environments. *International Journal of Artificial Life Research, 4*(1), 43–58. doi:10.4018/ijalr.2014010104

Laffey, J., Stichter, J., & Schmidt, M. (2010). Social orthotics for youth with ASD to learn in a collaborative 3D VLE. In S. Seok, E. Meyen, & B. DaCosta (Eds.), *Handbook of research on human cognition and assistive technology: Design, accessibility and transdisciplinary perspectives* (pp. 76–95). Hershey, PA: IGI Global. doi:10.4018/978-1-61520-817-3.ch005

Lai, S., & Han, H. (2014). Behavioral planning theory. In J. Wang (Ed.), *Encyclopedia of business analytics and optimization* (pp. 265–272). Hershey, PA: IGI Global. doi:10.4018/978-1-4666-5202-6.ch025

Lawson, D. (2013). Analysis and use of the life styles inventory 1 and 2 by human synergistics international. In M. Bocarnea, R. Reynolds, & J. Baker (Eds.), *Online instruments, data collection, and electronic measurements: Organizational advancements* (pp. 76–96). Hershey, PA: IGI Global. doi:10.4018/978-1-4666-2172-5.ch005

Lee, L., & Hung, J. C. (2011). Effect of teaching using whole brain instruction on accounting learning. In Q. Jin (Ed.), *Distance education environments and emerging software systems: New technologies* (pp. 261–282). Hershey, PA: IGI Global. doi:10.4018/978-1-60960-539-1.ch016

Levin, I., & Kojukhov, A. (2013). Personalization of learning environments in a post-industrial class. In M. Pătruţ & B. Pătruţ (Eds.), *Social media in higher education: Teaching in web 2.0* (pp. 105–123). Hershey, PA: IGI Global. doi:10.4018/978-1-4666-2970-7.ch006

Li, A., Li, H., Guo, R., & Zhu, T. (2013). MobileSens: A ubiquitous psychological laboratory based on mobile device. *International Journal of Cyber Behavior, Psychology and Learning, 3*(2), 47–55. doi:10.4018/ijcbpl.2013040104

Li, R. (2013). Traditional to hybrid: Social media's role in reshaping instruction in higher education. In A. Sigal (Ed.), *Advancing library education: Technological innovation and instructional design* (pp. 65–90). Hershey, PA: IGI Global. doi:10.4018/978-1-4666-3688-0.ch005

Li, X., Lin, Z., & Wu, J. (2014). Language processing in the human brain of literate and illiterate subjects. In *Computational linguistics: Concepts, methodologies, tools, and applications* (pp. 1391–1400). Hershey, PA: IGI Global. doi:10.4018/978-1-4666-6042-7.ch068

Li, X., Ouyang, Z., & Luo, Y. (2013). The cognitive load affects the interaction pattern of emotion and working memory. *International Journal of Cognitive Informatics and Natural Intelligence, 6*(2), 68–81. doi:10.4018/jcini.2012040104

Lin, T., Li, X., Wu, Z., & Tang, N. (2013). Automatic cognitive load classification using high-frequency interaction events: An exploratory study. *International Journal of Technology and Human Interaction, 9*(3), 73–88. doi:10.4018/jthi.2013070106

Linek, S. B. (2011). As you like it: What media psychology can tell us about educational game design. In P. Felicia (Ed.), *Handbook of research on improving learning and motivation through educational games: Multidisciplinary approaches* (pp. 606–632). Hershey, PA: IGI Global. doi:10.4018/978-1-60960-495-0.ch029

Linek, S. B., Marte, B., & Albert, D. (2014). Background music in educational games: Motivational appeal and cognitive impact. In J. Bishop (Ed.), *Gamification for human factors integration: Social, education, and psychological issues* (pp. 259–271). Hershey, PA: IGI Global. doi:10.4018/978-1-4666-5071-8.ch016

Logeswaran, R. (2011). Neural networks in medicine. In *Clinical technologies: Concepts, methodologies, tools and applications* (pp. 744–765). Hershey, PA: IGI Global. doi:10.4018/978-1-60960-561-2.ch308

Low, R. (2011). Cognitive architecture and instructional design in a multimedia context. In *Instructional design: Concepts, methodologies, tools and applications* (pp. 496–510). Hershey, PA: IGI Global. doi:10.4018/978-1-60960-503-2.ch301

Low, R., Jin, P., & Sweller, J. (2014). Instructional design in digital environments and availability of mental resources for the aged subpopulation. In *Assistive technologies: Concepts, methodologies, tools, and applications* (pp. 1131–1154). Hershey, PA: IGI Global. doi:10.4018/978-1-4666-4422-9.ch059

Lu, J., & Peng, Y. (2014). Brain-computer interface for cyberpsychology: Components, methods, and applications. *International Journal of Cyber Behavior, Psychology and Learning*, 4(1), 1–14. doi:10.4018/ijcbpl.2014010101

Ludvig, E. A., Bellemare, M. G., & Pearson, K. G. (2011). A primer on reinforcement learning in the brain: Psychological, computational, and neural perspectives. In E. Alonso & E. Mondragón (Eds.), *Computational neuroscience for advancing artificial intelligence: Models, methods and applications* (pp. 111–144). Hershey, PA: IGI Global. doi:10.4018/978-1-60960-021-1.ch006

Lützenberger, M. (2014). A driver's mind: Psychology runs simulation. In D. Janssens, A. Yasar, & L. Knapen (Eds.), *Data science and simulation in transportation research* (pp. 182–205). Hershey, PA: IGI Global. doi:10.4018/978-1-4666-4920-0.ch010

Mancha, R., Yoder, C. Y., & Clark, J. G. (2013). Dynamics of affect and cognition in simulated agents: Bridging the gap between experimental and simulation research. *International Journal of Agent Technologies and Systems*, 5(2), 78–96. doi:10.4018/jats.2013040104

Manchiraju, S. (2014). Predicting behavioral intentions toward sustainable fashion consumption: A comparison of attitude-behavior and value-behavior consistency models. In H. Kaufmann & M. Panni (Eds.), *Handbook of research on consumerism in business and marketing: Concepts and practices* (pp. 225–243). Hershey, PA: IGI Global. doi:10.4018/978-1-4666-5880-6.ch011

Mancilla, R. L. (2013). Getting smart about split attention. In B. Zou, M. Xing, Y. Wang, M. Sun, & C. Xiang (Eds.), *Computer-assisted foreign language teaching and learning: Technological advances* (pp. 210–229). Hershey, PA: IGI Global. doi:10.4018/978-1-4666-2821-2.ch012

Manrique-de-Lara, P. Z. (2013). Does discretionary internet-based behavior of instructors contribute to student satisfaction? An empirical study on 'cybercivism'. *International Journal of Cyber Behavior, Psychology and Learning, 3*(1), 50–66. doi:10.4018/ijcbpl.2013010105

Markov, K., Vanhoof, K., Mitov, I., Depaire, B., Ivanova, K., Velychko, V., & Gladun, V. (2013). Intelligent data processing based on multi-dimensional numbered memory structures. In X. Naidenova & D. Ignatov (Eds.), *Diagnostic test approaches to machine learning and commonsense reasoning systems* (pp. 156–184). Hershey, PA: IGI Global. doi:10.4018/978-1-4666-1900-5.ch007

Martin, J. N. (2014). How can we incorporate relevant findings from psychology into systems methods? *International Journal of Systems and Society, 1*(1), 1–11. doi:10.4018/ijss.2014010101

Mayer, I., Bekebrede, G., Warmelink, H., & Zhou, Q. (2014). A brief methodology for researching and evaluating serious games and game-based learning. In T. Connolly, T. Hainey, E. Boyle, G. Baxter, & P. Moreno-Ger (Eds.), *Psychology, pedagogy, and assessment in serious games* (pp. 357–393). Hershey, PA: IGI Global. doi:10.4018/978-1-4666-4773-2.ch017

Mazumdar, B. D., & Mishra, R. B. (2011). Cognitive parameter based agent selection and negotiation process for B2C e-commerce. In V. Sugumaran (Ed.), *Intelligent, adaptive and reasoning technologies: New developments and applications* (pp. 181–203). Hershey, PA: IGI Global. doi:10.4018/978-1-60960-595-7.ch010

McLaren, I. (2011). APECS: An adaptively parameterised model of associative learning and memory. In E. Alonso & E. Mondragón (Eds.), *Computational neuroscience for advancing artificial intelligence: Models, methods and applications* (pp. 145–164). Hershey, PA: IGI Global. doi:10.4018/978-1-60960-021-1.ch007

McMurray, B., Zhao, L., Kucker, S. C., & Samuelson, L. K. (2013). Pushing the envelope of associative learning: Internal representations and dynamic competition transform association into development. In L. Gogate & G. Hollich (Eds.), *Theoretical and computational models of word learning: Trends in psychology and artificial intelligence* (pp. 49–80). Hershey, PA: IGI Global. doi:10.4018/978-1-4666-2973-8.ch003

Mena, R. J. (2014). The quest for a massively multiplayer online game that teaches physics. In T. Connolly, T. Hainey, E. Boyle, G. Baxter, & P. Moreno-Ger (Eds.), *Psychology, pedagogy, and assessment in serious games* (pp. 292–316). Hershey, PA: IGI Global. doi:10.4018/978-1-4666-4773-2.ch014

Misra, S. (2011). Cognitive complexity measures: An analysis. In A. Dogru & V. Biçer (Eds.), *Modern software engineering concepts and practices: Advanced approaches* (pp. 263–279). Hershey, PA: IGI Global. doi:10.4018/978-1-60960-215-4.ch011

Mok, J. (2010). Social and distributed cognition in collaborative learning contexts. In S. Dasgupta (Ed.), *Social computing: Concepts, methodologies, tools, and applications* (pp. 1838–1854). Hershey, PA: IGI Global. doi:10.4018/978-1-60566-984-7.ch121

Moore, J. E., & Love, M. S. (2013). An examination of prestigious stigma: The case of the technology geek. In B. Medlin (Ed.), *Integrations of technology utilization and social dynamics in organizations* (pp. 48–73). Hershey, PA: IGI Global. doi:10.4018/978-1-4666-1948-7.ch004

Moore, M. J., Nakano, T., Suda, T., & Enomoto, A. (2013). Social interactions and automated detection tools in cyberbullying. In L. Caviglione, M. Coccoli, & A. Merlo (Eds.), *Social network engineering for secure web data and services* (pp. 67–87). Hershey, PA: IGI Global. doi:10.4018/978-1-4666-3926-3.ch004

Moseley, A. (2014). A case for integration: Assessment and games. In T. Connolly, T. Hainey, E. Boyle, G. Baxter, & P. Moreno-Ger (Eds.), *Psychology, pedagogy, and assessment in serious games* (pp. 342–356). Hershey, PA: IGI Global. doi:10.4018/978-1-4666-4773-2.ch016

Mpofu, S. (2014). Memory, national identity, and freedom of expression in the information age: Discussing the taboo in the Zimbabwean public sphere. In A. Solo (Ed.), *Handbook of research on political activism in the information age* (pp. 114–128). Hershey, PA: IGI Global. doi:10.4018/978-1-4666-6066-3.ch007

Mulvey, F., & Heubner, M. (2014). Eye movements and attention. In *Assistive technologies: Concepts, methodologies, tools, and applications* (pp. 1030–1054). Hershey, PA: IGI Global. doi:10.4018/978-1-4666-4422-9.ch053

Munipov, V. (2011). Psychological and social problems of automation and computerization. In D. Haftor & A. Mirijamdotter (Eds.), *Information and communication technologies, society and human beings: Theory and framework (Festschrift in honor of Gunilla Bradley)* (pp. 136–146). Hershey, PA: IGI Global. doi:10.4018/978-1-60960-057-0.ch012

Najjar, M., & Mayers, A. (2012). A cognitive computational knowledge representation theory. In *Machine learning: Concepts, methodologies, tools and applications* (pp. 1819–1838). Hershey, PA: IGI Global. doi:10.4018/978-1-60960-818-7.ch708

Nakamura, H. (2011). Cognitive decline in patients with Alzheimer's disease: A six-year longitudinal study of mini-mental state examination scores. In J. Wu (Ed.), *Early detection and rehabilitation technologies for dementia: Neuroscience and biomedical applications* (pp. 107–111). Hershey, PA: IGI Global. doi:10.4018/978-1-60960-559-9.ch013

Nankee, C. (2010). Switch technologies. In S. Seok, E. Meyen, & B. DaCosta (Eds.), *Handbook of research on human cognition and assistive technology: Design, accessibility and transdisciplinary perspectives* (pp. 157–168). Hershey, PA: IGI Global. doi:10.4018/978-1-61520-817-3.ch010

Nap, H. H., & Diaz-Orueta, U. (2014). Rehabilitation gaming. In J. Bishop (Ed.), *Gamification for human factors integration: Social, education, and psychological issues* (pp. 122–147). Hershey, PA: IGI Global. doi:10.4018/978-1-4666-5071-8.ch008

Naranjo-Saucedo, A. B., Suárez-Mejías, C., Parra-Calderón, C. L., González-Aguado, E., Böckel-Martínez, F., Yuste-Marco, A., … Marco, A. (2014). Interactive games with robotic and augmented reality technology in cognitive and motor rehabilitation. In Robotics: Concepts, methodologies, tools, and applications (pp. 1233-1254). Hershey, PA: IGI Global. doi:10.4018/978-1-4666-4607-0.ch059

Ndinguri, E., Machtmes, K., Hatala, J. P., & Coco, M. L. (2014). Learning through immersive virtual environments: An organizational context. In J. Keengwe, G. Schnellert, & K. Kungu (Eds.), *Cross-cultural online learning in higher education and corporate training* (pp. 185–199). Hershey, PA: IGI Global. doi:10.4018/978-1-4666-5023-7.ch010

Ninaus, M., Witte, M., Kober, S. E., Friedrich, E. V., Kurzmann, J., Hartsuiker, E., … Wood, G. (2014). Neurofeedback and serious games. In T. Connolly, T. Hainey, E. Boyle, G. Baxter, & P. Moreno-Ger (Eds.), Psychology, pedagogy, and assessment in serious games (pp. 82-110). Hershey, PA: IGI Global. doi:10.4018/978-1-4666-4773-2.ch005

Nobre, F. S. (2012). The roles of cognitive machines in customer-centric organizations: Towards innovations in computational organizational management networks. In F. Nobre, D. Walker, & R. Harris (Eds.), *Technological, managerial and organizational core competencies: Dynamic innovation and sustainable development* (pp. 653–674). Hershey, PA: IGI Global. doi:10.4018/978-1-61350-165-8.ch035

Norris, S. E. (2014). Transformative curriculum design and program development: Creating effective adult learning by leveraging psychological capital and self-directedness through the exercise of human agency. In V. Wang & V. Bryan (Eds.), *Andragogical and pedagogical methods for curriculum and program development* (pp. 118–141). Hershey, PA: IGI Global. doi:10.4018/978-1-4666-5872-1.ch007

Norris, S. E., & Porter, T. H. (2013). Self-monitoring scale. In M. Bocarnea, R. Reynolds, & J. Baker (Eds.), *Online instruments, data collection, and electronic measurements: Organizational advancements* (pp. 118–133). Hershey, PA: IGI Global. doi:10.4018/978-1-4666-2172-5.ch007

O'Connell, R. M. (2014). Mind mapping for critical thinking. In L. Shedletsky & J. Beaudry (Eds.), *Cases on teaching critical thinking through visual representation strategies* (pp. 354–386). Hershey, PA: IGI Global. doi:10.4018/978-1-4666-5816-5.ch014

Okrigwe, B. N. (2010). Cognition and learning. In S. Seok, E. Meyen, & B. DaCosta (Eds.), *Handbook of research on human cognition and assistive technology: Design, accessibility and transdisciplinary perspectives* (pp. 388–400). Hershey, PA: IGI Global. doi:10.4018/978-1-61520-817-3.ch027

Ong, E. H., & Khan, J. Y. (2013). Cognitive cooperation in wireless networks. In M. Ku & J. Lin (Eds.), *Cognitive radio and interference management: Technology and strategy* (pp. 179–204). Hershey, PA: IGI Global. doi:10.4018/978-1-4666-2005-6.ch010

Orlova, M. (2014). Social psychology of health as a social-psychological situation. In Ş. Erçetin & S. Banerjee (Eds.), *Chaos and complexity theory in world politics* (pp. 331–335). Hershey, PA: IGI Global. doi:10.4018/978-1-4666-6070-0.ch024

Orr, K., & McGuinness, C. (2014). What is the "learning" in games-based learning? In T. Connolly, T. Hainey, E. Boyle, G. Baxter, & P. Moreno-Ger (Eds.), Psychology, pedagogy, and assessment in serious games (pp. 221-242). Hershey, PA: IGI Global. doi:10.4018/978-1-4666-4773-2.ch011

Ortiz Zezzatti, C. A., Martínez, J., Castillo, N., González, S., & Hernández, P. (2012). Improve card collection from memory alpha using sociolinguistics and Japanese puzzles. In C. Ortiz Zezzatti, C. Chira, A. Hernandez, & M. Basurto (Eds.), *Logistics management and optimization through hybrid artificial intelligence systems* (pp. 310–326). Hershey, PA: IGI Global. doi:10.4018/978-1-4666-0297-7.ch012

Ota, N., Maeshima, S., Osawa, A., Kawarada, M., & Tanemura, J. (2011). Prospective memory impairment in remembering to remember in mild cognitive impairment and healthy subjects. In J. Wu (Ed.), *Early detection and rehabilitation technologies for dementia: Neuroscience and biomedical applications* (pp. 98–106). Hershey, PA: IGI Global. doi:10.4018/978-1-60960-559-9.ch012

Ouwehand, K., van Gog, T., & Paas, F. (2013). The use of gesturing to facilitate older adults' learning from computer-based dynamic visualizations. In R. Zheng, R. Hill, & M. Gardner (Eds.), *Engaging older adults with modern technology: Internet use and information access needs* (pp. 33–58). Hershey, PA: IGI Global. doi:10.4018/978-1-4666-1966-1.ch003

Özel, S. (2012). Utilizing cognitive resources in user interface designs. In B. Khan (Ed.), *User interface design for virtual environments: Challenges and advances* (pp. 115–123). Hershey, PA: IGI Global. doi:10.4018/978-1-61350-516-8.ch007

Parsons, T. D., & Courtney, C. G. (2011). Neurocognitive and psychophysiological interfaces for adaptive virtual environments. In M. Ziefle & C. Röcker (Eds.), *Human-centered design of e-health technologies: Concepts, methods and applications* (pp. 208–233). Hershey, PA: IGI Global. doi:10.4018/978-1-60960-177-5.ch009

Peden, B. F., & Tiry, A. M. (2013). Using web surveys for psychology experiments: A case study in new media technology for research. In N. Sappleton (Ed.), *Advancing research methods with new technologies* (pp. 70–99). Hershey, PA: IGI Global. doi:10.4018/978-1-4666-3918-8.ch005

Perakslis, C. (2014). Willingness to adopt RFID implants: Do personality factors play a role in the acceptance of uberveillance? In M. Michael & K. Michael (Eds.), *Uberveillance and the social implications of microchip implants: Emerging technologies* (pp. 144–168). Hershey, PA: IGI Global. doi:10.4018/978-1-4666-4582-0.ch006

Pereira, G., Brisson, A., Dias, J., Carvalho, A., Dimas, J., Mascarenhas, S., ... Paiva, A. (2014). Non-player characters and artificial intelligence. In T. Connolly, T. Hainey, E. Boyle, G. Baxter, & P. Moreno-Ger (Eds.), Psychology, pedagogy, and assessment in serious games (pp. 127-152). Hershey, PA: IGI Global. doi:10.4018/978-1-4666-4773-2.ch007

Pereira, R., Hornung, H., & Baranauskas, M. C. (2014). Cognitive authority revisited in web social interaction. In M. Pańkowska (Ed.), *Frameworks of IT prosumption for business development* (pp. 142–157). Hershey, PA: IGI Global. doi:10.4018/978-1-4666-4313-0.ch010

Phebus, A. M., Gitlin, B., Shuffler, M. L., & Wildman, J. L. (2014). Leading global virtual teams: The supporting role of trust and team cognition. In E. Nikoi & K. Boateng (Eds.), *Collaborative communication processes and decision making in organizations* (pp. 177–200). Hershey, PA: IGI Global. doi:10.4018/978-1-4666-4478-6.ch010

Plunkett, D., Banerjee, R., & Horn, E. (2010). Supporting early childhood outcomes through assistive technology. In S. Seok, E. Meyen, & B. DaCosta (Eds.), *Handbook of research on human cognition and assistive technology: Design, accessibility and transdisciplinary perspectives* (pp. 339–359). Hershey, PA: IGI Global. doi:10.4018/978-1-61520-817-3.ch024

Prakash, S., Vaish, A., Coul, N., Saravana, G. K., Srinidhi, T. N., & Botsa, J. (2014). Child security in cyberspace through moral cognition. In *Cyber behavior: Concepts, methodologies, tools, and applications* (pp. 1946–1958). Hershey, PA: IGI Global. doi:10.4018/978-1-4666-5942-1.ch102

Prescott, J., & Bogg, J. (2013). Self, career, and gender issues: A complex interplay of internal/external factors. In *Gendered occupational differences in science, engineering, and technology careers* (pp. 79–111). Hershey, PA: IGI Global. doi:10.4018/978-1-4666-2107-7.ch004

Prescott, J., & Bogg, J. (2013). Stereotype, attitudes, and identity: Gendered expectations and behaviors. In *Gendered occupational differences in science, engineering, and technology careers* (pp. 112–135). Hershey, PA: IGI Global. doi:10.4018/978-1-4666-2107-7.ch005

Pressey, A., Salciuviene, L., & Barnes, S. (2013). Uncovering relationships between emotional states and higher-order needs: Enhancing consumer emotional experiences in computer-mediated environment. *International Journal of Online Marketing*, *3*(1), 31–46. doi:10.4018/ijom.2013010103

Qin, X., Li, C., Chen, H., Qin, B., Du, X., & Wang, S. (2014). In memory data processing systems. In J. Wang (Ed.), *Encyclopedia of business analytics and optimization* (pp. 1182–1191). Hershey, PA: IGI Global. doi:10.4018/978-1-4666-5202-6.ch109

Ramos, I., & Oliveira e Sá, J. (2014). Organizational memory: The role of business intelligence to leverage the application of collective knowledge. In H. Rahman & R. de Sousa (Eds.), *Information systems and technology for organizational agility, intelligence, and resilience* (pp. 206–223). Hershey, PA: IGI Global. doi:10.4018/978-1-4666-5970-4.ch010

Ratten, V. (2013). The development of social e-enterprises, mobile communication and social networks: A social cognitive perspective of technological innovation. *Journal of Electronic Commerce in Organizations, 11*(3), 68–77. doi:10.4018/jeco.2013070104

Reddy, Y. B. (2013). Nanocomputing in cognitive radio networks to improve the performance. In N. Meghanathan & Y. Reddy (Eds.), *Cognitive radio technology applications for wireless and mobile ad hoc networks* (pp. 173–193). Hershey, PA: IGI Global. doi:10.4018/978-1-4666-4221-8.ch010

Redien-Collot, R., & Lefebvre, M. R. (2014). SMEs' leaders: Building collective cognition and competences to trigger positive strategic outcomes. In K. Todorov & D. Smallbone (Eds.), *Handbook of research on strategic management in small and medium enterprises* (pp. 143–158). Hershey, PA: IGI Global. doi:10.4018/978-1-4666-5962-9.ch008

Remmele, B., & Whitton, N. (2014). Disrupting the magic circle: The impact of negative social gaming behaviours. In T. Connolly, T. Hainey, E. Boyle, G. Baxter, & P. Moreno-Ger (Eds.), *Psychology, pedagogy, and assessment in serious games* (pp. 111–126). Hershey, PA: IGI Global. doi:10.4018/978-1-4666-4773-2.ch006

Renaud, P., Chartier, S., Fedoroff, P., Bradford, J., & Rouleau, J. L. (2011). The use of virtual reality in clinical psychology research. In *Clinical technologies: Concepts, methodologies, tools and applications* (pp. 2073–2093). Hershey, PA: IGI Global. doi:10.4018/978-1-60960-561-2.ch805

Revett, K. (2012). Cognitive biometrics: A novel approach to continuous person authentication. In I. Traore & A. Ahmed (Eds.), *Continuous authentication using biometrics: Data, models, and metrics* (pp. 105–136). Hershey, PA: IGI Global. doi:10.4018/978-1-61350-129-0.ch006

Rødseth, I. (2011). A motive analysis as a first step in designing technology for the use of intuition in criminal investigation. In A. Mesquita (Ed.), *Sociological and philosophical aspects of human interaction with technology: Advancing concepts* (pp. 276–298). Hershey, PA: IGI Global. doi:10.4018/978-1-60960-575-9.ch015

Rothblatt, M. (2014). Mindclone technoselves: Multi-substrate legal identities, cyber-psychology, and biocyberethics. In *Cyber behavior: Concepts, methodologies, tools, and applications* (pp. 1199–1216). Hershey, PA: IGI Global. doi:10.4018/978-1-4666-5942-1.ch062

Rückemann, C. (2013). Integrated information and computing systems for advanced cognition with natural sciences. In C. Rückemann (Ed.), *Integrated information and computing systems for natural, spatial, and social sciences* (pp. 1–26). Hershey, PA: IGI Global. doi:10.4018/978-1-4666-2190-9.ch001

Rudnianski, M., & Kravcik, M. (2014). The road to critical thinking and intelligence analysis. In T. Connolly, T. Hainey, E. Boyle, G. Baxter, & P. Moreno-Ger (Eds.), *Psychology, pedagogy, and assessment in serious games* (pp. 47–61). Hershey, PA: IGI Global. doi:10.4018/978-1-4666-4773-2.ch003

Rufer, R., & Adams, R. H. (2012). Adapting three-dimensional-virtual world to reach diverse learners in an MBA program. In H. Yang & S. Yuen (Eds.), *Handbook of research on practices and outcomes in virtual worlds and environments* (pp. 606–619). Hershey, PA: IGI Global. doi:10.4018/978-1-60960-762-3.ch033

Saadé, R. G. (2010). Cognitive mapping decision support for the design of web-based learning environments. *International Journal of Web-Based Learning and Teaching Technologies*, *5*(3), 36–53. doi:10.4018/jwltt.2010070103

Saeed, N., & Sinnappan, S. (2014). Comparing learning styles and technology acceptance of two culturally different groups of students. In T. Issa, P. Isaias, & P. Kommers (Eds.), *Multicultural awareness and technology in higher education: Global perspectives* (pp. 244–264). Hershey, PA: IGI Global. doi:10.4018/978-1-4666-5876-9.ch012

Samuelson, L. K., Spencer, J. P., & Jenkins, G. W. (2013). A dynamic neural field model of word learning. In L. Gogate & G. Hollich (Eds.), *Theoretical and computational models of word learning: Trends in psychology and artificial intelligence* (pp. 1–27). Hershey, PA: IGI Global. doi:10.4018/978-1-4666-2973-8.ch001

Sanjram, P. K., & Gupta, M. (2013). Task difficulty and time constraint in programmer multitasking: An analysis of prospective memory performance and cognitive workload. *International Journal of Green Computing*, *4*(1), 35–57. doi:10.4018/jgc.2013010103

Sato, Y., Ji, Z., & van Dijk, S. (2013). I think I have heard that one before: Recurrence-based word learning with a robot. In L. Gogate & G. Hollich (Eds.), *Theoretical and computational models of word learning: Trends in psychology and artificial intelligence* (pp. 327–349). Hershey, PA: IGI Global. doi:10.4018/978-1-4666-2973-8.ch014

Scalzone, F., & Zontini, G. (2013). Thinking animals and thinking machines in psychoanalysis and beyond. In F. Orsucci & N. Sala (Eds.), *Complexity science, living systems, and reflexing interfaces: New models and perspectives* (pp. 44–68). Hershey, PA: IGI Global. doi:10.4018/978-1-4666-2077-3.ch003

Schafer, S. B. (2013). Fostering psychological coherence: With ICTs. In M. Cruz-Cunha, I. Miranda, & P. Gonçalves (Eds.), *Handbook of research on ICTs for human-centered healthcare and social care services* (pp. 29–47). Hershey, PA: IGI Global. doi:10.4018/978-1-4666-3986-7.ch002

Scheiter, K., Wiebe, E., & Holsanova, J. (2011). Theoretical and instructional aspects of learning with visualizations. In *Instructional design: Concepts, methodologies, tools and applications* (pp. 1667–1688). Hershey, PA: IGI Global. doi:10.4018/978-1-60960-503-2.ch710

Seo, K. K., Byk, A., & Collins, C. (2011). Cognitive apprenticeship inspired simulations. In *Gaming and simulations: Concepts, methodologies, tools and applications* (pp. 346–358). Hershey, PA: IGI Global. doi:10.4018/978-1-60960-195-9.ch202

Serenko, N. (2014). Informational, physical, and psychological privacy as determinants of patient behaviour in health care. In V. Michell, D. Rosenorn-Lanng, S. Gulliver, & W. Currie (Eds.), *Handbook of research on patient safety and quality care through health informatics* (pp. 1–20). Hershey, PA: IGI Global. doi:10.4018/978-1-4666-4546-2.ch001

Shibata, T. (2013). A human-like cognitive computer based on a psychologically inspired VLSI brain model. In J. Wu (Ed.), *Technological advancements in biomedicine for healthcare applications* (pp. 247–266). Hershey, PA: IGI Global. doi:10.4018/978-1-4666-2196-1.ch027

Shirkhodaee, M., & Rezaee, S. (2013). Evaluating the persuasive and memory effects of viral advertising. *International Journal of Online Marketing*, *3*(3), 51–61. doi:10.4018/ijom.2013070104

Simzar, R., & Domina, T. (2014). Attending to student motivation through critical practice: A recommendation for improving accelerated mathematical learning. In S. Lawrence (Ed.), *Critical practice in P-12 education: Transformative teaching and learning* (pp. 66–116). Hershey, PA: IGI Global. doi:10.4018/978-1-4666-5059-6.ch004

Smart, P. R., Engelbrecht, P. C., Braines, D., Strub, M., & Giammanco, C. (2010). The network-extended mind. In D. Verma (Ed.), *Network science for military coalition operations: Information exchange and interaction* (pp. 191–236). Hershey, PA: IGI Global. doi:10.4018/978-1-61520-855-5.ch010

Smith, M. A. (2011). Functions of unconscious and conscious emotion in the regulation of implicit and explicit motivated behavior. In D. Gökçay & G. Yildirim (Eds.), *Affective computing and interaction: Psychological, cognitive and neuroscientific perspectives* (pp. 25–55). Hershey, PA: IGI Global. doi:10.4018/978-1-61692-892-6.ch002

Soliman, F. (2014). Could knowledge, learning, and innovation gaps be spiralling? In F. Soliman (Ed.), *Learning models for innovation in organizations: Examining roles of knowledge transfer and human resources management* (pp. 1–29). Hershey, PA: IGI Global. doi:10.4018/978-1-4666-4884-5.ch001

Somyürek, S. (2012). Interactive learning in workplace training. In J. Jia (Ed.), *Educational stages and interactive learning: From kindergarten to workplace training* (pp. 498–514). Hershey, PA: IGI Global. doi:10.4018/978-1-4666-0137-6.ch027

Spadaro, L., Timpano, F., Marino, S., & Bramanti, P. (2013). Telemedicine and Alzheimer disease: ICT-based services for people with Alzheimer disease and their caregivers. In V. Gulla, A. Mori, F. Gabbrielli, & P. Lanzafame (Eds.), *Telehealth networks for hospital services: New methodologies* (pp. 191–206). Hershey, PA: IGI Global. doi:10.4018/978-1-4666-2979-0.ch013

Spiegel, T. (2014). An overview of cognition roles in decision-making. In J. Wang (Ed.), *Encyclopedia of business analytics and optimization* (pp. 74–84). Hershey, PA: IGI Global. doi:10.4018/978-1-4666-5202-6.ch008

Stachon, Z., & Šašinka, C. (2012). Human cognition: People in the world and world in their minds. In T. Podobnikar & M. Čeh (Eds.), *Universal ontology of geographic space: Semantic enrichment for spatial data* (pp. 97–122). Hershey, PA: IGI Global. doi:10.4018/978-1-4666-0327-1.ch005

Stefurak, J. R., Surry, D. W., & Hayes, R. L. (2011). Technology in the supervision of mental health professionals: Ethical, interpersonal, and epistemological implications. In D. Surry, R. Gray Jr, & J. Stefurak (Eds.), *Technology integration in higher education: Social and organizational aspects* (pp. 114–131). Hershey, PA: IGI Global. doi:10.4018/978-1-60960-147-8.ch009

Stieglitz, S. (2014). The American memory project. In J. Krueger (Ed.), *Cases on electronic records and resource management implementation in diverse environments* (pp. 106–116). Hershey, PA: IGI Global. doi:10.4018/978-1-4666-4466-3.ch006

Suárez, M. G., & Gumiel, C. G. (2014). The use of sensorial marketing in stores: Attracting clients through their senses. In F. Musso & E. Druica (Eds.), *Handbook of research on retailer-consumer relationship development* (pp. 258–274). Hershey, PA: IGI Global. doi:10.4018/978-1-4666-6074-8.ch014

Sugiura, M. (2013). A cognitive neuroscience approach to self and mental health. In J. Wu (Ed.), *Biomedical engineering and cognitive neuroscience for healthcare: Interdisciplinary applications* (pp. 1–10). Hershey, PA: IGI Global. doi:10.4018/978-1-4666-2113-8.ch001

Sujo-Montes, L. E., Armfield, S. W., Yen, C., & Tu, C. (2014). The use of ubiquitous learning for children with Down Syndrome. In F. Neto (Ed.), *Technology platform innovations and forthcoming trends in ubiquitous learning* (pp. 160–176). Hershey, PA: IGI Global. doi:10.4018/978-1-4666-4542-4.ch009

Tamba, H. (2013). Workers' mental health problems and future perspectives in Japan: Psychological job stress research. In J. Wu (Ed.), *Biomedical engineering and cognitive neuroscience for healthcare: Interdisciplinary applications* (pp. 370–379). Hershey, PA: IGI Global. doi:10.4018/978-1-4666-2113-8.ch038

Tatachari, S., Manikandan, K. S., & Gunta, S. (2014). A synthesis of organizational learning and knowledge management literatures. In M. Chilton & J. Bloodgood (Eds.), *Knowledge management and competitive advantage: Issues and potential solutions* (pp. 122–147). Hershey, PA: IGI Global. doi:10.4018/978-1-4666-4679-7.ch008

Taxén, L. (2010). Cognitive grounding. In L. Taxen (Ed.), *Using activity domain theory for managing complex systems* (pp. 108–124). Hershey, PA: IGI Global. doi:10.4018/978-1-60566-192-6.ch006

Te'eni, D. (2012). Knowledge for communicating knowledge. In *Organizational learning and knowledge: Concepts, methodologies, tools and applications* (pp. 1656–1665). Hershey, PA: IGI Global. doi:10.4018/978-1-60960-783-8.ch501

Terras, M. M., & Ramsay, J. (2014). E-learning, mobility, and time: A psychological framework. In E. Barbera & P. Reimann (Eds.), *Assessment and evaluation of time factors in online teaching and learning* (pp. 63–90). Hershey, PA: IGI Global. doi:10.4018/978-1-4666-4651-3.ch003

Thapa, A. (2013). A study on worker's perceptions of psychological capital on their earnings. *International Journal of Applied Behavioral Economics, 2*(3), 27–42. doi:10.4018/ijabe.2013070103

Thatcher, A., & Ndabeni, M. (2013). A psychological model to understand e-adoption in the context of the digital divide. In *Digital literacy: Concepts, methodologies, tools, and applications* (pp. 1402–1424). Hershey, PA: IGI Global. doi:10.4018/978-1-4666-1852-7.ch074

Thompson, K., & Markauskaite, L. (2014). Identifying group processes and affect in learners: A holistic approach to assessment in virtual worlds in higher education. In S. Kennedy-Clark, K. Everett, & P. Wheeler (Eds.), *Cases on the assessment of scenario and game-based virtual worlds in higher education* (pp. 175–210). Hershey, PA: IGI Global. doi:10.4018/978-1-4666-4470-0.ch006

Titus, C. S. (2013). The use of developmental psychology in ethics: Beyond Kohlberg and Seligman? In F. Doridot, P. Duquenoy, P. Goujon, A. Kurt, S. Lavelle, N. Patrignani, ... A. Santuccio (Eds.), *Ethical governance of emerging technologies development* (pp. 266–286). Hershey, PA: IGI Global. doi:10.4018/978-1-4666-3670-5.ch018

Tiwary, U. S., & Siddiqui, T. J. (2014). Working together with computers: Towards a general framework for collaborative human computer interaction. In *Assistive technologies: Concepts, methodologies, tools, and applications* (pp. 141–162). Hershey, PA: IGI Global. doi:10.4018/978-1-4666-4422-9.ch008

Tomono, A. (2013). Display technology of images with scents and its psychological evaluation. In T. Nakamoto (Ed.), *Human olfactory displays and interfaces: Odor sensing and presentation* (pp. 429–445). Hershey, PA: IGI Global. doi:10.4018/978-1-4666-2521-1.ch022

Torres, G., Jaime, K., & Ramos, F. (2013). Brain architecture for visual object identification. *International Journal of Cognitive Informatics and Natural Intelligence, 7*(1), 75–97. doi:10.4018/jcini.2013010104

Trajkovski, G., Stojanov, G., Collins, S., Eidelman, V., Harman, C., & Vincenti, G. (2011). Cognitive robotics and multiagency in a fuzzy modeling framework. In G. Trajkovski (Ed.), *Developments in intelligent agent technologies and multi-agent systems: Concepts and applications* (pp. 132–152). Hershey, PA: IGI Global. doi:10.4018/978-1-60960-171-3.ch009

Tran, B. (2014). Rhetoric of play: Utilizing the gamer factor in selecting and training employees. In T. Connolly, T. Hainey, E. Boyle, G. Baxter, & P. Moreno-Ger (Eds.), *Psychology, pedagogy, and assessment in serious games* (pp. 175–203). Hershey, PA: IGI Global. doi:10.4018/978-1-4666-4773-2.ch009

Tran, B. (2014). The psychology of consumerism in business and marketing: The macro and micro behaviors of Hofstede's cultural consumers. In H. Kaufmann & M. Panni (Eds.), *Handbook of research on consumerism in business and marketing: Concepts and practices* (pp. 286–308). Hershey, PA: IGI Global. doi:10.4018/978-1-4666-5880-6.ch014

Travica, B. (2014). Homo informaticus. In *Examining the informing view of organization: Applying theoretical and managerial approaches* (pp. 34–66). Hershey, PA: IGI Global. doi:10.4018/978-1-4666-5986-5.ch002

Twomey, K. E., Horst, J. S., & Morse, A. F. (2013). An embodied model of young children's categorization and word learning. In L. Gogate & G. Hollich (Eds.), *Theoretical and computational models of word learning: Trends in psychology and artificial intelligence* (pp. 172–196). Hershey, PA: IGI Global. doi:10.4018/978-1-4666-2973-8.ch008

Ursyn, A. (2014). Cognitive processes involved in visual thought. In *Perceptions of knowledge visualization: Explaining concepts through meaningful images* (pp. 131–173). Hershey, PA: IGI Global. doi:10.4018/978-1-4666-4703-9.ch005

Ursyn, A. (2014). Communication through many senses. In *Perceptions of knowledge visualization: Explaining concepts through meaningful images* (pp. 25–60). Hershey, PA: IGI Global. doi:10.4018/978-1-4666-4703-9.ch002

Ursyn, A. (2014). Four trapped in an elevator. In *Computational solutions for knowledge, art, and entertainment: Information exchange beyond text* (pp. 322–329). Hershey, PA: IGI Global. doi:10.4018/978-1-4666-4627-8.ch016

Usart, M., & Romero, M. (2014). Time factor assessment in game-based learning: Time perspective and time-on-task as individual differences between players. In T. Connolly, T. Hainey, E. Boyle, G. Baxter, & P. Moreno-Ger (Eds.), *Psychology, pedagogy, and assessment in serious games* (pp. 62–81). Hershey, PA: IGI Global. doi:10.4018/978-1-4666-4773-2.ch004

Usoro, A., Majewski, G., & Bloom, L. (2012). Individual and collaborative approaches in e-learning design. In *Virtual learning environments: Concepts, methodologies, tools and applications* (pp. 1110–1130). Hershey, PA: IGI Global. doi:10.4018/978-1-4666-0011-9.ch514 van den Brink, J. C. (2014). How positive psychology can support sustainable project management. In *Sustainable practices: Concepts, methodologies, tools and applications* (pp. 958–973). Hershey, PA: IGI Global. doi:10.4018/978-1-4666-4852-4.ch053

van der Helden, J., & Bekkering, H. (2014). The role of implicit and explicit feedback in learning and the implications for distance education techniques. In T. Yuzer & G. Eby (Eds.), *Handbook of research on emerging priorities and trends in distance education: Communication, pedagogy, and technology* (pp. 367–384). Hershey, PA: IGI Global. doi:10.4018/978-1-4666-5162-3.ch025

van Mierlo, C. M., Jarodzka, H., Kirschner, F., & Kirschner, P. A. (2012). Cognitive load theory in e-learning. In Z. Yan (Ed.), *Encyclopedia of cyber behavior* (pp. 1178–1211). Hershey, PA: IGI Global. doi:10.4018/978-1-4666-0315-8.ch097

van Rosmalen, P., Wilson, A., & Hummel, H. G. (2014). Games for and by teachers and learners. In T. Connolly, T. Hainey, E. Boyle, G. Baxter, & P. Moreno-Ger (Eds.), *Psychology, pedagogy, and assessment in serious games* (pp. 243–269). Hershey, PA: IGI Global. doi:10.4018/978-1-4666-4773-2.ch012

Vega, J., Perdices, E., & Cañas, J. M. (2014). Attentive visual memory for robot localization. In Robotics: Concepts, methodologies, tools, and applications (pp. 785-811). Hershey, PA: IGI Global. doi:10.4018/978-1-4666-4607-0.ch038

Vinther, J. (2012). Cognitive skills through CALL-enhanced teacher training. In F. Zhang (Ed.), *Computer-enhanced and mobile-assisted language learning: Emerging issues and trends* (pp. 158–187). Hershey, PA: IGI Global. doi:10.4018/978-1-61350-065-1.ch008

Vogel, E. H., & Ponce, F. P. (2011). Empirical issues and theoretical mechanisms of Pavlovian conditioning. In E. Alonso & E. Mondragón (Eds.), *Computational neuroscience for advancing artificial intelligence: Models, methods and applications* (pp. 81–110). Hershey, PA: IGI Global. doi:10.4018/978-1-60960-021-1.ch005

Vragov, R. (2013). Detecting behavioral biases in mixed human-proxy online auction markets. *International Journal of Strategic Information Technology and Applications*, 4(4), 60–79. doi:10.4018/ijsita.2013100104

Wagner, C. L., & Delisi, J. (2010). Multi-sensory environments and augmentative communication tools. In S. Seok, E. Meyen, & B. DaCosta (Eds.), *Handbook of research on human cognition and assistive technology: Design, accessibility and transdisciplinary perspectives* (pp. 121–131). Hershey, PA: IGI Global. doi:10.4018/978-1-61520-817-3.ch008

Walk, A. M., & Conway, C. M. (2014). Two distinct sequence learning mechanisms for syntax acquisition and word learning. In *Computational linguistics: Concepts, methodologies, tools, and applications* (pp. 540–560). Hershey, PA: IGI Global. doi:10.4018/978-1-4666-6042-7.ch025

Wang, H. (2014). A guide to assistive technology for teachers in special education. In *Assistive technologies: Concepts, methodologies, tools, and applications* (pp. 12–25). Hershey, PA: IGI Global. doi:10.4018/978-1-4666-4422-9.ch002

Wang, J. (2012). Organizational learning and technology. In V. Wang (Ed.), *Encyclopedia of e-leadership, counseling and training* (pp. 154–170). Hershey, PA: IGI Global. doi:10.4018/978-1-61350-068-2.ch012

Wang, K. Y. (2014). Mixing metaphors: Sociological and psychological perspectives on virtual communities. In *Cross-cultural interaction: Concepts, methodologies, tools and applications* (pp. 116–132). Hershey, PA: IGI Global. doi:10.4018/978-1-4666-4979-8.ch008

Wang, Y. (2013). Neuroinformatics models of human memory: Mapping the cognitive functions of memory onto neurophysiological structures of the brain. *International Journal of Cognitive Informatics and Natural Intelligence*, 7(1), 98–122. doi:10.4018/jcini.2013010105

Wang, Y. (2013). The cognitive mechanisms and formal models of consciousness. *International Journal of Cognitive Informatics and Natural Intelligence*, 6(2), 23–40. doi:10.4018/jcini.2012040102

Wang, Y. (2013). Towards the synergy of cognitive informatics, neural informatics, brain informatics, and cognitive computing. In Y. Wang (Ed.), *Cognitive informatics for revealing human cognition: Knowledge manipulations in natural intelligence* (pp. 1–19). Hershey, PA: IGI Global. doi:10.4018/978-1-4666-2476-4.ch001

Wang, Y., Berwick, R. C., Haykin, S., Pedrycz, W., Kinsner, W., & Baciu, G. ... Gavrilova, M. L. (2013). Cognitive informatics and cognitive computing in year 10 and beyond. In Y. Wang (Ed.), Cognitive informatics for revealing human cognition: Knowledge manipulations in natural intelligence (pp. 140-157). Hershey, PA: IGI Global. doi:10.4018/978-1-4666-2476-4.ch010

Wang, Y., Fariello, G., Gavrilova, M. L., Kinsner, W., Mizoguchi, F., Patel, S., ... Tsumoto, S. (2013). Perspectives on cognitive computers and knowledge processors. *International Journal of Cognitive Informatics and Natural Intelligence*, 7(3), 1–24. doi:10.4018/ijcini.2013070101

Wang, Y., Patel, S., & Patel, D. (2013). The cognitive process and formal models of human attentions. *International Journal of Software Science and Computational Intelligence*, 5(1), 32–50. doi:10.4018/ijssci.2013010103

Wang, Y., Pedrycz, W., Baciu, G., Chen, P., Wang, G., & Yao, Y. (2012). Perspectives on cognitive computing and applications. In Y. Wang (Ed.), *Breakthroughs in software science and computational intelligence* (pp. 1–12). Hershey, PA: IGI Global. doi:10.4018/978-1-4666-0264-9.ch001

Wang, Y., Widrow, B. C., Zhang, B., Kinsner, W., Sugawara, K., Sun, F., ... Zhang, D. (2013). Perspectives on the field of cognitive informatics and its future development. In Y. Wang (Ed.), *Cognitive informatics for revealing human cognition: Knowledge manipulations in natural intelligence* (pp. 20–34). Hershey, PA: IGI Global. doi:10.4018/978-1-4666-2476-4.ch002

Was, C. A., & Woltz, D. J. (2013). Implicit memory and aging: Adapting technology to utilize preserved memory functions. In R. Zheng, R. Hill, & M. Gardner (Eds.), *Engaging older adults with modern technology: Internet use and information access needs* (pp. 1–19). Hershey, PA: IGI Global. doi:10.4018/978-1-4666-1966-1.ch001

Wei, H. (2013). A neural dynamic model based on activation diffusion and a micro-explanation for cognitive operations. *International Journal of Cognitive Informatics and Natural Intelligence*, 6(2), 1–22. doi:10.4018/jcini.2012040101

Wexler, R. H., & Roff-Wexler, S. (2013). The evolution and development of self in virtual worlds. *International Journal of Cyber Behavior, Psychology and Learning*, 3(1), 1–6. doi:10.4018/ijcbpl.2013010101

Wickramasinghe, N. (2012). Knowledge economy for innovating organizations. In *Organizational learning and knowledge: Concepts, methodologies, tools and applications* (pp. 2298–2309). Hershey, PA: IGI Global. doi:10.4018/978-1-60960-783-8.ch616

Widrow, B. C., & Aragon, J. (2012). Cognitive memory: Human like memory. In Y. Wang (Ed.), *Breakthroughs in software science and computational intelligence* (pp. 84–99). Hershey, PA: IGI Global. doi:10.4018/978-1-4666-0264-9.ch006

Widyanto, L., & Griffiths, M. (2013). An empirical study of problematic internet use and self-esteem. In R. Zheng (Ed.), *Evolving psychological and educational perspectives on cyber behavior* (pp. 82–95). Hershey, PA: IGI Global. doi:10.4018/978-1-4666-1858-9.ch006

Wilson, M. S., & Pascoe, J. (2010). Using software to deliver language intervention in inclusionary settings. In S. Seok, E. Meyen, & B. DaCosta (Eds.), *Handbook of research on human cognition and assistive technology: Design, accessibility and transdisciplinary perspectives* (pp. 132–156). Hershey, PA: IGI Global. doi:10.4018/978-1-61520-817-3.ch009

Wilson, S., & Haslam, N. (2013). Reasoning about human enhancement: Towards a folk psychological model of human nature and human identity. In R. Luppicini (Ed.), *Handbook of research on technoself: Identity in a technological society* (pp. 175–188). Hershey, PA: IGI Global. doi:10.4018/978-1-4666-2211-1.ch010

Wilson, S. G. (2014). Enhancement and identity: A social psychological perspective. In S. Thompson (Ed.), *Global issues and ethical considerations in human enhancement technologies* (pp. 241–256). Hershey, PA: IGI Global. doi:10.4018/978-1-4666-6010-6.ch014

Winsor, D. L. (2012). The epistemology of young children. In S. Blake, D. Winsor, & L. Allen (Eds.), *Child development and the use of technology: Perspectives, applications and experiences* (pp. 21–44). Hershey, PA: IGI Global. doi:10.4018/978-1-61350-317-1.ch002

Winsor, D. L., & Blake, S. (2012). Socrates and Descartes meet the E*Trade baby: The impact of early technology on children's developing beliefs about knowledge and knowing. In S. Blake, D. Winsor, & L. Allen (Eds.), *Child development and the use of technology: Perspectives, applications and experiences* (pp. 1–20). Hershey, PA: IGI Global. doi:10.4018/978-1-61350-317-1.ch001

Yakavenka, H. (2012). Developing professional competencies through international peer learning communities. In V. Dennen & J. Myers (Eds.), *Virtual professional development and informal learning via social networks* (pp. 134–154). Hershey, PA: IGI Global. doi:10.4018/978-1-4666-1815-2.ch008

Yamaguchi, M., & Shetty, V. (2013). Evaluating the psychobiologic effects of fragrances through salivary biomarkers. In T. Nakamoto (Ed.), *Human olfactory displays and interfaces: Odor sensing and presentation* (pp. 359–369). Hershey, PA: IGI Global. doi:10.4018/978-1-4666-2521-1.ch017

Yan, Z., & Zheng, R. Z. (2013). Growing from childhood into adolescence: The science of cyber behavior. In R. Zheng (Ed.), *Evolving psychological and educational perspectives on cyber behavior* (pp. 1–14). Hershey, PA: IGI Global. doi:10.4018/978-1-4666-1858-9.ch001

Yildirim, G., & Gökçay, D. (2011). Problems associated with computer-mediated communication cognitive psychology and neuroscience perspectives. In D. Gökçay & G. Yildirim (Eds.), *Affective computing and interaction: Psychological, cognitive and neuroscientific perspectives* (pp. 244–261). Hershey, PA: IGI Global. doi:10.4018/978-1-61692-892-6.ch011

Younan, Y., Joosen, W., Piessens, F., & Van den Eynden, H. (2012). Improving memory management security for C and C. In K. Khan (Ed.), *Security-aware systems applications and software development methods* (pp. 190–216). Hershey, PA: IGI Global. doi:10.4018/978-1-4666-1580-9.ch011

Yu, C., & Smith, L. B. (2013). A sensory-motor solution to early word-referent learning. In L. Gogate & G. Hollich (Eds.), *Theoretical and computational models of word learning: Trends in psychology and artificial intelligence* (pp. 133–152). Hershey, PA: IGI Global. doi:10.4018/978-1-4666-2973-8.ch006

Yu, J., Chen, Z., Lu, J., Liu, T., Zhou, L., Liu, X., . . . Chui, D. (2013). The important role of lipids in cognitive impairment. In Bioinformatics: Concepts, methodologies, tools, and applications (pp. 268-272). Hershey, PA: IGI Global. doi:10.4018/978-1-4666-3604-0.ch014

Yu, Y., Yang, J., & Wu, J. (2013). Cognitive functions and neuronal mechanisms of tactile working memory. In J. Wu (Ed.), *Biomedical engineering and cognitive neuroscience for healthcare: Interdisciplinary applications* (pp. 89–98). Hershey, PA: IGI Global. doi:10.4018/978-1-4666-2113-8.ch010

Zelinski, E. M. (2013). How interventions might improve cognition in healthy older adults. *International Journal of Gaming and Computer-Mediated Simulations*, *5*(3), 72–82. doi:10.4018/jgcms.2013070105

Zhang, J., Luo, X., Lu, L., & Liu, W. (2013). An acquisition model of deep textual semantics based on human reading cognitive process. *International Journal of Cognitive Informatics and Natural Intelligence*, *6*(2), 82–103. doi:10.4018/jcini.2012040105

Zheng, R. Z. (2013). Effective online learning for older people: A heuristic design approach. In R. Zheng, R. Hill, & M. Gardner (Eds.), *Engaging older adults with modern technology: Internet use and information access needs* (pp. 142–159). Hershey, PA: IGI Global. doi:10.4018/978-1-4666-1966-1.ch008

Zhou, M., & Xu, Y. (2013). Challenges to use recommender systems to enhance meta-cognitive functioning in online learners. In *Data mining: Concepts, methodologies, tools, and applications* (pp. 1916–1935). Hershey, PA: IGI Global. doi:10.4018/978-1-4666-2455-9.ch099

Ziaeehezarjeribi, Y., & Graves, I. (2013). Behind the MASK: Motivation through avatar skills and knowledge. In R. Ferdig (Ed.), *Design, utilization, and analysis of simulations and game-based educational worlds* (pp. 225–239). Hershey, PA: IGI Global. doi:10.4018/978-1-4666-4018-4.ch014

Zoss, A. M. (2014). Cognitive processes and traits related to graphic comprehension. In M. Huang & W. Huang (Eds.), *Innovative approaches of data visualization and visual analytics* (pp. 94–110). Hershey, PA: IGI Global. doi:10.4018/978-1-4666-4309-3.ch005

Compilation of References

Abdullah, T., & Brown, T. (2011). Mental illness and ethnocultural beliefs, values, and norms: An integrative review. *Clinical Psychology Review, 31*(6), 934–948. doi:10.1016/j.cpr.2011.05.003 PMID:21683671

Abe-Kim, J., Takeuchi, D., Hong, S., Zane, N., Sue, S., & Alegría, M. (2007). Use of mental health-related services among immigrant and U.S.-born Asian Americans: Results from the national Latino and Asian American study. *American Journal of Public Health, 97*(1), 91–98. doi:10.2105/AJPH.2006.098541 PMID:17138905

Abe-Kim, J., Takeuchi, D., & Hwang, W. C. (2002). Predictors of help seeking for emotional distress among Chinese Americans: Family matters. *Journal of Counseling and Clinical Psychology, 70*(5), 1186–1190. doi:10.1037/0022-006X.70.5.1186 PMID:12362969

African American Mental Health. (n.d.). Retrieved from https://www.nami.org/Find-Support/ Diverse-Communities/African-American-Mental-Health

Aggarwal, N. K., Cedeño, K., Guarnaccia, P., Kleinman, A., & Lewis-Fernández, R. (2016). The meanings of cultural competence in mental health: An exploratory focus group study with patients, clinicians, and administrators. *SpringerPlus, 5*(1), 384. doi:10.118640064-016-2037-4 PMID:27065092

Agnetti, G. (2007). Arrivano i consumatori: dove andiamo? *Psichiatria di comunità, 6*(2), 73-79.

Alegría, M., Takeuchi, D., Canino, G., Duan, N., Shrout, P., Meng, X. L., ... Gong, F. (2004). Considering context, place and culture: The National Latino and Asian American Study. *International Journal of Methods in Psychiatric Research, 13*(4), 208–222. doi:10.1002/mpr.178 PMID:15719529

Ali, S. (2014). Identification and approach t treatment of mental health disorders in A0.sian American population. In R. Parekh (Ed.), The Massachusetts general hospital textbook on diversity and cultural sensitivity in mental health (pp. 31-59). Humana Press.

Allport, G. W. (1954). *The nature of prejudice*. New York, NY: Perseus.

American Counseling Association. (2014). *2014 ACA code of ethics: As approved by the ACA governing council*. Retrieved from http://counseling.org/docs/ethics/2014-aca-code-of-ethics. pdf?sfvrsn=4

Anderson, K. M., & Wallace, B. (2015). Digital storytelling as a trauma narrative intervention for children exposed to domestic violence. *Film and video-based therapy*, 95-107.

Anderson, J. E., & Lowen, C. A. (2010). Connecting youth with health services Systematic review. *Canadian Family Physician Medecin de Famille Canadien, 56*, 778–784. PMID:20705886

Andrews, G., Issakidis, C., & Carter, G. (2001). Shortfall in mental health service utilization. *The British Journal of Psychiatry, 179*(05), 417–425. doi:10.1192/bjp.179.5.417 PMID:11689399

Angermeyer, M. C., & Matschinger, H. (2003). The stigma of mental illness: Effects of labelling on public attitudes towards people with mental disorder. *Acta Psychiatrica Scandinavica, 108*(4), 304–309. doi:10.1034/j.1600-0447.2003.00150.x PMID:12956832

Angermeyer, M., & Dietrich, S. (2006). Public beliefs about and attitudes towards people with mental illness: A review of population studies. *Acta Psychiatrica Scandinavica, 113*(3), 163–179. doi:10.1111/j.1600-0447.2005.00699.x PMID:16466402

Anil, A. (2014, August 20). *Facebook Users in Nepal*. Retrieved April 12, 2017, from Aakarpost: http://tech.aakarpost.com/2014/08/facebook-users-in-nepal.html

Anthony, W. (2000). A recovery-oriented service system: Setting some system level standards. *Psychiatric Rehabilitation Journal, 24*(2), 159–169. doi:10.1037/h0095104

Arcidiacono, C., Gelli, B., & Putton, A. (1999). *Empowerment sociale. Il futuro della solidarietà: modelli di psicologia di comunità*. Milano: FrancoAngeli.

Arkell, J., Osborn, D., Ivens, D., & King, M. (2006). Factors associated with anxiety in patients attending a sexually transmitted infection clinic: Qualitative survey. *International Journal of STD & AIDS, 17*(5), 299–303. doi:10.1258/095646206776790097 PMID:16643678

Atagün, M. İ., Balaban, Ö. D., Atagün, Z., Elagöz, M., & Özpolat, A. Y. (2011). Burden on the caregivers in chronic diseases. *Psikiyatride Güncel Yaklasimlar, 3*(3), 513–552. doi:10.5455/cap.20110323

Awad, A. G., & Voruganti, L. N. (2008). The burden of schizophrenia on caregivers. *PharmacoEconomics, 26*(2), 149–162. doi:10.2165/00019053-200826020-00005 PMID:18198934

Azar, S., Benjet, C., Fuhrmann, G., & Cavallero, L. (1995). Child maltreatment and termination of parental rights: Can behavioral research help Solomon? *Behavior Therapy, 26*(4), 599–623. doi:10.1016/S0005-7894(05)80035-8

Badiee, J., Moore, D. J., Atkinson, J. H., Vaida, F., Gerard, M., Duarte, N. A., ... Grant, I. (2012). Lifetime suicidal ideation and attempt are common among HIV+ individuals. *Journal of Affective Disorders, 136*(3), 993–999. doi:10.1016/j.jad.2011.06.044 PMID:21784531

Bahora, M., Hanafi, S., Chien, V. H., & Compton, M. T. (2008). Preliminary evidence of effects of crisis intervention team training on self-efficacy and social distance. *Administration and Policy in Mental Health*, *35*(3), 159–167. doi:10.100710488-007-0153-8 PMID:18040771

Baker, F. M., & Takeshita, J. (2002). The ethnic minority elderly. In W. S. Tseng & J. Streltzer (Eds.), *Culture and psychotherapy: A guide to clinical practice* (pp. 209–222). Washington, DC: American Psychiatric Press.

Baral, A. (2017, January 14). *Canada Nepal*. Retrieved April 8, 2017, from Rapper Yama Buddha committed suicide: http://www.ecanadanepal.com/2017/01/rapper-yama-buddha-committed-suicide.html

Barney, L. J., Griffiths, K. M., Jorm, A. F., & Christensen, H. (2006). Stigma about depression and its impact on help-seeking intentions. *The Australian and New Zealand Journal of Psychiatry*, *40*(1), 51–54. doi:10.1080/j.1440-1614.2006.01741.x PMID:16403038

Barrera, M., & Castro, F. G. (2006). A heuristic framework for the cultural adaptation of interventions. *Clinical Psychology: Science and Practice*, *13*(4), 311–316. doi:10.1111/j.1468-2850.2006.00043.x

Barth, K., Cook, R., Downs, S., Switzer, G., & Fischhoff, B. (2002). Social stigma and negative consequences: Factors that influence college students' decisions to seek testing for sexually transmitted infections. *Journal of American College Health*, *50*(4), 153–159. doi:10.1080/07448480209596021 PMID:11910948

Bartol, G. M., Moon, E., & Linton, M. (1994). Nursing assistance for families of patients. *Journal of Psychosocial Nursing*, *32*(12), 27–29. PMID:7714849

Baruth, L. G., & Manning, M. L. (2003). *Multicultural counseling and psychotherapy: A lifespan perspective*. Dallas, TX: Pearson.

Baum, F. E., & Ziersch, A. M. (2003). A glossary of social capital. *Journal of Epidemiology and Community Health*, *57*(5), 320–323. doi:10.1136/jech.57.5.320 PMID:12700212

BBC. (2017, April 26). *Editorial Guidelines*. Retrieved April 26, 2017, from BBC: http://www.bbc.co.uk/editorialguidelines/guidelines/harm-and-offence/suicide

Bedregal, L., O'Connell, M., & Davidson, L. (2006). The Recovery Knowledge Inventory: Assessment of mental health staff knowledge and attitudes about recovery. *Psychiatric Rehabilitation Journal*, *30*(2), 96–103. doi:10.2975/30.2006.96.103 PMID:17076052

Beltran, R. O., Scanlan, J. N., Hancock, N., & Luckett, T. (2007). The effect of first year mental health fieldwork on attitudes of occupational therapy students towards people with mental illness. *Australian Occupational Therapy Journal*, *54*(1), 42–48.

Bender, S., & Hill, K. (2017). *The Experience of STI Exposure Discovery in the Context of Monogamous Relationships*. Manuscript in Preparation.

Benedict, R. (1934). Anthropology and the abnormal. *Journal of General Psychiatry, 10*(1), 59–80. doi:10.1080/00221309.1934.9917714

Bentall, R. (2003). *Madness explained: Psychosis and human nature.* London: Penguin.

Beretta, V., Roten, Y., Stigler, M., Drapeau, M., Fischer, M., & Despland, J. N. (2005). The influence of patients' personal schemas on early alliance building. *Swiss Journal of Psychology, 64*(1), 13–20. doi:10.1024/1421-0185.64.1.13

Bernal, G., Bonilla, J., & Bellido, C. (1995). Ecological validity and cultural sensitivity for outcome research: Issues for the cultural adaptation and development o psychosocial treatments wit Hispanics. *Journal of Abnormal Child Psychology, 23*(1), 67–82. doi:10.1007/BF01447045 PMID:7759675

Bernal, G., Jiménez Chafey, M. I., & Rodríguez, M. M. D. (2009). Culturally adaptations of treatments: A resource for considering culture in evidence-based practice. *Professional Psychology, Research and Practice, 40*(4), 361–368. doi:10.1037/a0016401

Berninger, A., Webber, M. P., Cohen, H. W., Gustave, J., Lee, R., Niles, J. K., ... Prezant, D. J. (2010). Trends of elevated PTSD risk in firefighters exposed to the World Trade Center disaster: 2001–2005. *Public Health Reports, 125*(4), 556–566. doi:10.1177/003335491012500411 PMID:20597456

Bernstein, R. & Seltzer, T. (2003). Criminalization of people with mental illnesses: The role of mental health courts in system reform. *University of the District of Columbia Law Review, 143.*

Berry, J. (1997). Immigration, acculturation and adaption. *Applied Psychology, 46*(1), 5–34.

Bertotti, M., Watts, P., Netuveli, G., Yu, G., Schmidt, E., Tobi, P., ... Renton, A. (2013). Types of Social Capital and Mental Disorder in Deprived Urban Areas: A Multilevel Study of 40 Disadvantaged London Neighbourhoods. *PLoS One, 8*(12), e80127. doi:10.1371/journal. pone.0080127 PMID:24312459

Bharadwaj, P., Pai, M. M., & Suziedelyte, A. (2015). *Mental health stigma* (National Bureau of Economic Research). Retrieved from http://economics.ucr.edu/seminars_colloquia/201415/ applied_economics/Suzie elyte%20paper%20for%206%205%2015%20seminar.pdf

Blow, A. J., Gorman, L., Ganoczy, D., Kees, M., Kashy, D. A., Valenstein, M., ... Chermack, S. (2013). Hazardous drinking and family functioning in National Guard veterans and spouses postdeployment. *Journal of Family Psychology, 27*(2), 303–313. doi:10.1037/a0031881 PMID:23544925

Bordin, E. S. (1979). The generalizability of the psychoanalytic concept of the working alliance. *Psychotherapy (Chicago, Ill.), 16*(3), 252–260. doi:10.1037/h0085885

Bos, A. E. R., Pryor, J. B., Reeder, G. D., & Stutterheim, S. E. (2013). Stigma: Advances in Theory and Research. *Basic and Applied Social Psychology, 35*(1), 1–9. doi:10.1080/0197353 3.2012.746147

Bosco, N., Petrini, F., Giaccherini, S., & Meringolo, P. (2014). Theater as instrument to promote inclusion of mental health patients: an innovative experience in a local community. In C. Pracana (Eds.), Psychology Applications & Developments (pp. 55-66). Lisbon: InSciencePress.

Bosco, N., Guazzini, A., Guidi, E., Giaccherini, S., & Meringolo, P. (2016). Self-Stigma in mental health: planning effective programs for teenagers. In C. Pracana, & M. Wang (Eds.), *International Psychological Applications Conference and Trends* (pp. 36-39). Lisbon: W.I.A.R.S.

Brohan, E., Elgie, R., Sartorius, N., & Thornicroft, G. (2010). Self-stigma, empowerment and perceived discrimination among people with schizophrenia in 14 European countries: The GAMIAN-Europe study. *Schizophrenia Research*, *122*(1-3), 232–238. doi:10.1016/j. schres.2010.02.1065 PMID:20347271

Brown, J., & Isaacs, D. (2005). *The World Café: Shaping the World Through Conversations that Matter*. Berret-Kohler Publishers Inc.

Bulut, C., Eren, H., & Halac, D. S. (2013). Social innovation and psychometric analysis. *Procedia: Social and Behavioral Sciences*, *82*, 122–130. doi:10.1016/j.sbspro.2013.06.235

Bunnell, B. E., Davidson, T. M., Hamblen, J. L., Cook, D. L., Grubaugh, A. L., Lozano, B. E., ... & Ruggiero, K. J. (2017). Protocol for the evaluation of a digital storytelling approach to address stigma and improve readiness to seek services among veterans. *Pilot and Feasibility Studies, 3*(1), 7.

Bureau of European Policy Advisors (BEPA). (2011). *Empowering people, driving change: Social innovation in the European Union*. Luxembourg: BEPA.

Burke, P. J., & Stets, J. E. (2009). *Identity theory*. Oxford University Press. doi:10.1093/acprof :oso/9780195388275.001.0001

Buzan, B., Waever, O., & Wilde, J. d. (1997). *Security: A New Framework for Analysis*. London: Lynne Rienner Publishers.

Byrne, P. (1997). Psychiatric stigma: Past, passing and to come. *Journal of the Royal Society of Medicine*, *90*(11), 618–620. doi:10.1177/014107689709001107 PMID:9496274

Byrne, P. (2000). Stigma of mental illness and ways of diminishing it. *Advances in Psychiatric Treatment*, *6*(1), 65–72. doi:10.1192/apt.6.1.65

CACREP Annual Reports. (2016). Retrieved from http://www.cacrep.org/about- cacrep/ publications/cacrep-annual-reports/

Calabrese, J., & Corrigan, P. (2005). Beyond dementia praecox: Findings from long-term follow-up studies of schizophrenia. In R. Ralph & P. Corrigan (Eds.), *Recovery in Mental Illness: Broadening Our Understanding of Wellness* (pp. 60–72). Washington, DC: American Psychological Association. doi:10.1037/10848-003

Caracci, G., & Mezzich, J. E. (2001). Culture and urban mental health. *The Psychiatric Clinics of North America*, *24*(3), 581–593. doi:10.1016/S0193-953X(05)70249-5 PMID:11593865

Carnevale, F. A. (2007). Revisiting Goffman's Stigma: The social experience of families with children requiring mechanical ventilation at home. *Journal of Child Health Care, 11*(1), 7–18. doi:10.1177/1367493507073057 PMID:17287220

Castillo, R. J. (2002). *Lessons from Folk healing practices.* Washington, DC: American Psychiatric Press.

Castro, F. P., Barrera, M. Jr, & Holleran-Steiker, L. K. (2010). Issues and challenges in the design of culturally adapted evidence-based interventions. *Annual Review of Clinical Psychology, 6*(1), 213–239. doi:10.1146/annurev-clinpsy-033109-132032 PMID:20192800

Center for Disease Control (CDC). (2016). *Reported STDs in the United States: 2015 National Data for Chlamydia, Gonorrhea, and Syphilis.* Retrieved from: https://www.cdc.gov/nchhstp/newsroom/2016.std-suvelliance-report

Cheng, J. K. Y., Fancher, T. L., Ratanasen, M., Conner, K. R., Duberstein, P. R., Sue, S., & Takeuchi, D. (2010). Lifetime suicidal ideation and suicide attempts in Asian Americans. *Asian American Journal of Psychology, 1*(1), 8–30. doi:10.1037/a0018799 PMID:20953306

Chen, S., Sullivan, N. Y., Lu, Y. E., & Shibusawa, T. (2003). Asian Americans and mental health services: A study of utilization patterns in the 1990s. *Journal of Ethnic & Cultural Diversity in Social Work, 12*(2), 19–42. doi:10.1300/J051v12n02_02

Chen, Y., Wu, J., Yi, Q., Huang, G., & Wong, T. (2008). Depression associated with sexually transmitted infection in Canada. *Sexually Transmitted Infections, 84*(7), 535–540. doi:10.1136ti.2007.029306 PMID:18550695

Cheung, F. K., & Snowden, L. R. (1990). Community mental health and ethnic minority populations. *Community Mental Health Journal, 26*(3), 277–291. doi:10.1007/BF00752778 PMID:2354624

Christens, B. D., Speer, P. W., & Peterson, N. A. (2011). Social class as moderator of the relationship between (dis)empowering processes and psychological empowerment. *Journal of Community Psychology, 39*(2), 170–182. doi:10.1002/jcop.20425

Chu, J. P., Huynh, L., & Arean, P. A. (2012). Cultural adaptation of evidence-based practice utilizing an iterative stakeholder process and theoretical framework: Problem solving therapy for Chinese older adults. *International Journal of Geriatric Psychiatry, 27*(1), 97–106. doi:10.1002/gps.2698 PMID:21500283

Chu, J. P., & Sue, S. (2011). Asian American mental health: What we know and what we don't know. *Online Readings in Psychology and Culture, 3*(1). doi:10.9707/2307-0919.1026

Clark, C. S. (1993). Mental illness. *CQ Researcher, 3,* 673-696. Retrieved April 11, 2009 from http://library.cqpress.com/cqresearcher/cqresrre1993080600

Clark, W., Welch, S., Berry, S., Collentine, A., Collins, R., Lebron, D., & Shearer, A. (2013). Reducing stigma: Self-stigma. California's historic effort to reduce the stigma of mental illness: The Mental Health Services Act. *American Journal of Public Health, 103*(5), 786–794. doi:10.2105/AJPH.2013.301225

Clayton, A., O'Connell, M. J., Bellamy, C., Benedict, P., & Rowe, M. (2013). The Citizenship Project Part II: Impact of a Citizenship Intervention on Clinical and Community Outcomes for Persons with Mental Illness and Criminal Justice Involvement. *American Journal of Community Psychology*, *51*(1-2), 114–122. doi:10.100710464-012-9549-z PMID:22869206

Clement, S., Schauman, O., Graham, T., Maggioni, F., Evans-Lacko, S., Bezborodovs, N., ... Thornicroft, G. (2015). What is the impact of mental health related stigma on help-seeking? A systematic review of quantitative and qualitative studies. *Psychological Medicine*, *45*(1), 11–27. doi:10.1017/S0033291714000129 PMID:24569086

Coaffee, J. (2008). Sport, Culture and the Modern State: Emerging Themes in Stimulating urban Regeneration in the UK. *International Journal of Cultural Policy*, *14*(4), 377–397. doi:10.1080/10286630802445856

Cohen, B. E., Gima, K., Bertenthal, D., Kim, S., Marmar, C. R., & Seal, K. H. (2010). Mental health diagnoses and utilization of VA non-mental health medical services among returning Iraq and Afghanistan Veterans. *Journal of General Internal Medicine*, *25*(1), 18–24. doi:10.100711606-009-1117-3 PMID:19787409

Conner, K. O., McKinnon, S. A., Ward, C. J., Reynolds, C. F. III, & Brown, C. (2015). Peer education as a strategy for reducing internalized stigma among depressed older adults. *Psychiatric Rehabilitation Journal*, *38*(2), 186–193. doi:10.1037/prj0000109 PMID:25915057

Corrigan, P. W. (1999). Mental health stigma as social attribution: Implications for research methods and attitude change. *Clinical Psychology: Science and Practice*, *7*(1), 48–67. doi:10.1093/clipsy.7.1.48

Corrigan, P. W. (2004). How stigma interferes with mental health care. *The American Psychologist*, *59*(7), 614–625. doi:10.1037/0003-066X.59.7.614 PMID:15491256

Corrigan, P. W. (2011). Best practices: Strategic stigma change (SSC): Five principles for social marketing campaigns to reduce stigma. *Psychiatric Services (Washington, D.C.)*, *62*(8), 824–826. doi:10.1176/ps.62.8.pss6208_0824 PMID:21807820

Corrigan, P. W., & Boyle, M. G. (2003). What works for mental health system change: Evolution or revolution? *Administration and Policy in Mental Health*, *30*(5), 379–395. doi:10.1023/A:1024619913592 PMID:12940682

Corrigan, P. W., Larson, J. E., & Rusch, N. (2009). Self-stigma and the "why try" effect: impact on life goals and evidence based practices. *World Psychiatry; Official Journal of the World Psychiatric Association (WPA)*, *8*(2), 75–81. doi:10.1002/j.2051-5545.2009.tb00218.x PMID:19516923

Corrigan, P. W., & Matthews, A. (2003). Stigma and disclosure: Implications for coming out of the closet. *Journal of Mental Health (Abingdon, England)*, *12*(3), 235–248. doi:10.1080/0963823031000118221

Corrigan, P. W., Michaels, P. J., Vega, E., Gause, M., Watson, A. C., & Rüsch, N. (2012). *Self-stigma* of mental illness scale-short form: Reliability and validity. *Psychiatry Research*, *199*(1), 65–69. doi:10.1016/j.psychres.2012.04.009 PMID:22578819

Corrigan, P. W., & Miller, F. E. (2004). Shame, blame, and contamination: A review of the impact of mental illness stigma on family members. *Journal of Mental Health (Abingdon, England)*, *13*(6), 537–548. doi:10.1080/09638230400017004

Corrigan, P. W., Morris, S. B., Michaels, P. J., Rafacz, J. D., & Rüsch, N. (2012). Challenging the public stigma of mental illness: A meta-analysis of outcome studies. *Psychiatric Services (Washington, D.C.)*, *63*(10), 963–973. doi:10.1176/appi.ps.201100529 PMID:23032675

Corrigan, P. W., & Penn, D. L. (1999). Lessons from social psychology on discrediting psychiatric stigma. *The American Psychologist*, *54*(9), 765–776. doi:10.1037/0003-066X.54.9.765 PMID:10510666

Corrigan, P. W., & Rao, D. (2012). On the self-stigma of mental illness: Stages, disclosure, and strategies for change. *Canadian Journal of Psychiatry*, *57*(8), 464–469. doi:10.1177/070674371205700804 PMID:22854028

Corrigan, P. W., River, L. P., Lundin, R. K., Uphoff Wasowski, K., Campion, J., Mathisen, J., & ... . (2000). Stigmatizing attributions about mental illness. *Journal of Community Psychology*, *28*(1), 91–102. doi:

Corrigan, P. W., & Watson, A. C. (2002). The paradox of self-stigma and mental illness. *Clinical Psychology: Science and Practice*, *9*(1), 35–53. doi:10.1093/clipsy.9.1.35

Corrigan, P. W., & Watson, A. C. (2002). Understanding the impact of stigma on people with mental illness. *World Psychiatry; Official Journal of the World Psychiatric Association (WPA)*, *1*(1), 16–20. PMID:16946807

Corrigan, P. W., Watson, A. C., & Miller, F. E. (2006). The impact of mental illness and drug dependence stigma on family members. *Journal of Family Psychology*, *20*(2), 239–246. doi:10.1037/0893-3200.20.2.239 PMID:16756399

Corrigan, P., Druss, B., & Perlick, D. (2014). The impact of mental illness stigma on seeking and participating in mental health care. *Psychological Science in the Public Interest*, *15*(2), 37–70. doi:10.1177/1529100614531398 PMID:26171956

Corrigan, P., & Gelb, B. (2006). Three programs that use mass approaches to challenge the stigma of mental illness. *Psychiatric Services (Washington, D.C.)*, *57*(3), 393–398. doi:10.1176/appi.ps.57.3.393 PMID:16524999

Corrigan, P., Markowitz, F., & Watson, A. (2004). Structural levels of mental illness stigma and discrimination. *Schizophrenia Bulletin*, *30*(3), 481–491. doi:10.1093/oxfordjournals.schbul.a007096 PMID:15631241

Cottrell, A. B. (1990). Cross-national marriages: A review of the literature. *Journal of Comparative Family Studies*, *21*(2), 151–169.

Crandall, C. S., & Eshleman, A. (2003). A justification-suppression model of the expression and experience of prejudice. *Psychological Bulletin, 129*(3), 414–446. doi:10.1037/0033-2909.129.3.414 PMID:12784937

Crapanzano, K., & Vath, R. J. (2015). Observations: Confronting physician attitudes towards the mentally ill: A challenge to medical educators. *Journal of Graduate Medical Education, 7*(4), 686. doi:10.4300/JGME-D-15-00256.1 PMID:26692993

Crawford, M. J., Rutter, D., Manley, C., Weaver, T., Bhui, K., Fulop, N., & Tyrer, P. (2002). Systematic review of involving patients in the planning and development of health care. *British Medical Journal, 325*(7375), 1263. doi:10.1136/bmj.325.7375.1263 PMID:12458240

Crenshaw, K. (2016). *The urgency of intersectionality.* Retrieved from https://www.ted.com/talks/kimberle_crenshaw_the_urgency_of_intersectionalityedWomen2016

Creswell, J. W. (2003). *Research design: Qualitative, quantitative, and mixed methods approaches* (2nd ed.). Thousand Oaks, CA: Sage.

Crisp, A. H., Gelder, M. G., Rix, S., Meltzer, H. I., & Rowlands, O. J. (2000). Stigmatization of people with mental illness. *The British Journal of Psychiatry, 177*(1), 4–7. doi:10.1192/bjp.177.1.4 PMID:10945080

Crowe, A., & Averett, P. (2015). Attitudes of Mental Health Professionals toward Mental Illness: A Deeper Understanding. *Journal of Mental Health Counseling, 37*(1), 47–62. doi:10.17744/mehc.37.1.l23251h783703q2v

Curtis, J., Walkins, A., Rosenbaum, U. M. S., Teasdale, S., Kalucy, M., Samaras, K., & Ward, F. B. (2016). Evaluating an individualized lifestyle and life skills interventions to prevent antipsychotic-induced weight gain in first-episode psychosis. *Early Intervention in Psychiatry, 10*(3), 267–276. doi:10.1111/eip.12230 PMID:25721464

Dardas, L. A., & Simmons, L. A. (2015). The stigma of mental illness in Arab families: A concept analysis. *Journal of Psychiatric and Mental Health Nursing, 22*(9), 668–679. doi:10.1111/jpm.12237 PMID:26118332

Darroch, J., Myers, L., & Cassell, J. (2003). Sex differences in the experiences of testing positive for genital chlamydia infection: A qualitative study with implications for public health and for a national screening programme. *Sexually Transmitted Infections, 79*(5), 372–376. doi:10.1136ti.79.5.372 PMID:14573831

Davidson, L. (2006). Recovery guides: An emerging model of community-based care for adults with psychiatric disabilities. In A. Lightburn & P. Sessions (Eds.), *Handbook of community-based clinical practice* (pp. 476–502). Oxford, UK: Oxford University Press.

de Barros, V. V., Martins, L., Saitz, R., Bastos, R. R., & Ronzani, T. (2013). Mental health conditions, individual and job characteristics and sleep disturbances among firefighters. *Journal of Health Psychology, 18*(3), 350–358. doi:10.1177/1359105312443402 PMID:22517948

De Silva, M. J., McKenzie, K., Harpham, T., & Huttly, S. R. A. (2005). Social Capital and mental illness: A systematic review. *Journal of Epidemiology and Community Health*, *59*(8), 619–627. doi:10.1136/jech.2004.029678 PMID:16020636

Deegan, P. (1988). Recovery: The lived experience of rehabilitation. *Psychosocial Rehabilitation Journal*, *11*(4), 11–19. doi:10.1037/h0099565

Deegan, P. (1996). Recovery as a journey of the heart. *Psychiatric Rehabilitation Journal*, *19*(3), 91–98. doi:10.1037/h0101301

Devine, P. G., Plant, E. A., & Harrison, K. (1999). The problem of "us" versus "them" and AIDS stigma. *The American Behavioral Scientist*, *42*(7), 1212–1228. doi:10.1177/00027649921954732

Dewey, C. (2014, August 12). *Suicide contagion and social media: The dangers of sharing 'Genie, you're free'*. Retrieved April 20, 2017, from The Washington Post: https://www.washingtonpost.com/news/the-intersect/wp/2014/08/12/suicide-contagion-and-social-media-the-dangers-of-sharing-genie-youre-free/?utm_term=.c20fcac2338f

Dickstein, B. D., Vogt, D. S., Handa, S., & Litz, B. T. (2010). Targeting self-stigma in returning military personnel and veterans: A review of intervention strategies. *Military Psychology*, *22*(2), 224–236. doi:10.1080/08995600903417399

Dohrenwend, B. P., Turner, J. B., Turse, N. A., Adams, B. G., Koenen, K. C., & Marshall, R. (2006). The psychological risks of Vietnam for US veterans: A revisit with new data and methods. *Science*, *313*(5789), 979–982. doi:10.1126cience.1128944 PMID:16917066

Dovidio, J. F., Major, B., & Crocker, J. (2000). Stigma: Introduction and overview. In The social psychology of stigma (pp. 1-28). New York: Guilford Press.

Dovidio, J. F., Major, B., & Crocker, J. (2000). *The social psychology of stigma*. New York: Guilford Press.

Dovidio, J. R., Pagotto, L., & Hebl, M. R. (2011). Implicit attitudes and discrimination against people with disabilities. In R. L. Wiener & S. L. Wilborn (Eds.), *Disability and age discrimination: Perspectives in law and psychology* (pp. 157–184). New York, NY: Springer; doi:10.1007/978-1-4419-6293-5_9

Duncan, B., Hart, G., Scoular, A., & Bigrigg, A. (2001). Qualitative analysis of psychosocial impact of diagnosis of chlamydia trachomatis: Implication for screening. *British Medical Journal*, *27*(7280), 195–199. doi:10.1136/bmj.322.7280.195 PMID:11159612

Eack, S. M., & Newhill, C. E. (2008). What influences social workers' attitudes toward working with severe mental illness? *The Journal of Contemporary Social Services*, *89*(3), 419–428. PMID:24353397

Ehsan, A. M., & De Silva, M. J. (2015). Social capital and common mental disorder: A systematic review. *Journal of Epidemiology and Community Health*, *69*(10), 1021–1028. doi:10.1136/jech-2015-205868 PMID:26179447

Eisenberg, D., Downs, M. F., Golberstein, E., & Zivin, K. (2009). Stigma and help seeking for mental health among college students. *Medical Care Research and Review: MCRR, 66*(5), 522–541. doi:10.1177/1077558709335173 PMID:19454625

Ellis, A. (1994). *Reason and emotion in psychotherapy. Revised and updated.* Secaucus, NJ: Carol Publishing Group.

Fabrega, H. Jr. (1991). The culture and history of psychiatric stigma in early modern and modern western societies: A review of recent literature. *Comprehensive Psychiatry, 32*(2), 97–119. doi:10.1016/0010-440X(91)90002-T PMID:2022119

Faulkner, G., & Biddle, S. (1999). Exercise as an adjunct treatment for schizophrenia: A review of the literature. *Journal of Mental Health (Abingdon, England), 23*, 355–359.

Feldman, D. B., & Crandall, C. S. (2007). Dimensions of mental illness stigma: What about mental illness causes social rejection? *Journal of Social and Clinical Psychology, 26*(2), 137–154. doi:10.1521/jscp.2007.26.2.137

Field, J. (2003). *Social capital.* London: Routledge.

Finkelstein, J., Lapshin, O., & Wasserman, E. (2008). Randomized study of different anti-stigma media. *Patient Education and Counseling, 71*(2), 204–214. doi:10.1016/j.pec.2008.01.002 PMID:18289823

Fink, P. J., & Tasman, A. (1992). *Stigma and Mental Illness.* Washington, DC: American Psychiatric Press.

Firth, J., Cottr, J., Jerome, I., Elliott, R., French, P., & Yung, A. R. (2015). A systematic review and meta-analysis of exercise interventions in schizophrenic patients. *Psychological Medicine, 45*(07), 1343–1361. doi:10.1017/S0033291714003110 PMID:25650668

Firth, J., Rosenbaum, S., Strubbs, B., Gorcynski, P., Yung, A. R., & Vancampfort, D. (2016). Motivating factors and barriers towards exercise in severe mental illness: A systematic review and meta-analysis. *Psychological Medicine, 46*(14), 2869–2881. doi:10.1017/S0033291716001732 PMID:27502153

Fisher, W. H., Silver, E., & Wolff, N. (2006). Beyond criminalization: Toward a criminologically informed framework for mental health policy and services research. *Administration and Policy in Mental Health, 33*(5), 544–557. doi:10.100710488-006-0072-0 PMID:16791518

Forsman, A. K., Nordmyr, J., & Wahlbeck, K. (2011). Psychosocial interventions for the promotion of mental health and the prevention of depression among older adults. *Health Promotion International, 26*(suppl_1), S85–S107. doi:10.1093/heapro/dar074 PMID:22079938

Forsman, A. K., Nyqvist, F., Schierenbeck, I., Gustafson, Y., & Wahlbeck, K. (2013). Structural and cognitive social capital and depression among older adults in two Nordic regions. *Aging & Mental Health, 16*(6), 771–779. doi:10.1080/13607863.2012.667784 PMID:22486561

Foster, L., & Byers, E. (2008). Predictors of stigma and shame related to sexually transmitted infections: Attitudes, education, and knowledge. *The Canadian Journal of Human Sexuality*, *17*(4), 193–202.

Freud, S. (1911). The case of Schreber, papers on technique, and other works. In *The standard edition of the complete psychological works of Sigmund Freud* (Vol. 12). London, UK: The Hogarth Press and the Institute of Psychoanalysis.

Fuller Torrey, W. (2006). *Surviving schizophrenia: A manual for families, patients and providers*. New York, NY: Harper Collins.

Gaebel, W., Muijen, M., Baumann, A. E., Bhugra, D., Wasserman, D., Van Der Gaag, R. J., ... Zielesek, J. (2014). EPA guidance on building trust in mental health service. *European Psychiatry*, *29*(2), 83–100. doi:10.1016/j.eurpsy.2014.01.001 PMID:24506936

Garrido-Hernansaiz, H., Heylen, E., Bharat, S., Ramakrishna, J., & Ekstrand, M.L. (2016). Stigmas, symptom severity and perceived social support predict quality of life for PLHIC in urban Indian Context. *Health Quality Life Outcomes, 3*(14), 152. doi: 10.1186/s12955-016-0556-x

Gary, F. A. (2009). Stigma: Barrier to mental health care among ethnic minorities. *Issues in Mental Health Nursing*, *26*(10), 979–999. doi:10.1080/01612840500280638 PMID:16283995

Ghimire, B. (2017, January 16). *Rest in beats Yama Buddha*. Retrieved April 8, 2017, from Sharing my opinion with the world: http://barunghimire.blogspot.com/2017/01/rest-in-beats-yama-buddha.html

Gist, R., Taylor, V. H., & Raak, S. (2011). *Suicide surveillance, preven- tion, and intervention measures for the US Fire Service: Findings and recommendations for the Suicide and Depression Summit* [White paper]. Retrieved from http://lifesafetyinitiatives.com/13/suicide_whitepaper.pdf

Glaser, B. G., & Strauss, A. L. (1967). *The Discovery of Grounded Theory: Strategies for Qualitative Research*. Chicago: Aldine.

Goffma, E. (1963). *Stigma: Notes from the Management of a Spoiled Identity*. London: Penguin Books.

Goffman, E. (1961). *Asylums: Essays on the social situation of mental patient and other inmates*. New York, NY: Anchor Books.

Goffman, E. (1963). *Stigma: Notes on the management of spoiled identity*. Englewood Cliffs, NJ: Prentice Hall.

Goffman, E. (1963). *Stigma: Notes on the Management of Spoiled Identity*. New York, New York: Simon & Schuster.

Goodman, R., & Newman, D. (2014). Testing a digital storytelling intervention to reduce stress in adolescent females. *Storytelling, Self, Society*, *10*(2), 177–193. doi:10.13110torselfsoci.10.2.0177

Granovetter, M. (1983). The strength of weak ties: A network theory revisited. *Sociological Theory*, *1*, 201–233. doi:10.2307/202051

Greenwood, K., Carroll, C., Crowter, L., Jamieson, K., Ferraresi, L., Jones, A. M., & Brown, R. (2016). Early intervention for stigma towards mental illness? Promoting positive attitudes towards severe mental illness in primary school children. *Journal of Public Mental Health*, *15*(4), 188–199. doi:10.1108/JPMH-02-2016-0008

Griner, D., & Smith, T. B. (2006). Culturally adapted mental health intervention: A meta-analytic review. *Psychotherapy (Chicago, Ill.)*, *43*(4), 531–548. doi:10.1037/0033-3204.43.4.531 PMID:22122142

Grob, G. (1994). *The mad among us: A history of the care of America's mentally ill*. New York, NY: The Free Press.

Gulliver, A., Griffiths, K. M., & Christensen, H. (2010). Perceived barriers and facilitators to mental health help-seeking in young people: A systematic review. *BMC Psychiatry*, *10*(1), 113. doi:10.1186/1471-244X-10-113 PMID:21192795

Gülseren, L. (2002). Schizophrenia and family: Challenges, feelings, needs. *Türk Psikiyatri Dergisi*, *13*(2), 143–151. PMID:12794667

Gülseren, L., Çam, B., Karakoç, B., Yiğit, T., Danacı, A. E., Çubukçuoğlu, Z., ... Mete, L. (2010). The factors affecting the burden n the family in schizophrenia. *Turkish Journal of Psychiatry*, *21*, 203–212. PMID:20818508

Habamoment.com. (2017, January 20). *Yama Buddha and three other Nepali celebrities who committed suicide*. Retrieved March 26, 2017, from Habamoment.com: http://habamoment.com/yama-buddha-and-three-other-nepali-celebrities-who-suicided/

Haigh, C., & Hardy, P. (2011). Tell me a story—a conceptual exploration of storytelling in healthcare education. *Nurse Education Today*, *31*(4), 408–411. doi:10.1016/j.nedt.2010.08.001 PMID:20810195

Hailamariam, M., Fecadu, A., Prince, M., & Hanlon, C. (2017). Engaging and staying engaged: A phenomenological study of barriers to equitable access to mental health care for people with severe mental disorders in a rural African setting. *International Journal for Equity in Health*, *16*(1), 156. doi:10.118612939-017-0657-0 PMID:28851421

Haller, B. (2010). *Representing disability in an ableist world*. Louisville, KY: The Advocado Press.

Hamblen, J., Grubaugh, A., Davidson, T. M., Borkman, A. L., Bunnell, B., Tuerk, P. W., & Ruggiero, K. J. (2018). A feasibility and pilot evaluation of an online peer-to-peer educational campaign to reduce stigma and improve help seeking in veterans with PTSD. *Telemedicine and eHealth*.

Han, B., Hedden, S. L., Lipari, R., Copello, E. A. P., & Kroutil, L. A. (2015). *Receipt of services for behavioral health problems: results from the 2014 National Survey on Drug Use and Health*. Rockville, MD: Substance Abuse and Mental Health Services Administration.

Han, M., & Pong, H. (2015). Mental health help-seeking behaviors among Asian American community college students: The effect of stigma, cultural barriers, and acculturation. *Journal of College Student Development*, *56*(1), 1–14. doi:10.1353/csd.2015.0001

Hansson, L., Jormfeldt, H., Svedberg, P., & Swensson, B. (2011). Mental health professionals' attitudes towards people with mental illness: Do they differ from attitudes held by people with mental illness? *International Journal of Social Psychology*, *59*(1), 48–54. doi:10.1177/0020764011423176 PMID:21954319

Harding, C. M., Brooks, G., Ashikaga, T., Stauss, J., & Breier, A. (1987). The Vermont longitudinal study of persons with severe mental illness. *The American Journal of Psychiatry*, *144*(6), 718–735. doi:10.1176/ajp.144.6.718 PMID:3591991

Harpham, T., Grant, E., & Thomas, E. (2002). Measuring social capital within health surverys: Key issues. *Health Policy and Planning*, *17*(1), 106–111. doi:10.1093/heapol/17.1.106 PMID:11861592

Hartmann, D. (2003). Theorizing sport as social intervention: A view from the grassroots. *Quest.*, *55*(2), 118–140. doi:10.1080/00336297.2003.10491795

Haslam, S. A., Jetten, J., Postmes, T., & Haslam, C. (2009). Social Identity, Health and Well-Being: An Emerging Agenda for Applied Psychology. *Applied Psychology*, *58*(1), 1–23. doi:10.1111/j.1464-0597.2008.00379.x

Health, N. M. (2014). *Supporting Fact Sheet: Suicide and the Media*. Retrieved March 26, 2017, from Conversations Matter: http://www.conversationsmatter.com.au/LiteratureRetrieve. aspx?ID=4631

Hebl, M. R., Tickle, J., & Heatherton, T. F. (2000). Awkward moments in interactions between nonstigmatized and stigmatized individuals. In T. F. Heatherton, R. E. Kleck, M. R. Hebl, & J. G. Hull (Eds.), *The social psychology of stigma* (pp. 243–272). New York: Guilford Press.

Hedden, S. L., Kenner, J., Lipari, R., Medley, G., Tice, P., Copello, E. A. P., & Kroutil, L. A. (2015). *Behavioral health trends in the United States: Results from the 2014 National Survey on Drug Use and Health*. Rockville, MD: Center for Behavioral Statistics and Quality, Substance Abuse and Mental Health Services Administration.

Henderson, C., Noblett, J., Parke, H., Clement, S., Caffrey, A., Gale-Grant, O., ... Thornicroft, G. (2014). Mental health-related stigma in health care and mental health-care settings. *The Lancet. Psychiatry*, *1*(6), 467–482. doi:10.1016/S2215-0366(14)00023-6 PMID:26361202

Hinton, D. E., Pich, V., Chhean, D., Hofmann, S. G., & Pollack, M. H. (2006). Somatic-focused therapy for traumatized refugees: Treating posttraumatic stress disorder and comorbid neck-focused panic attacks among Cambodian refugees. *Psychotherapy (Chicago, Ill.)*, *43*(4), 491–505. doi:10.1037/0033-3204.43.4.491 PMID:22122139

Hinton, L., Tran, J. N., Tran, C., & Hinton, D. (2008). Religious and spiritual dimensions of the Vietnamese dementia caregiving experience. *Hallym International Journal of Aging*, *10*(2), 139–160. doi:10.2190/HA.10.2.e PMID:20930949

Hofstede, G. (1997). *Cultures and Organizations: Software of the mind.* New York: McGraw Hill.

Hoge, C. W., Auchterlonie, J., & Milliken, C. (2006). Mental health problems, use of mental health services, attrition from military service after returning from deployment to Iraq or Afghanistan. *Journal of the American Medical Association, 295*(9), 1023–1032. doi:10.1001/jama.295.9.1023 PMID:16507803

Hoge, C. W., Castro, C. A., Messer, S. C., McGurk, D., Cotting, D. I., & Koffman, R. L. (2004). Combat duty in Iraq and Afghanistan, mental health, barriers to care. *The New England Journal of Medicine, 351*(1), 13–22. doi:10.1056/NEJMoa040603 PMID:15229303

Hopper, K., & Wanderling, J. (2000). Revisiting the developed versus developing distinction in course and outcome in schizophrenia: Results from ISoS, the WHO collaborative follow-up project. International Study of Schizophrenia. *Schizophrenia Bulletin, 26*(4), 835–846. doi:10.1093/oxfordjournals.schbul.a033498 PMID:11087016

Howarth, C. (2006). Race as stigma: Positioning the stigmatized as agents, not objects. *Journal of Community & Applied Social Psychology, 16*(6), 442–451. doi:10.1002/casp.898

Howley, E. T. (2001). Type of activity: Resistance, aerobic and leisure versus occupational physical activity. *Medicine and Science in Sports and Exercise, 33*(Supplement), 364–369. doi:10.1097/00005768-200106001-00005 PMID:11427761

Hsu, E., Dabies, C. A., & Hansen, D. J. (2011). *Understanding mental health needs of Southeast Asian refugees: Historical, cultural, and contextual challenges.* Lincoln, NE: University of Nebraska. Available at http://digitalcommons.unl.edu/psychfacpub/86

Huang, W. Y., & Lin, C. Y. (2015). The relationship between *Self-stigma* and quality of life among people with mental illness who participated in a community program. *Journal of Nature and Science, 1*(7), e135.

Hwang, W. (2007). Acculturative family distancing: Theory research and clinical practice. *Psychotherapy (Chicago, Ill.), 43*(4), 397–409. doi:10.1037/0033-3204.43.4.397 PMID:22122132

Ivey, A. E., Ivey, M. B., & Simek-Morgan, L. (1997). *Counseling and psychotherapy: A multicultural perspective.* Needham Heights, MA: Allyn & Bacon.

James, P. (Ed.). (2003). *International encyclopedia of marriage and family.* New York, NY: Macmillan.

Jang, Y., Chiriboga, D. A., & Okazaki, S. (2009). Attitudes toward mental health services: Age group differences in Korean American adults. *Aging & Mental Health, 13*(1), 127–134. doi:10.1080/13607860802591070 PMID:19197698

Jenks, A. C. (2011). From 'lists of traits' to 'openmindedness": Emerging issues in cultural competence education. *Culture, Medicine, and Psychiatry. An International Journal of Cross-Cultural Health Research, 35*, 209–235. doi:10.100711013-011-9212-4 PMID:21560030

Jeste, D., & Vahia, I. (2008). Comparison of the conceptualization of wisdom in ancient Indian literature with modern views: Focus on the Bhagavad Gita. *Psychiatry, 71*(3), 197–208. doi:10.1521/psyc.2008.71.3.197 PMID:18834271

Jones, E., Farina, A., Hastorf, A., Markus, H., Miller, D. T., & Scott, R. (1984). *Social Stigma: The Psychology of Marked Relationships*. New York, NY: Freeman.

Kadushin, A., & Harkness, D. (2014). *Supervision in social work*. New York, NY: Columbia University Press. doi:10.7312/kadu15176

Kahneman, D. (2011). *Thinking, fast and slow*. New York, NY: Farar, Straus, and Giroux.

Kamal, R. (2013). *A Narrative Study of the Lived Experiences of Family Caregivers Through Different Stages of Mental Illness* (Unpublished Doctoral Dissertation). Department of Counselor Education, New Mexico.

Kessler, R. C., Berglund, P. A., Bruce, M. L., Koch, J. R., Laska, E. M., Leaf, P. J., ... Wang, P. S. (2001). The prevalence and correlates of untreated serious mental illness. *Health Services Research, 36*(6 Pt 1), 987. PMID:11775672

Khan, M. R., Kaufman, J. S., Pence, B. W., Gaynes, B. N., Adimora, A. A., Weir, S. S., & Miller, W. C. (2009). Depression, sexually transmitted infection, and sexual risk behavior among young adults in the United States. *Archives of Pediatrics & Adolescent Medicine, 163*(7), 644–652. doi:10.1001/archpediatrics.2009.95 PMID:19581548

Kim, B. S. K., Ahn, A. J., & Lam, N. A. (2009). Theories and research on acculturation and enculturation experiences among Asian American families. In N. H. Trinh, Y. C. Rho, F. G. Lu, & K. M. Sanders (Ed.), Handbook of mental health and acculturation in Asian American families (pp. 25-43). Humana Press. doi:10.1007/978-1-60327-437-1_2

Kimby, D., Vakhrushev, J., Bartels, M. N., Armstrong, H. F., Ballon, J. S., Khan, S., ... Ayanruoh, I. (2015). The impact of aerobic exercise on brain-derived neurothropic factor and neurocognition in individuals with schizoprenia: A single-blind randomized clinical trial. *Schizophrenia Bulletin, 41*(4), 859–868. doi:10.1093chbulbv022 PMID:25805886

Kimotho, S., Miller, A. N., & Ngure, P. (2015). Managing communication surrounding tungiasis stigma in Kenya. *Communicatio, 41*(4), 523–542. doi:10.1080/02500167.2015.1100646

Kim, P. Y., & Kendall, D. L. (2015). Etiology beliefs moderate the influence of emotional self-control on willingness to see a counselor through help-seeking attitudes among Asian American students. *Journal of Counseling Psychology, 62*(2), 148–158. doi:10.1037/cou0000015 PMID:24635590

Kim, P. Y., Thomas, J. L., Wilk, J. E., Castro, C. A., & Hoge, C. W. (2010). Stigma, barriers to care, and use of mental health services among active duty and National Guard soldiers after combat. *Psychiatric Services (Washington, D.C.), 61*(6), 582–588. doi:10.1176/ps.2010.61.6.582 PMID:20513681

Kingdon, D., Sharma, T., & Hart, D. (2004). What attitudes do psychiatrist hold towards people with mental illness? *Psychiatric Bulletin, 28*(11), 401–406. doi:10.1192/pb.28.11.401

Kingori, C., Ice, G. H., Hassan, Q., Elmi, A., & Perko, E. (2016). 'If I went to mom with that information, I'm dead': Sexual health knowledge barriers among immigrant and refugee Somali young adults in Ohio. *Ethnicity & Health*, *22*(4), 1–14. doi:10.1080/13557858.2016.1263285 PMID:27350450

Kirk, S. (2005). *Mental disorders in the social environment*. New York, NY: Columbia University Press.

Knifton, L., & Quinn, N. (2008, February). Media, Mental Health and Discrimination: A Frame for Reference for Understanding Reporting Trends. *International Journal of Mental Health Promotion*, *10*(1), 23–31. doi:10.1080/14623730.2008.9721754

Kok, B. C., Herrell, R. K., Thomas, J. L., & Hoge, C. W. (2012). Posttraumatic stress disorder associated with combat service in Iraq or Afghanistan: Reconciling prevalence differences between studies. *The Journal of Nervous and Mental Disease*, *200*(5), 444–450. doi:10.1097/NMD.0b013e3182532312 PMID:22551799

Kowalski, R. M., Morgan, M., & Taylor, K. (2016). Stigma of mental and physical illness and the use of mobile technology. *The Journal of Social Psychology*, 1–9. PMID:27841705

Krogh, J., Nordentolf, M., Sterne, J. A., & Lawlor, D. A. (2011). The effect of exercise in clinically depressed adults: Systematic review and meta-analysis of randomized contolled trials. *The Journal of Clinical Psychiatry*, *72*(04), 529–538. doi:10.4088/JCP.08r04913blu PMID:21034688

Kulhara, P., & Chakrabarti, S. (2001). Culture and schizophrenia and other psychotic disorders. *The Psychiatric Clinics of North America*, *24*(3), 449–464. doi:10.1016/S0193-953X(05)70240-9 PMID:11593856

Kung, W. (2004). Cultural and practical barriers to seeking mental health treatment for Chinese Americans. *Journal of Community Psychology*, *32*(1), 27–43. doi:10.1002/jcop.10077

Kurzban, R., & Leary, M. R. (2001). Evolutionary origins of stigmatization: The functions of social exclusion. *Psychological Bulletin*, *127*(2), 187–208. doi:10.1037/0033-2909.127.2.187 PMID:11316010

Langle, G., Siemssen, G., & Hornberger, S. (2000). The role of sport in the treatment and rehabilitation of schizophrenic patients. *Rehabilitation*, *39*(5), 276–282. doi:10.1055-2000-7863 PMID:11089261

Laposa, J. M., & Alden, L. E. (2003). Posttraumatic stress disorder in the emergency room: Exploration of a cognitive model. *Behaviour Research and Therapy*, *41*(1), 49–65. doi:10.1016/S0005-7967(01)00123-1 PMID:12488119

Larson, J. E., & Corrigan, P. (2008). The stigma of families with mental illness. *Academic Psychiatry*, *32*(2), 87–91. doi:10.1176/appi.ap.32.2.87 PMID:18349326

Lasalvia, A., Zoppei, S., Van Bortel, T., Bonetto, C., Cristofalo, D., Wahlbeck, K., & Germanavicius, A. (2013). Global pattern of experienced and anticipated discrimination reported by people with major depressive disorder: A cross-sectional survey. *Lancet, 381*(9860), 55–62. doi:10.1016/S0140-6736(12)61379-8 PMID:23083627

Lee, S., Juon, H., Martinez, G., Hsu, C., Robinson, E., Bawa, J., & Ma, G. X. (2009). Model minority at risk: Expressed needs of mental health by Asian American young adults. *Journal of Community Health: The Publications for Health Promotion and Disease Prevention, 34*(2), 144–152. doi:10.100710900-008-9137-1 PMID:18931893

Lee, S., & Kleinman, A. (2007). Are somatoform disorders changing over time? The case of neurasthenia in China. *Psychosomatic Medicine, 69*(9), 846–849. doi:10.1097/PSY.0b013e31815b0092 PMID:18040092

Lefley, H. P. (1990). Culture and chronic mental illness. *Hospital & Community Psychiatry, 41*(3), 277–286. PMID:2179100

Leiberman, R., & Kopelowicz, A. (2002). Recovery from schizophrenia: A challenge for the 21st century. *International Review of Psychiatry (Abingdon, England), 14*(4), 245–255. doi:10.1080/0954026021000016897

Leong, F. T. L., & Zachar, P. (1999). Gender and opinions about mental illness as predictors of attitudes toward seeking professional psychological help. *British Journal of Guidance & Counselling, 27*(1), 123–132. doi:10.1080/03069889908259720

Lichentenstein, B. (2003). Stigma as a barrier treatment of sexually transmitted infection in the American Deep South: Issues of races, gender, and poverty. *Social Science & Medicine, 57*(12), 2435–2445. doi:10.1016/j.socscimed.2003.08.002 PMID:14572849

Lichtenstein, B., Neal, T. M., & Brodsky, S. L. (2008). The stigma of sexually transmitted infections: Knowledge, attitudes, and an educationally-based intervention. *Health Educ. Monogr. ser, 25*, 28-33.

Liegghio, M. (2013). *The Stigma of Mental of Illness: Learning from the Situated Knowledge of Psychiatrized Youth, Caregivers, and Young Siblings* (Unpublished doctoral thesis). Wilfrid Laurier University, Canada.

Linehan, M. (1994). *Cognitive behavioral treatment of borderline personality disorder.* New York, NY: Guilford Press.

Link, B. G., Mirotznik, J., & Cullen, F. (1991). The Effectiveness of Stigma Coping Orientations: Can Negative Consequences of Mental Illness Labeling be Avoided? *Journal of Health and Social Behavior, 32*(3), 302–320. doi:10.2307/2136810 PMID:1940212

Link, B. G., & Phelan, J. C. (2001). Conceptualizing stigma. *Annual Review of Sociology, 27*(1), 363–385. doi:10.1146/annurev.soc.27.1.363

Link, B. G., Yang, L. H., Phelan, J. C., & Collins, P. Y. (2004). Measuring mental illness stigma. *Schizophrenia Bulletin*, *30*(3), 511–541. doi:10.1093/oxfordjournals.schbul.a007098 PMID:15631243

Lin, N. (1999). Building a Network Theory of Social Capital. *Connections*, *22*(1), 28–51.

Long, F. T. L., & Lee, S. H. (2006). A cultural accommodation model for cross-cultural psychotherapy: Illustrated with the case of Asian Americans. *Psychotherapy (Chicago, Ill.)*, *43*(4), 410–423. doi:10.1037/0033-3204.43.4.410 PMID:22122133

Lopez, R. A., & Yamazato, M. (2003). On growing old in America: Perceptions of an Okinawan War Bride. *Journal of Women & Aging*, *4*(2/3), 17–31. doi:10.1300/J074v15n04_03 PMID:14750587

Loury, G. C. (2003). Racial stigma: Toward a new paradigm for discrimination theory. *The American Economic Review*, *93*(2), 334–337. doi:10.1257/000282803321947308

Lu, F. G. (2010). Asian Americans and Pacific Islanders. In P. Ruiz & A. Primm (Ed.), Disparities in psychiatric care: Clinical and cross cultural perspectives (pp. 40-51). Baltimore, MD: Lippincott Williams & Wilkins.

Luitel, N. P., Jordans, M. J., & Adhikari, A., Upadhyay, Nawaraj, Hanlon, C., . . . Komproe, I. H. (2015). Mental health care in Nepal: Current situation and challenges for development of a district mental health care plan. *Conflict and Health*, *9*(3), 1–11. doi:10.118613031-014-0030-5 PMID:25694792

Lukes, S. (2005). *Power: A radical view*. Hampshire, UK: Palgrave McMillan. doi:10.1007/978-0-230-80257-5

Lundberg, B., Hansson, L., Wentz, E., & Björkman, T. (2008). Stigma, discrimination, empowerment and social networks: A preliminary investigation of their influence on subjective quality of life in a Swedish sample. *The International Journal of Social Psychiatry*, *54*(1), 47–55. doi:10.1177/0020764007082345 PMID:18309758

Madianos, M., Economou, M., Dafni, O., Koukia, E., Palli, A., & Rogakou, E. (2004). Family disruption, economic hardship and psychological distress in schizophrenia: Can they be measured? *European Psychiatry*, *19*(7), 408–414. doi:10.1016/j.eurpsy.2004.06.028 PMID:15504647

Magliano, L., Fiorillo, A., De Rosa, C., Malangone, C., & Maj, M. (2004). Beliefs about schizophrenia in Italy" A comparative nationwide survey of the general public, mental health professionals, and patients' relatives. *Canadian Journal of Psychiatry*, *49*(5), 323–331. doi:10.1177/070674370404900508 PMID:15198469

Mahat, G., Ann Scoloveno, M., & Ayres, C. (2011). HIV/AIDS knowledge and self-efficacy among Nepalese adolescents: A peer education program. *Research and Theory for Nursing Practice*, *25*(4), 271–283. doi:10.1891/1541-6577.25.4.271 PMID:22329081

Major, B., & O'Brien, L. T. (2005). The Social Psychology of Stigma. *Annual Review of Psychology*, *56*(1), 393–421. doi:10.1146/annurev.psych.56.091103.070137 PMID:15709941

Masuda, A., Anderson, P., Twohig, M., Feinstein, A., Chou, Y., Wendell, J., & Stormo, A. (2009). Help-seeking experiences and attitudes among African American, Asian American, and European American college students. *International Journal for the Advancement of Counseling, 31*(3), 168–180. doi:10.100710447-009-9076-2

Matsuoka, J. K., Breaux, C., & Ryujin, D. H. (1997). National utilization of mental health services by Asian Americans/Pacific Islanders. *Journal of Community Psychology, 25*(2), 141–145. doi:

Ma, Z. (2017). How the media cover mental illnesses: A review. *Health Education, 117*(1), 90–109. doi:10.1108/HE-01-2016-0004

McGinty, E. E., Webster, D. W., & Barry, C. L. (2013). Effects of news media messages about mass shootings on attitudes toward persons with serious mental illness and public support for gun control policies. *The American Journal of Psychiatry, 170*(5), 494–501. doi:10.1176/appi. ajp.2013.13010014 PMID:23511486

McKenzie, K., Whitley, R., & Weich, S. (2002). Social capital and mental health. *The British Journal of Psychiatry, 181*(04), 280–283. doi:10.1192/bjp.181.4.280 PMID:12356653

McNamee, I., Mead, G., MacGillivrey, S., & Lawrie, S. M. (2013). Schizophrenia, poor physical health and physical activity: Evidence-based interventions are required to reduce major health inequalities. *The British Journal of Psychiatry, 203*(04), 912–918. doi:10.1192/bjp.bp.112.125070 PMID:24085733

Mead, S., & Copeland, M. (2000). What recovery means to us: Consumer's perspectives. *Community Mental Health Journal, 36*(3), 315–328. doi:10.1023/A:1001917516869 PMID:10933247

Medicine, U. (2017, January 29). *Update Medicine.* Retrieved March 26, 2017, from Unanswered Questions on Yama Buddha's death: http://updatemedicine.com/yama-buddha-death-mystery/

Medicine, P. (2009). Media Portrayals of Suicide. *PLoS Medicine, 1-2.* doi:10.1371/journal. pmed.1000051 PMID:19296719

Medley, A., Kennedy, C., O'Reilly, K., & Sweat, M. (2009). Effectiveness of peer education interventions for HIV prevention in developing countries: A systematic review and meta-analysis. *AIDS Education and Prevention, 21*(3), 181–206. doi:10.1521/aeap.2009.21.3.181 PMID:19519235

Meisenbach, R. J. (2010). Stigma management communication: A theory and Agenda for applied research on how individuals manage moments of stigmatized identity. *Journal of Applied Communication Research, 38*(3), 268–292. doi:10.1080/00909882.2010.490841

Meurk, C., Whiteford, H., Head, B., Hall, W., & Carah, N. (2015, June). Media and evidence-informed policy development: The case of mental health in Australia. *Contemporary Social Science: Journal of the Academy of Social Sciences, 10*(2), 160–170. doi:10.1080/21582041.2 015.1053970

Mitani, S., Fujita, M., Nakata, K., & Shirakawa, T. (2006). Impact of post-traumatic stress disorder and job-related stress on burnout: A study of fire service workers. *The Journal of Emergency Medicine, 31*(1), 7–11. doi:10.1016/j.jemermed.2005.08.008 PMID:16798146

Monteiro, N. M. (2015). Addressing mental illness in Africa: Global health challenges and local opportunities. *Community Psychology in Global Perspective, 1*(2), 78–95.

Montero, M. (2010). Fortalecimiento de la Ciudadanía y Transformación Social: Área de Encuentro entre la Psicología Política y la Psicología Comunitaria. *Psykhe (Santiago), 19*(2), 51–63. doi:10.4067/S0718-22282010000200006

Morgan, A. J., Parker, A. G., Alvarez-Jimenez, A., & Jorm, A. F. (2013). Exercise and mental Health: An exercise and sport science Australia commisioned review. *Journal of Exercise Physiology, 16*(4), 64–73.

Morgan, C., Burns, T., Fitzpatrick, R., Pinfold, V., & Priebe, S. (2007). Social exclusion and mental health: Conceptual and methodological review. *The British Journal of Psychiatry, 191*(06), 477–483. doi:10.1192/bjp.bp.106.034942 PMID:18055950

Murray, C. J. L., & Lopez, A. D. (1996). *Global burden of disease: A comprehensive assessment of morality and disability from diseases, injuries, and risk factors 4 in 1990 and projected to 2020.* Cambridge, MA: Harvard School of Public Health.

Naslund, J. A., Aschbrenner, K. A., Marsch, L. A., & Bartels, S. J. (2016). The future of mental health care: Peer-to-peer support and social media. *Epidemiology and Psychiatric Sciences, 25*(02), 113–122. doi:10.1017/S2045796015001067 PMID:26744309

Natan, M., Drori, T., & Hochman, O. (2017). The impact of mental health reform on mental illness stigmas in Israel. *Archives of Psychiatric Nursing, 31*(6), 610–613. doi:10.1016/j.apnu.2017.09.001 PMID:29179829

National Association of Social Workers. (n.d.). *Code of Ethics.* Retrieved from http://www.naswdc.org/pubs/code/code.asp

National Institute of Childhood and Human Development (NICHD). (2017). *What are some types of sexually transmitted diseases or sexually transmitted infections (STDs/STIs)?* Retrieved from: https://www.nichd.nih.gov/topics/stds/conditioninfo/pages

National Research Council and Institute of Medicine. (2000). From neurons to neighborhoods: The science of early childhood development. Committee on integrating the science of early childhood development. In J. P. Shonkoff & D. A. Phillips (Eds.), *Board on children, youth, and families, commission on behavioral and social sciences and education.* Washington, DC: National Academy Press.

Nepal, A. (2017, January 29). *XNepali.net.* Retrieved March 18, 2017, from Why did Yama Buddha committed suicide, Anil is cremated at Pashupati Aryaghat: http://xnepali.net/why-did-yama-buddha-committed-suicide-anil-is-cremated-at-pashupati-aryaghat/

Nepal, N. N. (2017, January 30). *Yama Buddha Death Secret*. Retrieved April 7, 2017, from Youtube: https://www.youtube.com/watch?v=EHaUdfcdvds

Neuberg, S. L., Smith, D. M., & Asher, T. (2000). Why people stigmatize: Toward a biocultural framework. In T. F. Heatherton, R. E. Kleck, M. R. Hebl, & J. G. Hull (Eds.), *The social psychology of stigma* (pp. 31–61). New York: Guilford Press.

Neupane, S. (2017, January 17). *Letters: Causes of Suicide*. Retrieved March 25, 2017, from The Himalayan Times: https://thehimalayantimes.com/opinion/letters-causes-of-suicide/

Ng, C. H. (1997). The stigma of mental illness in Asian cultures. *Australian and New Zealand Journal of Psychology*, *31*(3), 382–390. doi:10.3109/00048679709073848 PMID:9226084

Nguyen, Q. C., & Anderson, L. P. (2005). Vietnamese Americans' attitudes toward seeking mental health services: Relation to cultural variables. *Journal of Community Psychology*, *33*(2), 213–231. doi:10.1002/jcop.20039

Nicadao, E. G., Hong, S., & Takeuchi, D. T. (2007). Prevalence and correlates of eating disorders from Asian Americans: Results from the national Latino and Asian American study. *International Journal of Eating Disorders*, *11*(4), 22–26. doi:10.1002/eat.20450 PMID:17879986

Noordsy, D., Torrey, W., Mueser, K., Mead, S., O'Keefe, C., & Fox, L. (2002). Recovery from severe mental illness: An intrapersonal and functional outcome definition. *International Review of Psychiatry (Abingdon, England)*, *14*(4), 318–326. doi:10.1080/0954026021000016969

Norwood, P., & Rascati, J. (2012). Recognizing and combating firefighter stress. *Fire Engineering*, *165*, 87–90.

O'Reilly, C., Bell, J. S., & Chen, T. (2012). Mental health consumers and caregivers as instructors for health professional students: A qualitative study. *Social Psychiatry and Psychiatric Epidemiology*, *47*(4), 607–613. doi:10.100700127-011-0364-x PMID:21384120

Office of Minority Mental Health. (2016). Retrieved from http://minorityhealth.hhs.gov/templates/content.aspx?ID=6476

Onwuegbuzie, A. J., Dickinson, W. B., Leech, N. L., Annmarie, G., & Zoran, P. (2009). A qualitative framework for collecting and analyzing: Data in focus group research. *International Journal of Qualitative Methods*, *8*(3), 87–111. doi:10.1177/160940690900800301

Orbell, S., & Henderson, C. J. (2016). Automatic effects of illness schema activation on behavioral manifestations of illness. *Health Psychology*, *35*(10), 1144–1153. doi:10.1037/hea0000375 PMID:27253428

Osborn, D. P. J., King, M. B., & Weir, M. (2002). Psychiatric health in a sexually transmitted infections clinic: Effect on reattendence. *Journal of Psychosomatic Research*, *52*(4), 267–272. doi:10.1016/S0022-3999(01)00299-9 PMID:11943245

Overton, S. L., & Medina, S. L. (2008). The stigma of mental illness. *Journal of Counseling and Development*, *86*(2), 143–151. doi:10.1002/j.1556-6678.2008.tb00491.x

Öztürk, O. (2001). *Mental Health and Disorders. Eight edition.* Ankara: Feryal Printing House.

Pahwah, R., Brekke, J., Rice, E., & Fulginiti, J. (2017). Mental illness disclosure decision making. *The American Journal of Orthopsychiatry, 87*(5), 575–584. doi:10.1037/ort0000250 PMID:28394157

Pan, D., Huey, S. J., & Hernandez, D. (2011). Culturally adapted versus standard exposure treatment for phobic Asian Americans: Treatment efficacy, moderators, and predictors. *Cultural Diversity & Ethnic Minority Psychology, 17*(1), 11–22. doi:10.1037/a0022534 PMID:21341893

Parcesepe, A. M., & Cabassa, L. J. (2013). Public stigma of mental illness in the United States: A systematic literature review. *Administration and Policy in Mental Health, 40*(5), 384–399. doi:10.100710488-012-0430-z PMID:22833051

Pawluk, S., & Zolezzi, M. (2017). Health care professionals perspectives on a mental health educational campaign for the public. *Health Education Journal, 76*(4), 479–491. doi:10.1177/0017896917696121

Pedersen, E., & Paves, A. (2014). Comparing perceived public stigma and personal stigma of mental health treatment seeking in a young adult sample. *Psychiatry Research, 219*(1), 143–150. doi:10.1016/j.psychres.2014.05.017 PMID:24889842

Penn, D. L., Guynan, K., Daily, T., Spaulding, W. D., Garbin, C. P., & Sullivan, M. (1994). Dispelling the stigma of schizophrenia: What sort of information is best? *Schizophrenia Bulletin, 20*(3), 567–578. doi:10.1093chbul/20.3.567 PMID:7973472

Pescosolido, B. A. (1991). Illness careers and network ties: A conceptual model of utilization and compliance. In G. L. Albrecht & J. A. Levy (Eds.), *Advances in medical sociology* (pp. 161–184). Greenwich, CT: JAI Press.

Pescosolido, B. A. (2006). Of pride and prejudice: The role of sociology and social networks in integrating the health sciences. *Journal of Health and Social Behavior, 47*(3), 189–208. doi:10.1177/002214650604700301 PMID:17066772

Pescosolido, B. A., Martin, J. K., Link, B. G., Kikuzawa, S., Burgos, G., & Swindle, R. (2000). *Americans' view of mental illness and health at century's end: Continuity and change. Public report on the MacArthur Mental health module, 1996 general social survey.* Bloomington, IN: Indiana Consortium for Mental Health Services Research.

Pescosolido, B. A., Olafsdottir, S., Martin, J. K., & Long, J. S. (2008). Cross-cultural aspects of the stigma of mental illness. In J. Arboleda-Flórez & N. Sartorius (Eds.), *Understanding the Stigma of Mental Illness: Theory and Interventions* (pp. 19–35). John Wiley & Sons. doi:10.1002/9780470997642.ch2

Pew Research. (2012). *The rise of Asian Americans.* Retrieved on April 9, 2017, available at http://www.pewsocialtrends.org/2012/06/19/the-rise--of-asian-americans/3

Phelan, J. C. (2002). Genetic bases of mental illness–a cure for stigma? *Trends in Neurosciences, 25*(8), 430–431. doi:10.1016/S0166-2236(02)02209-9 PMID:12127761

Phelan, J. C., Link, B. G., & Dovidio, J. F. (2008). Stigma and prejudice: One animal or two? *Social Science & Medicine, 67*(3), 358–367. doi:10.1016/j.socscimed.2008.03.022 PMID:18524444

Phongsavan, P., Chey, T., Bauman, A., Brooks, R., & Silove, D. (2006). Social capital, socio-economic status and psychological distress among Australian adults. *Social Science & Medicine, 63*(10), 2546–2561. doi:10.1016/j.socscimed.2006.06.021 PMID:16914244

Pinfold, V., Byrne, P., & Toulman, H. (2005). Challenging stigma and discrimination in communities: A focus group study identifying UK mental health services users? Main campaign priorities. *The International Journal of Social Psychiatry, 51*(2), 128–138. doi:10.1177/0020764005056760 PMID:16048242

Pinfold, V., Toulmin, H., Thornicroft, G., Huxley, P., Farmer, P., & Graham, T. (2003). Reducing psychiatric stigma and discrimination: Evaluation of educational interventions in UK secondary schools. *The British Journal of Psychiatry, 182*(4), 342–346. doi:10.1192/bjp.182.4.342 PMID:12668411

Pingani, L., Forghieri, M., Ferrari, S., Ben-Zeev, D., Artoni, P., Mazzi, F., ... Corrigan, P. W. (2012). Stigma and discrimination toward mental illness: Translation and validation of the Italian version of the Attribution Questionnaire-27 (AQ-27-I). *Social Psychiatry and Psychiatric Epidemiology, 47*(6), 993–999. doi:10.100700127-011-0407-3 PMID:21688158

Pinto-Foltz, M. D., Logsdon, M. C., & Myers, J. A. (2011). Feasibility, acceptability, and initial efficacy of a knowledge-contact program to reduce mental illness stigma and improve mental health literacy in adolescents. *Social Science & Medicine, 72*(12), 2011–2019. doi:10.1016/j.socscimed.2011.04.006 PMID:21624729

Pirkis, J., & Blood, W. (2010). *Suicide and the news information media.* Mindframe National Media Initiative. Retrieved April 6, 2017, from http://www.mindframe-media.info/__data/assets/pdf_file/0016/5164/Pirkis-and-Blood-2010,-Suicide-and-the-news-and-information-media.pdf

Plakum, E. M. (2008). Psychiatry in Tibetan Buddhism: Madness and its cure seen through the lens of religious and national history. *The American Academy of Psychoanalysis and Dynamic Psychiatry, 36*(3), 415–430. doi:10.1521/jaap.2008.36.3.415 PMID:18834281

Porta, M. (2014). *A dictionary of epidemiology.* Oxford University Press. doi:10.1093/acref/9780199976720.001.0001

President's New Freedom Commission on Mental Health. (2003). *Achieving the promise: Transforming mental health care in America. Final Report.* Department of Health and Human Services Publication No. SMA-03-3831. Rockville, MD: DHHS.

Programme, R. F. (2003). *Suicide and the Media: Pitfalls and Prevention.* Reuters Foundation Programme; University of Oxford Centre for Suicide Research. Retrieved February 26, 2017, from http://cebmh.warne.ox.ac.uk/csr/Suicide%20&%20the%20Media%20seminar.pdf

Rayan, A., & Obiadate, K. (2017). The correlates of quality of life among Jordanian patients with schizophrenia. *Journal of the American Psychiatric Nurses Association, 23*(6), 404–413. doi:10.1177/1078390317710498 PMID:28569084

Read, J., & Reynolds, J. (1997). *Speaking Our Minds—An Anthology*. London: MacMillan.

Re, E. (2005). L'associazionismo degli utenti psichiatrici tra difficoltà e possibilità. *Prospettive Sociali e Sanitarie, 35*, 1–3.

Reeves, T. J., & Bennett, C. E. (2004). *We the people: Asians in the United States, Census 2000 Special Reports*. Washington, DC: U.S. Census Bureau.

Remschmidt, H., Nurcombe, B., Belfer, M. L., Sartorius, N., & Okasha, A. (2007). *The mental health of children and adolescents: An area of global neglect*. Chichester, UK: Wiley. doi:10.1002/9780470512555

Rethrost, C. D., Wipfli, B. M., & Landers, D. M. (2009). The antidepressive effects of exsercise: A meta-analysis of Randomized trials. *Sports Medicine (Auckland, N.Z.), 39*, 491–511. PMID:19453207

Reviews, N. (2017, January 14). *Yama Buddha suicide letter*. Retrieved April 11, 2017, from Youtube: https://www.youtube.com/watch?v=GTuL4Evrbcc

Rho, Y., & Rho, K. (2009). Clinical considerations in working with Asian American children and adolescents. In N. Trinh, Y. Rho, F. Lu, & K. M. Sanders (Eds.), *Handbook of mental health and acculturation in Asian American families* (pp. 143–166). New York, NY: Humana Press. doi:10.1007/978-1-60327-437-1_8

Rickwood, D., Deane, F., Wilson, C., & Ciarrochi, J. (2005). Young people's help-seeking for mental health problems. *Australian e-Journal for the Advancement of Mental Health, 4*(3), 218–251. doi:10.5172/jamh.4.3.218

Robin, B. R. (2008). Digital storytelling: A powerful technology tool for the 21st century classroom. *Theory into Practice, 47*(3), 220–228. doi:10.1080/00405840802153916

Rogers, C. R. (1980). *A way of being*. Boston, MA: Houghton Mifflin.

Rosenbaum, S., Tiederman, A., Sherrington, C., Curtis, J., & Ward, P. B. (2014). Physical activity interventions for people with mental illness: A systematic review and meta-analyses. *The Journal of Clinical Psychiatry, 75*(09), 964–974. doi:10.4088/JCP.13r08765 PMID:24813261

Rosenfield, S. (1997). Labeling mental illness: The effects of received services and perceived stigma on life satisfaction. *American Sociological Review, 62*(4), 660–672. doi:10.2307/2657432

Ross, M.W., Larsson, M., Nyoni, J.E., Agardh, A. (2016). Prevalence of STI symptoms and high levels of stigma in STI healthcare among men who have sex with men in Dar es Salaam, Tanzania: a respondent-driven sampling study. *International Journal of STD and AIDS, 28*(9), 925-928. doi: 10.1177/0956462416683625

Rutz, W. (2001). Mental health in Europe: Problems, advances and challenges. *Acta Psychiatrica Scandinavica. Supplementum*, *410*(s410), 15–20. doi:10.1034/j.1600-0447.2001.1040s2015.x PMID:11863046

Ruzek, N. A., Nguyen, D. Q., & Herzog, D. C. (2011). Acculturation, enculturation, psychological distress and help-seeking preferences among Asian American college students. *Asian American Journal of Psychology*, *2*(3), 181–196. doi:10.1037/a0024302

Saha, S., Chant, D., & McGrat, J. (2007). A systematic review on mortality in schizophrenia: Is the differential mortality gap worsenig over time? *Archives of General Psychiatry*, *64*(10), 1123–1131. doi:10.1001/archpsyc.64.10.1123 PMID:17909124

Saint Martin, M. L. (1999). Running Amok: A modern perspective on a culture-bound syndrome. *Primary Care Companion to the Journal of Clinical Psychiatry*, *1*(3), 66–70. doi:10.4088/PCC. v01n0302 PMID:15014687

Sartorius, N. (1997). Fighting schizophrenia and its stigma. A new world psychiatric association educational programme. *The British Journal of Psychiatry*, *170*(4), 297. doi:10.1192/bjp.170.4.297 PMID:9246243

Sartorius, N. (1998). Stigma: What can psychiatrists do about it? *Lancet*, *352*(9133), 1058–1059. doi:10.1016/S0140-6736(98)08008-8 PMID:9759771

Sartorius, N. (2007). Stigma and mental health. *Lancet*, *370*(9590), 810–811. doi:10.1016/S0140-6736(07)61245-8 PMID:17804064

Sartorius, N., Gulbinat, W., Harrison, G., Laska, E., & Siegel, C. (1996). Long-term follow-up of schizophrenia in 16 countries. A description of the international study of schizophrenia conducted by the world health organization. *Social Psychiatry and Psychiatric Epidemiology*, *31*(5), 249–258. PMID:8909114

Sartorius, N., Jablensky, A., & Shapiro, R. (1978). Cross-cultural differences in the short-term prognosis of schizophrenic psychoses. *Schizophrenia Bulletin*, *4*(1), 102–113. doi:10.1093chbul/4.1.102 PMID:746359

Saunders, J. C., & Byrne, M. M. (2002). A thematic analysis of families living with schizophrenia. *Archives of Psychiatric Nursing*, *16*(5), 217–223. doi:10.1053/apnu.2002.36234 PMID:12434327

Scheim, A., & Travers, R. (2016). Barriers and facilitators to HIV and sexually transmitted infections testing for gay, bisexual, and other transgender men who have sex with men. *AIDS Care*, *27*, 1–6. doi:10.1080/09540121.2016.1271937 PMID:28027664

Seeman, N., Tang, S., Brown, A., & Ing, A. (2016). World survey of mental illness stigma. *Journal of Affective Disorders*, *190*(15), 115–121. doi:10.1016/j.jad.2015.10.011 PMID:26496017

Sellers, R. M., & Shelton, J. N. (2003). The role of racial identity in perceived racial discrimination. *Journal of Personality and Social Psychology*, *84*(5), 1079–1092. doi:10.1037/0022-3514.84.5.1079 PMID:12757150

Sercu, C., & Bracke, P. (2017). Stigma, social structure and the biomedical framework: Exploring the stigma experiences of in-patient service users in two different psychiatric hospitals. *Qualitative Health Research, 27*(8), 1249–1261. doi:10.1177/1049732316648112 PMID:27251609

Sharfstein, S. S. (2012). Status of stigma. *Psychiatric Services (Washington, D.C.), 63*(10), 953. doi:10.1176/appi.ps.631011 PMID:23032671

Sharma, C. (2017, January 15). *Famous rapper Yama Buddha no more.* Retrieved March 14, 2017, from My Republica: http://www.myrepublica.com/news/13100/

Shea, M., & Yeh, C. (2008). Asian American students' cultural values, stigma, and relational self-construal: Correlates and attitudes toward professional help seeking. *Journal of Mental Health Counseling, 30*(2), 157–172. doi:10.17744/mehc.30.2.g662g5l2r1352198

Shen, E. K., Alden, L. E., Söchting, I., & Tsang, P. (2006). Clinical observations of a Cantonese cognitive-behavioral treatment program for Chinese immigrants. *Psychotherapy (Chicago, Ill.), 43*(4), 518–530. doi:10.1037/0033-3204.43.4.518 PMID:22122141

Sherry, E., & O'May, F. (2013). Exploring the impact of sport participation in the Homeless World Cup on individuals with substance abuse or mental health disorders. *Journal of Sports for Development, 1*, 1-9.

Shibre, T., Negash, A., Kullgren, G., Kebede, D., Alem, A., Fekadu, A., ... Jacobsson, L. (2001). Perception of stigma among family members of individuals with schizophrenia and major affective disorders in rural Ethiopia. *Social Psychiatry and Psychiatric Epidemiology, 36*(6), 299–303. doi:10.1007001270170048 PMID:11583460

Shimotsu, S., Horikawa, N., Emora, R., Ishikawa, S. I., Nagao, A., Hiejima, S., & Hosomi, J. (2014). Effectiveness of Cognitive Behavioral Therapy in reducing self-stigma in Japanese Psychiatric Patients. *Asian Journal of Psychiatry, 10*, 39–44. doi:10.1016/j.ajp.2014.02.006 PMID:25042950

Shrivastava, A., Johnston, M., & Bureau, Y. (2012). Stigma of mental illness – 1: Clinical reflections. *MSM Mens Sana Monographs, 10*(1), 70–84. doi:10.4103/0973-1229.90181 PMID:22654383

Shrivastava, A., Johnston, M., & Bureau, Y. (2012). Stigma of mental illness – 2: Non-compliance and intervention. *MSM Mens Sana Monographs, 10*(1), 85–97. doi:10.4103/0973-1229.90276 PMID:22654384

Sickel, A. E., Seacat, J. D., & Nabors, N. A. (2014). Mental health stigma update: A review of consequences. *Advances in Mental Health, 12*(3), 202–215. doi:10.1080/18374905.2014.11081898

Simpson, E. L., & House, A. O. (2003). User and carer involvement in mental health services: From rhetoric to science. *The British Journal of Psychiatry, 183*(02), 89–91. doi:10.1192/bjp.183.2.89 PMID:12893657

Slu, T. (1989). Short-term prognosis of schizophrenia in developed and developing countries. WHO international study program. *Zhurnal Nevropatologii i Psikhiatrii Imeni S. S. Korsakova, 89*(5), 66–72. PMID:2781923

Smith, A. L., & Cahswell, C. S. (2010). Stigma and mental illness: Investigating attitudes of mental health and non-mental health professionals and trainees. *The Journal of Humanistic Counseling, Education and Development, 49*(2), 189–202. doi:10.1002/j.2161-1939.2010.tb00097.x

Smith, J., Mittal, D., Chekuri, L., Han, X., & Sullivan, G. (2017). A comparison of provider attitudes towards SMI across different health care disciplines. *Stigma and Health, 4*(2), 327–337. doi:10.1037ah0000064

Smith, R. (2007). Language of the lost: An explication of stigma Ccmmunication. *Communication Theory, 17*(4), 462–485. doi:10.1111/j.1468-2885.2007.00307.x

Smith, R. A. (2012). An experimental test of stigma communication content with a hypothetical infectious disease alert. *Communication Monographs, 79*(4), 522–538. doi:10.1080/03637751 .2012.723811

Solberg, V. S., Ritsma, S., Davis, B. L., Tata, S. P., & Jolly, A. (1994). Asian American students' severity of problems and willingness to seek help from university counseling centers: Role of previous counseling experience, gender, and ethnicity. *Journal of Counseling Psychology, 41*(3), 275–279. doi:10.1037/0022-0167.41.3.275

Sontag, S. (1989). *AIDS and its metaphors*. New York, NY: Picadur.

Soundy, A., Freeman, P., Stubbs, B., Probst, M., Roskell, C., & Vancampfort, D. (2015). The psychosocial consequences of sports participation for individuals with severe mental illness: a metasynthesis review. *Advances in Psychiatry*, 1-8.

Soundy, A., Freeman, P., Stubbs, R., Probst, M., Coffee, P., & Vancmpfort, D. (2014). The trascending benefits of physical activity for indoividuals with schizoprenia: A systematic review and meta ethnography. *Psychiatry Research, 220*(1-2), 11–19. doi:10.1016/j.psychres.2014.07.083 PMID:25149128

Stack, S. (2005). Suicide in the media: A quantitative review of studies based on non-fictional stories. *Suicide & Life-Threatening Behavior, 35*(2), 121–133. doi:10.1521uli.35.2.121.62877 PMID:15843330

Stanley, I. H., Hom, M. A., Hagan, C. R., & Joiner, T. E. (2015). Career prevalence and correlates of suicidal thoughts and behaviors among firefighters. *Journal of Affective Disorders, 187*, 163–171. doi:10.1016/j.jad.2015.08.007 PMID:26339926

Steele, C. M., & Aronson, J. (1995). Stereotype threat and the intellectual test performance of African Americans. *Journal of Personality and Social Psychology, 69*(5), 797–811. doi:10.1037/0022-3514.69.5.797 PMID:7473032

Stevenson, C. (1996). The Tao, social constructionism and psychiatric nursing practice and research. *Journal of Psychiatric and Mental Health Nursing, 3*(4), 217–224. doi:10.1111/j.1365-2850.1996. tb00115.x PMID:8997982

Stiglitz, J. E. (2009). Selected Works: Vol. 1. *Information and Economic Analysis*. Oxford, UK: Oxford University Press.

Strkalj-Ivezic, S. (2013). Stigma in clinical practice. *Psychiatria Danubina*, *25*, 200–202. PMID:23995176

Struening, E. L., Perlick, D. A., Link, B. G., Hellman, F., Herman, D., & Sirey, J. A. (2001). Stigma as a barrier to recovery: The extent to which caregivers believe most people devalue consumers and their families. *Psychiatric Services (Washington, D.C.)*, *52*(12), 1633–1638. doi:10.1176/appi.ps.52.12.1633 PMID:11726755

Stuart, H., & Arboleda-Flórez, J. (2001). Community attitudes toward persons with schizophrenia. *Canadian Journal of Psychiatry*, *46*(3), 245–252. doi:10.1177/070674370104600304 PMID:11320678

Stubbs, A. (2014). Reducing mental illness stigma in health care students and professionals: A review of the literature. *Australasian Psychiatry*, *22*(6), 579–584. doi:10.1177/1039856214556324 PMID:25371444

Stubbs, B., Firth, J., Berry, A., Schuch, F. B., Rosenbaum, S., Ward, P. B., ... Vacampfort, D. (2016). How much physical activities do people with schizophrenia engage in? A systematic review, comparative meta-analysis and meta-regression. *Schizophrenia Research*, *176*(2), 431–440. doi:10.1016/j.schres.2016.05.017 PMID:27261419

Sue, D. W., Bucceri, J., Lin, A. I., Nadal, K. L., & Torino, G. C. (2007). Racial microaggressions and the Asian American experience. *Cultural Diversity & Ethnic Minority Psychology*, *13*(1), 72–81. doi:10.1037/1099-9809.13.1.72 PMID:17227179

Sue, D. W., & Sue, D. (1999). *Counseling the culturally different: Theory and practice* (3rd ed.). New York: Wiley and Sons.

Sue, D. W., & Sue, D. (2016). *Counseling the Culturally Diverse: Theory and Practice* (7th ed.). Hoboken, NJ: John Wiley and Sons.

Sue, S. (1994). Mental health. In N. Zane, D. T. Takeuchi, & K. Young (Eds.), *Confronting critical health issues of Asian and Pacific Islander Americans* (pp. 266–288). Newbury Park, CA: Sage.

Sue, S., & McKinney, H. (1975). Asian Americans in the community mental health care system. *The American Journal of Orthopsychiatry*, *45*(1), 111–118. doi:10.1111/j.1939-0025.1975. tb01172.x PMID:1167437

Sue, S., Yan-Cheng, J. K., Saad, C. S., & Chu, J. P. (2012). Asian American mental health: A call to action. *The American Psychologist*, *67*(7), 532–544. doi:10.1037/a0028900 PMID:23046304

Sue, S., Zane, N., Hall, G. C. N., & Berger, L. K. (2009). The case for cultural competency in psychotherapeutic interventions. *Annual Review of Psychology*, *60*(1), 525–548. doi:10.1146/annurev.psych.60.110707.163651 PMID:18729724

Sullivan, M. A. (2005). Kum Ba Yah: The relevance of family systems theory for clinicians and clients of African descent. In M. Rastogi & E, Wieling (Eds.), Voices of Color (pp. 277-295). London: Sage.

Sullivan, H. S. (1962). *Schizophrenia as a human process*. New York, NY: WW Norton.

Sulovic, V. (2010, October 5). Meaning of Security and Theory of Securitization. *Belgrade Centre for Security Policy*. Retrieved April 15, 2017, from http://www.bezbednost.org/upload/document/sulovic_(2010)_meaning_of_secu.pdf

Summers, C. (2017, January 22). *Nepal mourns its 'voice of a generation' after the mysterious death of the country's most famous rapper who was found hanged at his wife's parents' home in a west London suburb*. Retrieved March 8, 2017, from MailOnline: http://www.dailymail.co.uk/news/article-4145452/Nepal-mourns-death-country-s-famous-rapper.html

Sundstrom, E. (2004). The Clogs. *Schizophrenia Bulletin*, *30*(1), 191–192. doi:10.1093/oxfordjournals.schbul.a007063 PMID:15176773

Tajfel, H. (1981). *Human groups and social categories: Studies in social psychology*. Cambridge, UK: Cambridge University Press.

Takaki, R. (1998). *Strangers from a different shore*. Boston, MA: Little, Brown, and Company.

Takayama, J. (2010). *Ecological systems theory of Asian American mental health service seeking* (School of Professional Psychology, paper 121). Retrieved on April 8, 2017, available at http://commons.pacificu.edu/spp/121

Task Force on DSM-IV. (2000). *Diagnostic and statistical manual of mental disorders: DSM-IV TR* (4th ed.). Washington, DC: American Psychiatric Publishing.

Teschinsky, U. (2000). Living with schizophrenia: The family illness experience. *Issues in Mental Health Nursing*, *21*(4), 387–396. doi:10.1080/016128400248004 PMID:11249357

Tew, J., Ramon, S., Slade, M., Bird, V., Melton, J., & Le Boutillier, C. (2012). Social factors and recovery from mental health difficulties: A review of the evidence. *British Journal of Social Work*, *42*(3), 443–460. doi:10.1093/bjsw/bcr076

The 2010 National Drug Use and Survey on Health. (2012). *SAMHSA*. Retrieved on April 9, 2017, available at http://www.samhsa.gov/data/nsduh/2k10nsduh/2k10results.html

Thoits, P. A. (2011). Resisting the stigma of mental illness. *Social Psychology Quarterly*, *74*(1), 6–28. doi:10.1177/0190272511398019

Thompson, M., & Thompson, T. (1997). *Discrimination Against People with Experiences of Mental Illness*. Wellington: Mental Health Commission.

Times, T. H. (2017, January 15). *Yama Buddha commits suicide.* Retrieved March 6, 2017, from The Himalayan Times: https://thehimalayantimes.com/entertainment/anil-adhikari-yama-buddha-commits-suicide/

Ting, J., & Hwang, W. C. (2009). Cultural influences on help-seeking attitudes in Asian American students. *American Journal of Public Health, 79*(1), 125–132. PMID:19290732

Tomita, A., & Burns, J. K. (2013). A multilevel analysis of association between neighbourhood social capital and depression: Evidence from the first South African National Income Dynamics Study. *Journal of Affective Disorders, 144*(1-2), 101–105. doi:10.1016/j.jad.2012.05.066 PMID:22858263

Townsend, J. M. (1975). Cultural conceptions, mental disorders, and social roles: A comparison of Germany and America. *American Sociological Review, 40*(6), 739–752. doi:10.2307/2094177 PMID:1211687

Tran, B. (2016). The impact of the model minority culture in higher education institutions: The cause of Asian Americans' psychological and mental health. In N. P. Ololube (Ed.), *Handbook of research on organizational justice and culture in higher education institutions* (pp. 282–323). Hersey, PA: IGI Global. doi:10.4018/978-1-4666-9850-5.ch012

Tran, B. (2017). *The impact of the model minority culture in higher education institutions: The cause of Asian Americans' psychological and mental health (Reprint Collection). In Gaming and technology addiction: Breakthroughs in research and practice* (Vol. 1, pp. 404–445). Hersey, PA: IGI Global.

Trust, M. (2007). *Sensitive Coverage Saves Lives.* Leeds, UK: MediaWise Trust. Retrieved March 3, 2017, from http://www.mediawise.org.uk/wp-content/uploads/2011/03/Sensitive-Coverage-Saves-Lives.pdf

Tseng, W., & Strelzer, J. (2001). *Culture and psychotherapy: A guide to clinical practice* (pp. 173–191). Washington, DC: American Psychiatric Press.

TV, E. (2017, January 15). *Kina Beltma Jhundiyeka Thiye Ta Yama Buddha? Rahasya Yesto.* Retrieved April 11, 2017, from Youtube: https://www.youtube.com/watch?v=KVEIMVcO_w4

TV, T. (2017, January 28). *Yama Buddha bakasma auda pitako halat yesto, Kathmanduma ruwabasi.* Retrieved April 13, 2017, from Youtube: https://www.youtube.com/watch?v=1zWxxaBiifk

Uba, L. (1994). *Asian American personality patterns, identity, and mental health.* New York: The Guilford Press.

United States Census. (2013a). *Facts for features: Asian /Pacific American heritage month.* Retrieved on April 9, 2017, available at http://www.census.gov/newsroom/releases/archives/facts_for_features_special_editins/cb13-ff09.html

United States Census. (2013b). *The Hispanic population: 2010 brief.* Retrieved on April 9, 2017, available at http://www.census.gov/prod/cen2010/briefs/c2010br-04.pdf

United States Department of Health & Human Services. (2000). *Healthy People 2010: Understanding and Improving Health* (2nd ed.). Washington, DC: U.S. Government Printing Office.

United States Department of Health and Human Services. (2001). *Mental health: Culture, race and ethnicity: A supplement to mental health: A report of the surgeon general.* Rockville, MD: Author.

United States National Institutes of Mental Health. (2001). *Mental health: Culture, race, and ethnicity. A supplement to mental health: A report of the surgeon general.* Rockville, MD: Author.

United States Office of the Surgeon General. (2001). *Mental health: Culture, race, and ethnicity. A supplement to mental health: A report of the surgeon general.* Rockville, MD: Author.

United States Substance Abuse and Mental Health Services Administration. (2001). *Mental health: Culture, race, and ethnicity. A supplement to mental health: A report of the surgeon general.* Rockville, MD: Author.

Uprety, S., & Lamichhane, B. (2016). *Mental Health in Nepal - A Backgrounder.* Kathmandu: HERD. Retrieved April 21, 2017, from http://www.herd.org.np/publications/27

Uprety, S., McGrath, N. A., McNerney, S., Ghimire, R., & Baral, S. (2016). *Media mentoring in Nepal: helping journalists write better stories on urban health issues.* HERD; COMDIS-HSD. Retrieved March 23, 2017, from http://comdis-hsd.leeds.ac.uk/resource/media-mentoring-nepal-helping-journalists-write-better-stories-urban-health-issues/

Van Brakel, W. H. (2006). Measuring health-related stigma—a literature review. *Psychology Health and Medicine, 11*(3), 307–334. doi:10.1080/13548500600595160 PMID:17130068

Vancampfort, D., De Hert, M., Skijevern, L. H., Lundvik Gyllensten, A., Parker, A., Mulders, N., ... Probst, M. (2012). International organization of physical therapy in mental health consensus on physical activity within multidisciplinary rehabilitation programmes for minimising cardio-metabolic risk in patients with schizophrenia. *Disability and Rehabilitation, 34*(1), 1–12. doi:10.3109/09638288.2011.587090 PMID:21957908

Veltman, A., Cameron, J. I., & Stewart, D. E. (2002). The experience of providing care to relatives with chronic mental illness. *The Journal of Nervous and Mental Disease, 190*(2), 108–114. doi:10.1097/00005053-200202000-00008 PMID:11889365

Vogel, D. L., Heimerdinger-Edwards, S. R., Hammer, J. H., & Hubbard, A. (2011). Boys Don't Cry": Examination of the Links Between Endorsement of Masculine Norms, *Self-stigma*, and Help-Seeking Attitudes for Men From Diverse Backgrounds. *Journal of Counseling Psychology, 58*(3), 368–382. doi:10.1037/a0023688 PMID:21639615

Vogel, D. L., Wade, N. G., & Haake, S. (2006). Measuring the *Self-stigma* Associated With Seeking Psychological Help. *Journal of Counseling Psychology*, *53*(3), 325–337. doi:10.1037/0022-0167.53.3.325

Wagner, S. L., McFee, J. A., & Martin, C. A. (2010). Mental health implications of fire service membership. *Traumatology*, *16*(2), 26–32. doi:10.1177/1534765610362803

Wahl, O. F. (1999). Mental health consumers' experience of stigma. *Schizophrenia Bulletin*, *25*(3), 467–478. doi:10.1093/oxfordjournals.schbul.a033394 PMID:10478782

Wakanyi-Kahindi, L. (2012). *The Agikuyu concept of THAHU and its bearing on the biblical concept of sin* (Doctoral dissertation).

Walpole, S. C., McMillan, D., House, A., Cottrell, D., & Ghazala, M. (2013). Interventions for treating depression in Muslim patients: A systematic review. *Journal of Affective Disorders*, *145*(1), 11–20. doi:10.1016/j.jad.2012.06.035 PMID:22854098

Walton, G. M., & Cohen, G. L. (2003). Stereotype life. *Journal of Experimental Social Psychology*, *39*(5), 456–467. doi:10.1016/S0022-1031(03)00019-2

Wang, P.S., Demler, O, & Kessler, R.C. (2002). Adequacy of treatment for serious mental illness in the United States. *American Journal of Public Health, 92*, 92-98. doi: 10.2105-AJPH.92.1.92

Warner, R. (2004). *Recovery from schizophrenia: Psychiatry and political economy*. New York, NY: Brunner-Routledge.

Watson, A. C., Corrigan, P. W., Larson, J. E., & Sells, M. (2007). *Self-stigma* in people with mental illness. *Schizophrenia Bulletin*, *33*(6), 1312–1318. doi:10.1093chbulbl076 PMID:17255118

White, S., Park, Y. S., Israel, T., & Cordero, E. D. (2009). Longitudinal evaluation of peer health education on a college campus: Impact on health behaviors. *Journal of American College Health*, *57*(5), 497–506. doi:10.3200/JACH.57.5.497-506 PMID:19254890

WHO. (2008). *Preventing Suicide: A Resource for Media Professionals*. Geneva: WHO. Retrieved March 25, 2017, from http://www.who.int/mental_health/prevention/suicide/resource_media.pdf

Wong, E., Marshall, G., Schell, T., Elliott, M., Hambarsoomians, K., Berthold, S. M., & Chun, C. (2006). Barriers to mental health are utilization for U.S. Cambodian refugees. *Journal of Counseling and Clinical Psychology*, *74*(6), 1116–1120. doi:10.1037/0022-006X.74.6.1116 PMID:17154740

World Health Organization. (2001). *Mental health: new understanding, new hope*. World Health Organization.

World Health Organization. (2005). *Mental health atlas*. Geneva: World Health Organization.

Wynaden, D., Chapman, R., Orb, A., McGowan, S., Zeeman, Z., & Yeak, S. H. (2005). Factors that influence Asian communities' access to mental health care. *International Journal of Mental Health Nursing*, *14*(2), 88–95. doi:10.1111/j.1440-0979.2005.00364.x PMID:15896255

Yang, C., Narayanasamy, A., & Chang, S. (2011). Transcultural spirituality: The spiritual journey of hospitalized patients with schizophrenia in Taiwan. *Journal of Advanced Nursing*, *68*(2), 358–367. doi:10.1111/j.1365-2648.2011.05747.x PMID:21707724

Yang, L. H., & Pearson, V. J. (2002). Understanding families in their own context: Schizophrenia and structural family therapy in Beijing. *Journal of Family Therapy*, *24*(3), 233–257. doi:10.1111/1467-6427.00214

Yang, Y. T. C., & Wu, W. C. I. (2012). Digital storytelling for enhancing student academic achievement, critical thinking, and learning motivation: A year-long experimental study. *Computers & Education*, *59*(2), 339–352. doi:10.1016/j.compedu.2011.12.012

Yanos, P. T., Roe, D., Markus, K., & Lysaker, P. H. (2008). Pathways between internalized stigma and outcomes related to recovery in schizophrenia spectrum disorders. *Psychiatric Services (Washington, D.C.)*, *59*(12), 1437–1442. doi:10.1176/ps.2008.59.12.1437 PMID:19033171

Yeung, A., Chan, R., Mischoulon, D., Sonawalla, S., Wong, E., Nierenberg, A. A., & Fava, M. (2004). Prevalence of major depressive disorder among Chinese-Americans in primary care. *General Hospital Psychiatry*, *26*(1), 24–30. doi:10.1016/j.genhosppsych.2003.08.006 PMID:14757299

Yıldız, M., Özten, E., Işık, S., Özyıldırım, İ., Karayün, D., Cerit, C., & Üçok, A. (2012). Self-stigmatisation of schizophrenia patients, relatives of the patients and patients with major depressive disorders. *Anatolian Journal of Psychiatry*, *13*(1), 1–7.

Yoo, S. K., Goh, M., & Yoon, E. (2005). Psychological and cultural influences on Koreans' help-seeking attitudes. *Journal of Mental Health Counseling*, *27*(3), 266–281. doi:10.17744/mehc.27.3.9kh5v6rec36egxlv

Zane, N. W., Sue, S., Chang, J., Huang, L., Huang, J., Lowe, S., ... Lee, E. (2005). Beyond ethnic match: Effects of client-therapist cognitive match in problem perception coping orientation, and therapy goals on treatment outcomes. *Journal of Community Psychology*, *33*(5), 569–585. doi:10.1002/jcop.20067

Zane, N., & Mak, W. (2002). Major approaches to the measurement of acculturation among ethnic minority populations: A content analysis and an alternative empirical strategy. In K. M. Chun, P. B. Organista, & G. Martin (Eds.), *Acculturations: Advances in theory, measurement, and applied research* (pp. 39–60). Baltimore, MD: United Book Press.

Zhang, A. Y., Snowden, L. R., & Sue, S. (1998). Differences between Asian and White Americans' help-seeking and utilization patterns in the Los Angeles area. *Journal of Community Psychology*, *26*(4), 317–326. doi:

Zieger, A., Mungee, A., Schomerus, G., Ta, T. M. T., Weyers, A., Boge, K., ... Hahn, E. (2017). Attitude towards psychiatrists and psychiatric medication: A survey from five metropolitan cities in India. *Indian Journal of Psychiatry*, *59*(3), 341. doi:10.4103/psychiatry.IndianJPsychiatry_190_17 PMID:29085094

Zoppei, S., Lasalvia, A., Bonetto, C., Van Bortel, T., Nyqvist, F., Webber, M., ... Wahlbeck, K. (2014). Social capital and reported discrimination among people with depression in 15 European countries. *Social Psychiatry and Psychiatric Epidemiology*, *49*(10), 1589–1598. doi:10.100700127-014-0856-6 PMID:24638892

About the Contributors

Brittany A. Canfield holds a Master of Science in Counseling Studies from Capella University and a Master of Art in Clinical Psychology from Fielding Graduate University. She is completing her Doctorate of Psychology in Clinical Psychology from California Southern University and will commence her doctoral students with the University of Birmingham in the United Kingdom in Sexuality and Gender Studies this year. She is adjunct faculty at Southern New Hampshire University and teaches Social Psychology through the university's online community. Ms. Canfield provides psychological services in Southern Arizona and has extensive experience working with trauma, cultural diversity, and underserved populations. Her research interests include trauma, stigma, gender issues and gender identification, semiotics, social psychology, critical theory, rural communities, critical psychology, cultural competency, and social justice.

* * *

Sara Bender is an Assistant Professor of Psychology at Central Washington University where she teaches a variety of undergraduate psychology and graduate counseling courses. Dr. Bender maintains several research interests including: Clinical supervision, the role of technology in mental health, understanding stigma, as well as the provision of mental health services to underserved populations.

Katrina Y. Billingsley holds a Doctorate of Philosophy in Counseling and Counselor Education from NC State University. She is a National Certified Counselor (NCC) and holds the NC certification as a Licensed Professional Counselor Associate (LPCA). Dr. Billingsley currently works as a clinician in private practice and in community mental health working with diverse populations. Additionally, Dr. Billingsley serves as an adjunct professor in Counseling for the clinical mental health track.

Nicolina Bosco, Community Psychologist, Ph.D. in Educational Science and Psychology at the University of Florence, her work is based on the promotion of mental health for young people. Her research is focused on stigma, with emphasis on self-stigma for seeking help.

Brian Bunnell is a NIMH F32-funded Postdoctoral Fellow at the at the Medical University of South Carolina (MUSC). During the past 4 years, he has served as Principal- and Co-Investigator on a number of grant-funded research efforts, the majority of which focus and have focused on technology-based solutions to improving the quality of health care across the developmental spectrum. His research experiences have varied in nature and have included studies focused on observational and experimental assessment of anxiety, PTSD, and related disorders; psychometric analysis and measurement development; open and randomized controlled treatment trials for mood and behavioral disorders; and most currently, the examination of intervention initiatives with a focus on the use of technology to facilitate and disseminate such interventions.

Stefano Castagnoli was born in Florence in 20/07/1964. Graduated in Medicine in 1991 and specialized in Psychiatry in 1995. He is the director of one of the Public Mental Health Service in the Florence area of Tuscany.

Donté Corey is an Assistant Professor at South University – High Point, NC in the Clinical Mental Health Counseling program. She is also a Licensed Professional Counselor Supervisor and has been in the mental health field working as a counselor since 2004. Dr. Corey also manages a part time counseling practice in Hillsborough, NC where she provides counseling services to children, adolescents, adults, and families as well as supervision for licensure.

Tatiana M. Davidson, Ph.D., is Assistant Professor and Co-Director of the Telehealth Resilience and Recovery Program (TRRP) at MUSC. Dr. Davidson serves as Chair for the Association of Behavioral and Cognitive Therapies' Hispanic Issues in Behavior Therapy (HIBT) Student Interest Group. She received her BS from the University of Washington and MA and PhD from Clark University, and completed her internship and NIMH postdoc at MUSC. Dr. Davidson's research has focused mainly on maximizing the reach and receipt of evidence-based mental health treatments among trauma-affected youth and their families through the development, evaluation, and dissemination of innovative, technology-based resources. Dr. Davidson is PI on an active Duke Endowment grant (through 2020) to implement TRRP in three partnering trauma centers across South Carolina. She serves as Co-Investigator on several federally-funded research grants focused on the development, evaluation and implementation of mHealth technologies (e.g., smartphone, tablet, computer) for providing best-practice mental health treatment to a wide range of traumatic stress populations, including disaster victims, child abuse victims, and first responders. A second major research focus is on addressing mental health care disparities among racial/ethnic minority populations through the development and evaluation of culturally-modified, evidence-based interventions. She has been awarded both external and internal grants to examine how cultural variables can influence formal mental health treatment seeking, access and completion among Latina/o populations, and to adapt evidence-based resources to mobile health delivery formats to reduce traditional barriers to mental health treatment among Latina/o youth and families.

Rajesh Ghimire is a seasoned media critic with over 25 years of experience in media research and development communications. Based in Kathmandu, Nepal, Rajesh specializes in media research on environment, health, children and various social aspects. Rajesh is Editorial Director for Aakhi Jhyal (a famous documentary on social development affairs that has been aired for more than 1000 episodes).

Susanna Giaccherini is a psychologist and psychotherapist. She is manager psychologist in public mental health service, where she is Chief of rehabilitation and prevention service. Her research is focused on stigma, health promotion, mental health treatment and rehabilitation

Elif Gökçearslan Çifci graduated from Social Services Academy of Hacettepe University in 1998. She served as a social worker in various departments (such as provincial directorate, nursery school etc.) of the Prime Ministry Social Services and Child Protection Agency between 1998 to 2001. She was a research assistant at Hacettepe University Social Services Department between 2002-2008 and received her doctoral degree in 2008. She was involved in observations and conducted various investigations at an institution where young drug addicts were treated in 2006 in Berlin, Germany. She worked at the Social Services Department of the Faculty of Health Sciences of Ankara University as research assistant in 2008, as teaching assistant in 2009, and she has served as associate professor since 2012. She officiated as Dean of the Faculty of Health Sciences of Ankara University between 2015-2017. Her research interests are child welfare, forensic social services, substance abuse and treatment methods, children in need of protection, institutional care, social exclusion, peer violence, juveniles pushed to crime and children with disabilities.

Jessica L. Hamblen is the Deputy for Education at the National Center for PTSD. She is an Associate Professor of Psychiatry at the Geisel School of Medicine at Dartmouth. She attended the State University of New York at Buffalo where she obtained her Ph.D in clinical psychology. She completed her pre-doctoral internship and post-doctoral fellowship at Dartmouth and the National Center for PTSD. Dr. Hamblen oversaw the development of the AboutFace website along with her colleagues at the National Center for PTSD. Her research interests are in developing, disseminating, and evaluating cognitive behavioral treatments for PTSD and related conditions. She was principal author of a 12-session cognitive behavioral intervention for postdisaster distress that was used in New York after 9/11, in Baton Rouge, LA after Hurricane Katrina, and most recently after the Boston Marathon Bombings. She recently completed a randomized controlled trial of a cognitive behavioral treatment for PTSD in veterans with co-morbid PTSD and substance use disorders.

Stephen Kimotho is a Communication Specialist, who holds a PhD in communication from Daystar University. He holds a wealth of knowledge and a vast experience in varied areas of communication discipline including: health communication and communication for social change; public policy lobbying and advocacy; Program specific strategic communication; Strategic crisis communication management; strategic communication during conflicts and disasters; media relations and media training; formulating media campaigns strategies; formulating digital media strategies; events management; and resource mobilization strategies among others. Dr. Kimotho has, published books, Journal articles, delivered lectures, presented papers in conferences on various communication subjects. He has worked as communication strategist, a rapporteur and editor for many local and international organizations. Currently, Dr. Kimotho is the Director of Journalism and Master of Communication Programs at United States International University – Africa (USIU-A). He previously worked as the Director of Communication at National Environment Trust Fund (NETFUND), Head of Business and Senior Editor at Lynka Communications, Senior Editor at Longhorn publishers, trainer and rapporteur with several local and international organizations.

Debra Kram-Fernandez spent the first ten years of her career working as a social worker and dance therapist with individuals, families and groups touched by a diagnosis of serious mental illness. Much of the focus of her work involved helping people develop coping skills and instilling hope. Next she worked for 2.5 years as the Study Coordinator for the New York State site of a SAMHSA funded multi-site study on Women, Co-occurring Disorders and Trauma. Following this experience, she worked for six years in child and family welfare. During the last two years of her child and family welfare work, prior to coming to Empire State College, she was the Sanctuary Implementation Coordinator for a family foster care unit of a child and family services agency. This work allowed her to participate in helping the agency to obtain Sanctuary certification. She is currently on faculty at SUNY Empire State College where she has the opportunity to offer a number of studies related to mental health, creative arts therapy and group work.

Patrizia Meringolo is Full Professor in Social and Community Psychology at Department of Education and Psychology of University of Florence, where is part of Research Unit in Research and Action for Psychosocial well-being and of Research Unit in Gender Pedagogy and Psychology. She is in charge for International Agreements between University of Florence and other Universities in European and non-European countries. She has carried out research, asked by Local Authorities, Health Public Services and NGO, and Projects funded by European Union. Her research in last years concerned issues about health promotion, gender differences, and psychosocial problems related to migration, risky behavior and substance use. She has produced, individually or within a research group, more than 280 essays.

Angela Moreland, Ph.D., is an Assistant Professor at the National Crime Victims Research and Treatment Center (NCVC) at the Medical University of South Carolina (MUSC). She earned her Ph.D. in clinical psychology from Purdue University in 2009 and completed her pre-doctoral clinical internship and post-doctoral research fellowship at the NCVC. Dr. Moreland has been utilizing and teaching graduate students, interns, postdoctoral fellows, and residents in CBT techniques for the past 11 years. She currently serves as the Director of CBT training in the Department of Psychiatry Residency Training Program, as well as carries her own caseload of children, adolescents, and adults. Dr. Moreland also conducts research on the effectiveness of evidence-based practice for victims of interpersonal violence, as well as primary and secondary prevention of child abuse and risk factors for maltreatment among parents of young children, with particular focus on high-risk, disadvantaged families.

Fausto Petrini is a community psychologist, Ph.D. in social psychology and temporary professor at the University of Florence, President of the Academic Spin-off social cooperative "LabCom Ricerca e Azione per il benessere psicosociale".

Ken Ruggiero, PhD, is Professor and Co-Director of the Technology Applications Center for Healthful Lifestyles (TACHL), as well as Director of the Telehealth Resilience and Recovery Program. He received his BA from the State University of New York at Buffalo and MA and PhD from West Virginia University, and completed his internship and NIMH postdoc at MUSC. Dr. Ruggiero's research centers on the development and evaluation of technology-based interventions. Most of his early research focused on brief, web-based self-help interventions for individuals affected by traumatic events. Over time, this work evolved into the use and evaluation of wholly technology based stepped care approaches for victims of disaster and serious injury. He is PI on an active NIH grant (through 2020) to conduct a randomized controlled trial of a stepped-care smartphone-based intervention for disaster survivors in partnership with the American Red Cross; as well as Co-PI on an active Duke Endowment grant (through 2020) to adapt and implement the Telehealth Resilience and Recovery Program in three partnering trauma centers across South Carolina. A second major line of research focuses on the development and evaluation of tablet-based resources to improve quality of care in child mental health treatment. This work aims specifically to improve child engagement and provider fidelity in delivery of best practices. He is PI on an active R01 (through 2021) to conduct a randomized controlled trial examining tablet-facilitated vs. standard evidence-based treatment with 120 providers and 360 families. Dr. Ruggiero has had continuous extramural funding from the National Institutes of Health since 2001. He has led as PI five NIH, four VA, and five Department of Homeland Securities grants, and has served as Co-I on numerous grants funded by DoD, NIDA, and SAMHSA. He has over 160 scholarly publications and 200 presentations, a high percentage of which were led by former interns, postdocs, and junior faculty members whom he has mentored. He was recently awarded the inaugural 2017 MUSC Population Health Award. He is a standing member of an NIMH review panel, and serves on four editorial boards. He has served as a formal mentor on NIAAA and NIMH T32s, an NIH F32, two NIMH R25s, an NIMH minority fellowship supplement, and NIH K23 and VA career development awards.

Ben Tran is a Senior Vocational Rehabilitation Counselor, Qualified Rehabilitation Professional, with the State of California's Department of Rehabilitation. Dr. Tran received his Doctor of Psychology (Psy.D.) in Organizational Psychology from California School of Professional Psychology at Alliant International University in San Francisco, California, United States of America. Dr. Tran's research interests include domestic and expatriate recruitment, selection, retention, evaluation, training, and disability and accommodation, assistive technology, gender, business and organizational ethics, organizational/international organizational behavior, knowledge management, and minorities in multinational organizations.

Sudeep Uprety is a Kathmandu based researcher specializing in security and development communications research. Sudeep has a Masters in Conflict, Peace and Development Studies from Tribhuvan University, Nepal and has carried out several studies related to media research on disaster response, crisis communications, health, among others. He is also Contributing Author for Research to Action, one of the premier global web portals for development communications and research. Sudeep currently works as Research Uptake and Impact Coordinator for Gender and Adolescence: Global Evidence (GAGE) programme, managed by Overseas Development Institute (ODI) based in London, UK. He also teaches Development Communications at National College, affiliated with Kathmandu University.

Jennifer Winkelmann is a program manager and mental health clinician in the College of Nursing at the Medical University of South Carolina. She received her B.A. in Psychology from the University of Wisconsin – Milwaukee in 2008 and in 2012 she earned a M.S. in Counseling and Clinical Health Psychology from the Philadelphia College of Osteopathic Medicine. Jennifer is currently a Licensed Professional Counselor – Intern working towards full licensure. One of her main roles is the treatment of patients after traumatic injury through the Trauma Resilience and Recovery Program. She also works on federally-funded research projects that focus on the development and evaluation of technology-based interventions for traumatic stress populations.

Index

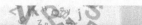
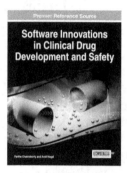
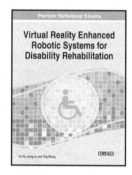
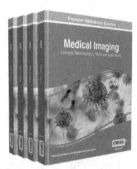
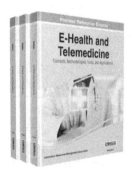
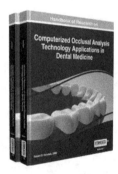
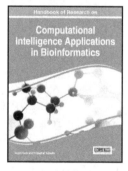 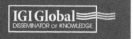

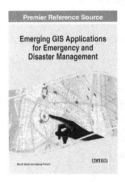
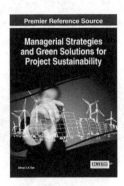
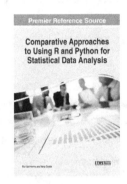
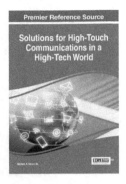

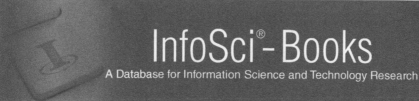
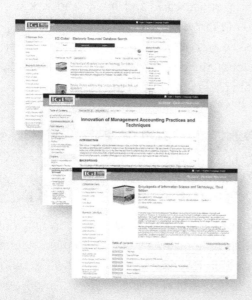
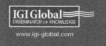

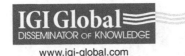
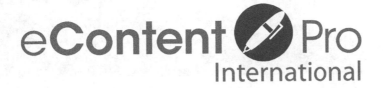
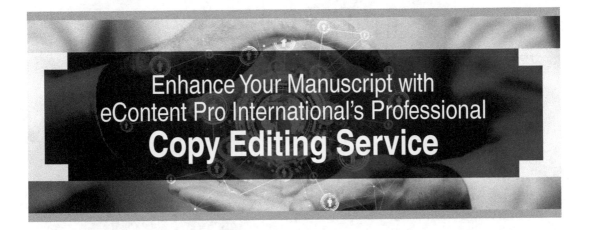

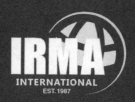
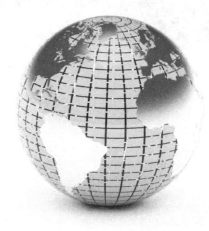

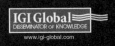
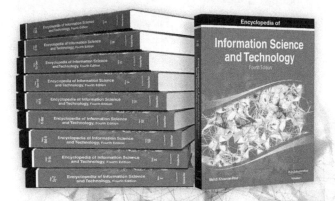